★ CABANIS ★

Enlightenment and Medical Philosophy
in the French Revolution

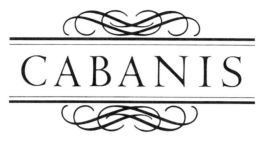

CABANIS

Enlightenment and Medical Philosophy
in the French Revolution

MARTIN S. STAUM

PRINCETON UNIVERSITY PRESS
PRINCETON, NEW JERSEY

Publication of this book has been aided by the Research Grants
Committee of the University of Calgary

Library of Congress Cataloging in Publication Data

Staum, Martin S
Cabanis.

Bibliography: p. 383
Includes index.
1. Cabanis, Pierre Jean Georges, 1757-1808.
2. Physicians—France—Biography.   3. Medicine—
France—History—18th century.   4. Philosophy, French—
18th century.   5. Enlightenment.   6. France—History—
Revolution, 1789-1799.
R507.C24S7   610'.92'4 [B]   79-3231
ISBN 0-691-05301-4

To My Mother and Father

Contents

★ CONTENTS ★

Preface

The profusion of competing theories and techniques in the social sciences lends a peculiar fascination to the quaint ideal of a single, all-encompassing "science of man." The works of a philosopher at the University of Strasbourg, Georges Gusdorf, in particular his *Introduction aux sciences humaines*, which appeared twenty years ago, first called my attention to the impressive aspirations of the "French Ideological School" and inspired my enthusiasm for the study of Cabanis. I have had access to Gusdorf's recent synthesis on *La conscience révolutionnaire, les Idéologues* only in time for final corrections to the manuscript. It is all the more gratifying, therefore, to ascertain that his interpretation of the reasons for the neglect of the Idéologues and his assessment of the monistic philosophy of Cabanis are thoroughly compatible with my own views. Readers of this book will find several perspectives different from those of Gusdorf. I have not denied the crucial impact of the Revolution and of Revolutionary circumstances on Idéologue thought, though I have tried to stress as well the Enlightenment heritage of a thinker such as Cabanis. And I have defined the Idéologue circle more narrowly than Gusdorf and thus given deliberately sharper emphasis to the differences among the principal spokesmen of the group rather than accepting the "unity in difference" of a wider circle. Despite my differences from Gusdorf in emphasis, readers should be able to find a remarkable degree of consensus in recent major interpretations of the Idéologues, including the invaluable work of Sergio Moravia and the first major special study of Destutt de Tracy by Emmet Kennedy.

My indebtedness to other French scholars is personal as well as intellectual. For a cordial welcome, for words of encouragement, for facilitating access to libraries, I am grateful to the historians of science, Professors Georges Canguilhem, René Taton, Mirko Grmek, and to the sociologist Bernard-Pierre Lécuyer, all from branches of the University of Paris. I especially appreciate several helpful conversations with M. Claude Lehec, editor of the *Oeuvres philosophiques* of Cabanis. Many librarians and archivists in France provided valuable aid in research. I would particularly like to thank M. Chazelas of the Archives de l'Académie des sciences morales et politiques, Mme Laffitte-Larnaudie of the Archives de l'Institut, M. Guy Quincy of the Archives départementales de la Corrèze, Mlle Marie-Rose Guillot of the Musée Ernest Rupin in Brive, Mlle Moureaux of the Archives de l'Ecole de médecine de Paris, M. César of the Archives nationales, and Mme Antoinette Becheau La Fonta, president of the Société historique d'Auteuil et de Passy.

For useful advice and a gracious reception, I should like to thank Professor Owsei Temkin, dean of American historians of medicine. And as this study has developed, I have especially appreciated the encouragement of colleagues such as Emmet Kennedy of George Washington University and Louis Greenbaum of the University of Massachusetts.

I wish to acknowledge the generous financial support of the Lehman Foundation of New York as well as the U. S. Public Health Service (Fellowship #1-F01-GH-39, 738-01) during 1967-1969, the period of research for my doctoral dissertation at Cornell University. I am also grateful to the Canada Council for additional funding in 1974 toward further research and revision of the manuscript. I very much appreciate the aid of the University of Calgary Research Grants Committee in support of publication.

Permission to quote portions of this study that have appeared earlier in "Cabanis and the Science of Man," *Journal of the History of the Behavioral Sciences* x (1974), 135-143 (Clinical Psychology Publishing Co., Brandon, Vermont) and "Medical Components of Cabanis's Science of Man," *Studies in History of Biology* (Johns Hopkins Press) II (1978), 1-31 is hereby acknowledged.

★ PREFACE ★

For the early supervision of research and writing on this subject and for an ideal of historical scholarship as a human study and the teaching of history as a human experience, I would like to thank Professor Henry Guerlac, still an active researcher who inspired many students in his years of teaching at Cornell University.

Any error of fact or interpretation remains solely my own responsibility.

Many thanks go to the typist, Mrs. Doreen Nordquist, whose speed and accuracy have been admirable.

Finally, a note of special gratitude is due to my wife, Sarah, who bravely endured the vicissitudes of our sojourn in France and whose encouragement has been crucial for the completion of this study.

July 1979

★ CABANIS ★

Enlightenment and Medical Philosophy
in the French Revolution

Introduction

At a session of the new Class of Moral and Political Sciences of the French National Institute in 1796, the physician and philosopher Pierre-Jean-Georges Cabanis exhorted his colleagues to establish the "science of man and society." In doing so, he claimed, they would follow the ancient Delphic injunction "Know thyself!" According to Cabanis, the new republican government of the Directory now created favorable circumstances for the transmission of the message of the "semaphore of science and reason" throughout Europe and to future generations.[1] Thus, a member of the intellectual elite of the Directory in France reaffirmed the urgency of a central goal of many Enlightenment philosophes—the formulation of the human sciences.

Cabanis's career and convictions offer a striking opportunity for studying the survival and modification of Enlightenment ideals in the turbulent period of the Revolution. As a man of theory, Cabanis was a philosopher who blended convictions in the unity of nature and the unity of scientific method with the physician's concern for the uniqueness of life and human diversity. Consideration of his thought compels our reexamination of eighteenth-century tendencies to metaphysical monism and transformism of living species as well as of physiologists' efforts to account for the phenomena of life and mind. On the one hand, Cabanis insisted on the unity of the physical and mental, "confounded at their source,"[2] and the unity of "analytic" method appropriate for all the sciences. On the other hand, he never reduced physical sensitivity, which accounted for mental phenomena, to the identical physicochemical forces active in nonliving matter. He also believed that procedures of the physical sciences would have to be changed in human studies. The ancient medical theory of temperament suggested

3

to him a means of affecting physical sensitivity to restore healthful equilibrium in the human body, to sharpen ideas, to moderate passions, or even to induce a more beneficial "acquired temperament."

In the Revolutionary era Cabanis's goal was to establish a "science of man," uniting physiology, "analysis of ideas," and ethics.[3] He shared these aspirations with a loosely defined group of philosophers and physicians known as "Ideologists" (from "Ideology," the science of ideas), or "Idéologues" to their enemies and to historians. As critical disciples of Condillac, the philosophers were concerned with empiricist principles of learning, the faculties of the mind, and methods of analysis. The physicians wished to integrate man into nature and make him an object of science by rigorous study of physical-mental relations.[4]

Neither the classic study of Picavet nor the recent works of Moravia have established clear-cut criteria for identifying an Idéologue. All students of the subject agree on the leaders of the Idéologue circle—Destutt de Tracy, who in 1796 invented and defined the term "Ideology" as a science of ideas, including the formation of ideas, their expression (grammar), and combination (logic); and his close friend Cabanis, the physician who provided the physiological basis for the psychology. Most studies also designate several friends of Cabanis and Tracy as Idéologues on the basis of contemporary testimony. Picavet and Gusdorf include a wider group than I think is justifiable. I shall base my definition of an Idéologue on the following criterion: authorship of a serious work in medical or philosophical Ideology, as defined above, or in the elements of ethics, politics, or economics. I will also require at least one of the following three conditions for peripheral members of the group and at least two of the three for the core members: regular appearance at the salon of Mme Helvétius, the Auteuil circle of Cabanis, or the salon of Mme de Condorcet in 1794-1809; participation as editor or reviewer in *La Décade philosophique*, a newspaper particularly sympathetic to the goals of Ideology; or a political commitment to a moderate republic after 1794, implying oppo-

4

sition to Bonaparte after 1801. The criteria are thus based on philosophical and political kinship as well as on direct personal relations.

As a man of practice, Cabanis was a politically active Idéologue—a hospital reformer, a deputy in the Council of Five Hundred who advocated standards for the medical profession, universal primary education, and national public assistance, and a conspirator in Bonaparte's coup of Brumaire (November 1799). While his political thought does not follow logically from his philosophy, nor does it determine his philosophical arguments, his politics do stress the principle of a dynamic equilibrium. Just as Cabanis the physician intervened to cure disease, so did Cabanis the social therapist intervene to establish a natural equilibrium in society. But a return to a previous state was not his intended prescription either for the individual or for society, for Cabanis believed in individual perfectibility and the imperative of achieving greater social harmony.

The interpretation of the thought of the Idéologues in general and of Cabanis in particular has been hindered by hostile critics in the nineteenth and early twentieth centuries. In the Idéologue project to establish "moral and political sciences," critics perceived challenges to such religious tenets as the uniqueness of man, the existence of absolute moral standards, and the authority of Revelation. The empiricist method and monist metaphysic certainly did imperil beliefs in the existence of God, the spiritual and immortal soul, and free will meriting external reward by divine Grace.

In his twelve memoirs of the *Rapports du physique et du moral de l'homme* (six read to the Institute in 1796-1797, published in 1798; six added for a separate edition in 1802), Cabanis related physical sensitivity to "ideas and passions" without mentioning a soul. He considered physical sensitivity the most refined manifestation of a single universal force of affinity, including gravitation and chemical affinity at simpler levels. His physical-mental correlations were hardly controversial, but clearly a monist metaphysic was heretical. Cabanis's anticlericalism did influence his belief in monism, and such ideas

5

were out of fashion by 1802, in a period of Catholic revival. Chateaubriand had attacked the Idéologues even during the Consulate for arid materialism—a view of man as a machine adrift in an indifferent cosmos and as a coldly calculating egoistic hedonist subversive of religion and morality. When Cabanis's preface to the *Rapports* announced merely "physiological inquiries," rather than metaphysical speculation or ethical imperatives, no orthodox believer could accept this disclaimer.[5]

In the Restoration Cabanis's political associations with the Revolution were also unacceptable. Conservative and Catholic writers saw the taint of disorder in even a moderate supporter of the Directory and a timid liberal opponent of Bonaparte after 1801. The accusations of heresy directed against Cabanis and his guilt by association with the Revolution did not invite subtle contrast of his thought with the works of other alleged materialists or atheists. Aimé-Martin, biographer of the Rousseauist novelist, botanist, and engineer Bernardin de Saint-Pierre, related Idéologue insolence when Saint-Pierre extolled the wisdom of God at the Institute in 1798. Cabanis allegedly stormed, "I wish that the name of God never be pronounced within these walls."[6] In view of Cabanis's moderate opinions later, and the fact that there is no unbiased record of this reaction to Saint-Pierre, such a blatantly atheist remark may be apocryphal. In general reference works, too, even careful scholars have designated Cabanis an atheist or a bold mechanical materialist who crassly compared the formation of thought in the brain to the digestion of food in the stomach.[7]

Misunderstandings of Cabanis's thought, apart from religious or political bias, have stemmed from an inattentive reading of the *Rapports* and underemphasis of Cabanis's medical works. In the *Rapports* Cabanis never declared that the world was material or that human beings were moral automata ruled by pleasure and pain. And in his early medical work *Degré de certitude de la médecine* (1788; published 1798), Cabanis's model of acceptable explanation stressed observed relationships among phenomena rather than understanding of the essence of objects. As Newton had refused to explain gravity, Cabanis felt no obligation to explain whether the force of physical sensitivity was spiritual or material. Thus, even in the *Rapports* he questioned whether gravitation might some day be identified as a kind of sensitivity rather than sensitivity being reduced to a higher-order gravitation.

In an unpublished "Letter on First Causes," written probably in 1806 to the young author Claude Fauriel, who was preparing a history of Stoicism, Cabanis privately advocated the probable existence of a universal intelligence from which all forces emanate and even the possible existence of an immortal soul. The metaphysic was still monist, though more akin to a panpsychism than to a mechanical materialism. Even in the *Rapports* Cabanis had not presented a fatalistic view of man in an indifferent universe. Rather, each simple level of the universal force foreshadowed human physical sensitivity, and physical sensitivity was itself the organic basis of innate moral sympathy. Thus, even the most elemental forces of the universe had at least a distant relationship to human moral purpose. The refusal to use the term "soul" in the *Rapports* neither denigrated human intelligence nor, in Cabanis's view, undermined morality. Sympathy, as much as pleasure, was a natural law and an added spur to social virtue.

The letter to Fauriel remained undiscovered in Cabanis's papers until 1824. When the Montpellier physician F.-E. Bérard published the letter, he concluded that Cabanis had masked his true opinions in the *Rapports* in deference to the anticlerical fashion of the Revolution. Another opponent of materialism, Jean-Philibert Damiron, hailed Cabanis's "remarkable conversion" at the time of the letter to Fauriel.[8] Other dualist physicians and philosophers still saw dangers in Cabanis's speculation about a universal intelligence. They argued that believers in God and the soul would only be exchanging one monist heresy—the ancient materialism of Lucretius—for another—the pantheism of Spinoza, which allegedly identified God and the world. Still other critics merely pointed out the blatant contradictions between Cabanis's "physiological determinism" and his claims of moral freedom.[9]

Cabanis's image as a materialist, long accepted by historians of philosophy, often seemed contradictory to the findings of historians of medicine, who noted his defense of vitalist physicians and his insistence on a distinct epistemological status for medicine.[10] Indeed, Cabanis's long historical and philosophical study *Coup d'oeil sur les révolutions et sur la réforme de la médecine* (1795; published 1804) outlined special features of medical "analysis" and the dangers of the subservience of medicine to physics, chemistry, and mathematics. Cabanis particularly agreed with the limited therapeutic role for anatomy and chemistry and the profound reverence for life characteristic of the Montpellier school of physicians. The medical tradition balanced the search for rigorous theory with recognition of the unclassifiable nature of some case histories.

A blending of medical and philosophical traditions is thus crucial to Cabanis's thought. The thorough study of Cabanis by Sergio Moravia has independently and concurrently traced the importance of vitalist medicine in the formation of Cabanis's ideas and has also noted that the bias of critics has often obscured the roots of Cabanis's thought. Yet even Moravia too often uses the term "materialism" interchangeably with "monism," underestimates the letter to Fauriel, and concludes, perhaps too boldly, that a science of anthropology necessarily required a materialist psychophysiology—as if dualist physicians could never have achieved similar knowledge by speaking of correlations.[11]

My argument will be that the monism of Cabanis was not mechanist, but distinctively biomedical. Such an interpretation must begin with a review of concepts of unity of nature and unity of the sciences in eighteenth-century thinkers who influenced Cabanis as well as a review of related concepts in medical literature, for the significance of Cabanis's thought is not merely his own special contribution but his unique synthesis of disparate eighteenth-century ideas. The particular importance of reviewing Cabanis's intellectual ancestry is the challenge it poses to the most common assumption about the revival of materialism in the eighteenth century—that the triumph of Descartes's mechanical philosophy in the physical sciences prepared its extension to the life sciences. In Descartes's philosophy there was a distinction between spiritual principles of motion—such as the human soul—and inert, passive matter—including even animal bodies. Descartes's model of the totally corporeal "beast-machine" could then be transformed, in this conventional view, by a dose of religious unorthodoxy (as in Hobbes or La Mettrie), to the totally corporeal, soulless "man-machine."[12]

Eighteenth-century thinkers such as La Mettrie in *L'homme machine* and Diderot in *Le Rêve de d'Alembert* did not present a purely mechanist materialism, however. Discoveries in natural history and experiments in physiology (such as Haller's work on irritability) made plausible the concepts of nonmechanical yet active physical forces in the animal body. "Mechanist" and "vitalist" physiologists differed in interpretation of these forces, but either view enriched the concept of motion in the body. And as mechanists and vitalists grew closer in their description of phenomena, an interpreter committed to monism could easily use, not a Cartesian mechanism, but an active physical force to account for all physical and mental behavior. Cabanis's use of physical sensitivity was profoundly indebted to Montpellier vitalists, and this vitalist legacy was decisive in his ultimate advocacy of panpsychism in his letter to Fauriel.

The second major portion of my argument will explore the relationships between Cabanis's philosophy and his politics in the context of the Revolution. His recommendations for revolutionary practice could not derive from his philosophical or medical doctrines, because his early works on hospitals and public assistance, which already expressed basic political choices, preceded the full elaboration of his philosophy. One possible exception was the claim by the Idéologues that scientific principles about human nature did in fact justify a political commitment to natural rights to liberty and equality before the law. But even here the belief in natural rights was independent of this line of reasoning as a justification.[13] Revolutionary political choices in this instance derived more from Enlightenment political ideals than from the findings of a "science" of politics.

A more tempting exercise is the derivation of Cabanis's medical and philosophical views from his social and political interests (to see "Ideology" as an ideology in the Marxist sense of a mask for interests of a social group or class).[14] Although the thought of the group of Idéologues was not at all monolithic, they did have definite social and political convictions. They faced the fundamental problems of any moderate revolutionaries—a new basis of legitimacy for political power and a new standard for moral and social behavior to replace the now unacceptable doctrines of Catholic morality and theology. Only with solidly grounded principles would citizens come to see the identity of self-interest and the public interest. "Enlightenment" would thus lead to "virtue."

The perspective of Idéologue "science" was thus undoubtedly colored by the politics of gradualist reform. The Idéologues had rallied to the ideals of 1789—constitutional government, civil and legal equality, and education of people in their rights and in basic skills. As individuals, the Idéologues could play an eminent role in politics and culture from 1789 to 1793 and, as a more self-conscious group, from 1794 to 1800. The misfortune of the Idéologues was that reform was ill-suited to an era in which demands for radical redistribution of property and for increased access to political power by all citizens were often predominant concerns. After 1793 the Idéologues thought that the imperative of order outweighed the need for direct popular participation in government. Like the majority of the Idéologues and like the Enlightenment philosophes, Cabanis was unsympathetic to direct universal suffrage and street violence and was confident in a natural hierarchy based on property and education rather than on birth and privilege.

Certainly the Idéologues were all men of property and standing who often found Adam Smith's liberal political economy congenial. They favored the removal of the relics of seigneurial privilege and the enhancement of commercial and industrial interests. Yet this evidence does not necessarily mean that one can derive their science from their social and political doctrines in any simplistic fashion. The commonplace conclusion is that the group exemplifies "bourgeois ideology," often with the connotation of laissez-faire liberalism.

If any prorevolutionary group that favored property, commerce, and industry and opposed popular democracy is defined as bourgeois, then the Idéologues fit that label and their thought can be called bourgeois ideology. However, at least in the case of Cabanis, the label mystifies more than it explains. My contention will be that the most important analogies between his philosophical and political thought occur on the issue of balancing the "natural" and the free with the "artificial" and the regulated. Thus, an emphasis on laissez-faire liberalism to the exclusion of other elements can result in distortions.

In Cabanis's medical and philosophical works, the idea of temperament as healthful equilibrium was a pervasive concept. In medical treatment, however, Cabanis argued that the physician must not await the healing force of nature but rather must intervene to aid the beneficial, and counteract the harmful, development of a disease. Similarly, in the science of man, the therapist must use changes in climate and regimen to help restore physical and mental health. The goals of such intervention were not merely restorative but directed at improvement of the individual and species. Even in medical method, there were analogies to the concept of intervention in the course of "natural" observation, for the "artificial" application of rational categories in the clinical journal would facilitate understanding of the raw data and meaningful diagnoses of subsequent cases.

In politics and society, Cabanis also believed in intervention to allow the operation of natural law. Because survivals of the ancien régime abounded, immediate application of laissez-faire liberalism would be an inadequate response. Public assistance had to help remove the "artificial" social inequalities created by privilege and monopoly without disturbing the "natural" inequalities promoting incentives to work. The idea of "natural" laws in society did not preclude Cabanis from advocating the right of the poor to health care and to employment, preferably at home, for the able-bodied. He also supported hospital reform to treat diseases without complicating their natural course and relatively small hospitals to attempt to re-create the salutary "natural" atmosphere of the home.

Revolutionary events did have an impact on the freedom-regulation balance in Cabanis's political and social thought. The overcrowding in public workhouses and the disorder he associated with outdoor public works made him more cautious about public assistance granted outside the home. Still, he supported a national public assistance fund as late as the Consulate and maintained the ideal of a more just distribution of wealth. Conversely, on other issues he became more reconciled to less "natural," or less liberal, approaches. Large hospitals seemed necessary to him in the large city as an aid to clinical research. His views on education also became more firmly interventionist; in 1791 he had shared Adam Smith's advocacy of free competition among private schoolmasters, but by 1799 he supported state-run schools at all levels to maintain secular and republican ideals. In the last two years of the Directory he participated in two political coups and called for repressive measures against the neo-Jacobin press and clubs, allegedly to save the Republic from a new outbreak of terror. And in supporting the Consulate constitution, he clearly preferred a government guided by notables to the dangers of direct popular sovereignty.

While Cabanis thus defended the salutary role of the "middle classes" (his own term), his position is not identical with laissez-faire liberalism. The term "bourgeois ideology" simply does not differentiate the position of Cabanis well enough from that of a host of contemporaries who showed no concern about further need to redistribute wealth or who were less sympathetic to education that insured a degree of social mobility. Cabanis's hope that society would evolve dynamically suggests none of the smugness and complacency of liberals of the 1830s. Certainly his commitments to public health and to public assist-

12

ance were intended to spread the benefits of the science of man beyond a limited sphere.

Yet undeniably Cabanis had what we may call the liberal illusion that once natural laws operated they would insure a just society without pervasive government regulation. No doubt some Marxist interpreters would label "false consciousness" the position of any thinker who believed that a generally liberal economic regime would bring prosperity and justice to an entire society without continuing government intervention. For the case of Cabanis, we must recall that he died in 1808, long before the grim reality behind the liberal illusion, the harshness of industrialization, came to most of France. We cannot reason from the works of other Idéologues who outlived Cabanis what his reaction might have been. But if we argue that whatever the sincerity of his hopes he was still objectively serving bourgeois interests, then we are defining false consciousness so as to make it a self-evident affliction of any thinker who was not a radical revolutionary or at least an advocate of the *sans-culottes*. In that case, we could be sure that Cabanis had false consciousness before even studying his thought. My objective here will be to demonstrate that the special features of Cabanis's political and social thought cannot be easily subsumed under vague general categories.

Finally, my text will not deal in a substantive manner with the provocative issues raised by some historians of medicine and by the philosopher Michel Foucault concerning the professional monopoly of knowledge in medicine. There are some empirically resolvable questions concerning the relationship of elite and popular medicine or concerning the charge that a self-interested elite usurped authority in order to assume social control and stifle the unwelcome competition of folk medicine.[15] There are also some questions that may never be resolved, such as the degree of competence in a science or social science that justifies the assumption of authority. Except for a brief reference in Chapter 10, I shall leave most of these questions to social historians and philosophers. Suffice it to say here that

13

Cabanis was certainly a believer in therapy administered by qualified professionals. A hierarchical relationship was implicit both in regard to the patient and in regard to the charlatan, who was to be repressed as a purveyor of superstition. To suggest that this position was part of a sinister conspiracy to "medicalize" the masses seems an excessive exaggeration of the evidence. On the other hand, there are considerable grounds for arguing that the confidence that contemporary physicians had in the beneficial results of their therapy was also exaggerated. Further discussion of these problems will no doubt appear in studies by other scholars of the condition of the medical profession as a whole in the era of the Revolution.

The Youth of Cabanis: Initiation to Enlightenment

Derived from the village of Chabannes in the province of Limousin, the Cabanis family name occurred throughout southern France. Since the late sixteenth century, the branch who were progenitors of Cabanis the physician-philosophe were comfortable proprietors and professional men—surgeons, physicians, men of the law.[16] Cabanis's grandfather had the title of *avocat au Parlement* as well as a nearly hereditary post as seigneurial court judge near Brive, the crossroads of the east-west route from Bordeaux to Clermont and the north-south route from Limoges to Toulouse. His son Jean-Baptiste (1725-1786) acquired the same title and in 1747 married a daughter of the local petty nobility, Marie-Hélène d'Escarolle de Souleyrac.[17] The dowry brought him the château of Salaignac (the birthplace of Pierre-Jean-Georges on 5 June 1757) in Cosnac parish just outside Brive in rolling countryside suitable both for cultivation and pasture. The elder Cabanis was one of those all-too-few enterprising proprietors who accelerated the progress of agriculture in eighteenth-century France. When the intendant of Limousin established the Brive branch of the Royal Society of Agriculture in 1759, the elder Cabanis was a founding member. From 1761 to 1774, the next intendant, Turgot, personally encouraged the elder Cabanis's experimentation in potato culture, in breeding of Spanish merino sheep, and in planting fruit orchards. In fact, Turgot arranged a competition at the Bordeaux Academy for which the elder Cabanis contributed a memoir on grafting and transplantation, duly awarded the prize in 1764 (published in 1776). Turgot's patronage was later of material importance in obtaining introductions for young Cabanis in Paris.[18]

Cabanis's upper-bourgeois family was thus both innovative in agricultural entrepreneurship and socially conservative. The early death of his mother when Cabanis was seven contributed to the rebellious temperament of his boyhood. First educated by local priests, Cabanis was not always an enthusiastic pupil. He allegedly engineered his own expulsion from the Doctrinaire *collège* at Brive, which he attended from 1767 to 1771. His exasperated father brought him to Paris that year with a letter of introduction from Turgot to his protégé, the young poet Antoine Roucher (1745-1794).[19]

At fourteen, Cabanis must have found the capital bewildering, but he certainly arrived with advantageous connections. Roucher inspired in him a taste for letters, and the elder Cabanis could not convince his son to return to the confining atmosphere of Brive. In 1773 Cabanis accepted the offer of a post as secretary to a Polish visitor, the prince-bishop Massalski of Vilna. Accompanying his patron to Poland, Cabanis, for reasons not clear, refused to teach in a Vilna seminary but at sixteen expounded French literature at the Academy of Warsaw. His correspondence conveyed horror at the political anarchy and corruption in Poland: "Our abuses are better than their laws."[20] Limited opportunities for advancement and a quarrel with the bishop induced Cabanis to return to France in 1775. Cabanis's file as a medical student records the award of the M.A. in Paris, 5 August 1775, though no collège is specified.

Roucher had received, through Turgot's efforts, the *charge* of *gabelle* collector in Montfort-l'Amaury (southwest of Paris). Cabanis spent much time at the Roucher salon, where he first met his close friend, the future Idéologue Dominique-Joseph Garat (1749-1833), the physicist and naturalist Bernard-

Germain-Etienne de la Ville-sur-Illon, comte de Lacépède (1756-1825), and the dynamic, vitriolic writer Nicolas Chamfort (1741-1794). Roucher persuaded Cabanis to enter an Académie française competition for the best translation of an excerpt of the *Iliad*. Voltaire himself complimented Cabanis for his efforts in 1778, and Roucher published a part of the translation in the second edition of *Les mois* (1780). For the rest of his life, Cabanis worked intermittently at translating cantos of the *Iliad*.[21]

Cabanis's own hopes for a *charge* in France fell with Turgot's ministry in 1776. Paternal pressure and ill health compelled him to seek a more secure career than that of a *littérateur*. In 1777 he resolved to study medicine with J.-B.-Léon Dubreuil (1748-1783), a Royal physician attached to the hospital of Saint-Germain-en-Laye.[22] Since Dubreuil had studied with the Montpellier physician and chemist G.-F. Venel, Cabanis undoubtedly received a thorough introduction to the Montpellier clinical school. Dubreuil's own clinical training was reputedly good; he was alleged to have practiced as a naval physician in Brest where there had been a Naval Surgical School since 1740. According to Cabanis, Dubreuil founded a clinical school in the Naval Hospital of Brest several years before his death, under the auspices of the Minister of the Navy, Maréchal de Castries. In 1783 the school officially became the School of Naval Practical Medicine. Cabanis probably lived with Dubreuil for some time, in the company of the writer Jean de Pechméja, now remembered as the author of vehement antislavery passages in Raynal's *Histoire des deux indes* (1770).[23] While some biographers claim that Cabanis studied with Dubreuil for several years, we have evidence only of Cabanis's subsequent formal training at the Paris Faculty. But Cabanis himself testified to the importance of Dubreuil's role as mentor.

Turgot and Roucher ensured that Cabanis's intellectual life was not bounded by medical studies, however. In the spring of 1778, they introduced him to the salon of Mme Helvétius, one of the most intellectually vibrant circles of the late Enlightenment (baptized by Garat the "Estates-General of the human mind"). Helvétius's widow had transferred the former habitués of her late husband's salon on the rue Sainte-Anne to a quiet suburban villa in Auteuil. The ambiance was anticlerical, favorable to social reform, and full of enthusiasm for the American Revolution. Prominent philosophes such as d'Alembert, Condillac, and Turgot were occasional guests, while the *coterie holbachique* was always welcome, including the Baron himself, Diderot, the poet and dramatist Marmontel, the ally of the Physiocrats Morellet, the anticlerical J.-F. Saint-Lambert, and the theorist of public happiness Marquis de Chastellux. Other literary and administrative figures, such as the *parlementaire* Dupaty, the writers Chamfort and Thomas, and the young anticlerical student of exotic customs and empires Constantin-François Chassebeuf de Boisgiray, who took the pseudonym Volney (1757-1820), also made their appearances. After the outbreak of revolution, important political figures such as Siéyès, Talleyrand, and Mirabeau were guests. Most notably, however, this was the period in which the future Idéologues or patrons of Idéologues began to gather at Auteuil: the mathematician and legislator Marie-Jean-Antoine-Nicolas Caritat, marquis de Condorcet (1743-1794), the literary critic Pierre-Louis Ginguené (1748-1816), the Oratorian philosophy teacher Pierre-Claude-François Daunou (1761-1840), the philosopher Pierre Laromiguière (1786-1837), and, after 1792, the military officer Antoine-Louis-Claude Destutt de Tracy (1754-1836).[24]

While Cabanis's autobiographical sketch describing his encounters has been lost, at least three biographers who had access to it insist that Cabanis conversed with Condillac and met Diderot and d'Holbach. And there is no doubt that he established immediate rapport with the charming hostess of the Auteuil salon, Mme Helvétius. Though the gracious, aristocratic Mme Helvétius was "of a certain age" (born 1719), she was still declining marriage proposals from Turgot and her exotic guest Benjamin Franklin, who lived nearby in Passy from 1776 to 1785. Her maternal fondness for Cabanis led her to insist that he move into an apartment adjoining her villa (probably in 1778). Along with the secularized Benedictine abbé Martin

Lefebvre de La Roche (later editor of Helvétius's works), Cabanis became her perpetual house guest. And he impressed Franklin so favorably that the American Philosophical Society elected him to foreign membership on 21 July 1786 even before he completed any major written work.[25]

At the same time, Roucher introduced Cabanis to another society of scholars closely associated with the salon of Mme Helvétius. In 1776 the astronomer Jérome Lalande had founded the Masonic Loge des neuf soeurs, a unique circle of men of letters; it had been envisaged by Helvétius himself before his death and now sometimes met at his widow's villa. Upon Voltaire's triumphant return to Paris in 1778, the Loge initiated him amid elaborate ceremony including an ode by Roucher, who was not yet a member. Franklin, the Venerable Master from 1779 to 1781, Cabanis, Roucher, and Garat all became affiliates a few months later. It is here that Cabanis probably first met several future Idéologues: Daunou, Ginguené, Tracy, and the dramatist Marie-Joseph Chénier (1764-1811). Other associates of Cabanis, such as Volney, Lacépède, the physician Victor de Sèze, the influential lawyer Pastoret, and the lawyer and dramatist François de Neufchâteau were also members, and Condorcet joined later. Several of the members were of major importance in Cabanis's life and thought. Mirabeau employed Cabanis as speechwriter and physician, Siéyès provided some of the leading premises of Cabanis's political thought, and Pierre-Samuel Du Pont de Nemours (1739-1817) was a physiocratic economist with well-defined ideas on hospital and public assistance reform.

Unfortunately, there is little evidence concerning the degree of Cabanis's association with most of his lodge brothers. It is not clear whether or not the Neuf Soeurs was somehow essential for the development of Idéologue aspirations. Certainly the founders of the Loge offended the Court by admitting Voltaire and placing less emphasis on Masonic ritual than on discussions of general cultural and scientific questions. They celebrated the spirit of enlightenment and artistic creativity, admitted women to some meetings, and quarreled with other Masons as well as with the Parlement of Paris. Moreover, the members did support humanitarian ideals, including benevolence to the poor and universal brotherhood. But all members swore to say nothing against religion, morals, and the state, although many were freethinkers and social critics. The Loge was hardly a springboard for attacks on abuses of the ancien régime or for social leveling. Aside from the potential of lists of names for spreading ideas after the outbreak of revolution, neither the Neuf Soeurs nor the Masonic network generally was a coordinated protest group; indeed, many lodges included conservative members of the royal family and high nobility. The philosophes and future Idéologues did not require Masonry to find flaws in the existing order or enthusiasm for revolution.[26]

More important than his association with the Loge des neuf soeurs was Cabanis's participation in groups where prominent individuals could privately guide him, if they wished, to the most avant-garde Enlightenment principles. These principles, particularly as expressed by Diderot and d'Holbach, included a view of the unity of nature and of knowledge. Reading the naturalists would heighten Cabanis's inclination to accept that view.

CHAPTER I

The Late Enlightenment: Chain of Being, Chain of Truths

The Unity of Nature

eparating the influence of the philosophes at the Auteuil salon and of physicians in clinical practice on Cabanis's thought is at best an artificial exercise. The Enlightenment and medical components in Cabanis's education were concurrent. In fact, the most complete Enlightenment anticipation of Cabanis's thought, in the works of Diderot, is itself as much the product of medical theories as of Encyclopedist aspirations. Yet, for analytical purposes, I shall structure my discussion around the evident polarities in Cabanis's viewpoint—his scientific and Enlightenment quest for uniformity, theory, and method against his medical concern for individuality, eccentricity, and exceptional case history.

NEWTONIAN FORCES AND NEWTONIAN EXPLANATION

Eighteenth-century Enlightenment thinkers freshly posed the perennial problem of reconciling unity and diversity in nature. Several principal figures of the Scientific Revolution retained their fascination with the Neoplatonic and mystical search for the One in the All or for the hierarchy of interrelated spheres of beings. But the new philosophy, even in Kepler and Newton, was no latter-day occultism; rather, it was an enshrinement of a new method that found unity through mathematics, observation, and experiment rather than through the symbolic network of correspondences of alchemists, astrologers, and magi.[1]

Since the new laws were universal, accounting for disparate phenomena both in heaven and earth, the Scientific Revolution inspired both a new faith in God's Providence, whether general or special, and a revival of the heretical ancient Epicurean ideas that matter and motion (without the action of capricious spirits) were sufficient to explain phenomena. For Descartes, a mechanism of matter and motion alone explained observable physical processes.[2]

Yet mechanical philosophers, including Descartes and Boyle, safeguarded religious orthodoxy and the dignity of the human soul by postulating an absolute difference between active spirit and inert matter. God endowed matter with its ordinary properties—extension, inertia, and mobility—at the Creation, and conserved motion; matter on its own could not move or act, much less think. For Cartesian-style philosophies, the activation of matter by a willing spirit, especially in living organisms, was still a difficult problem.

By the late seventeenth century, Newton agreed that God was the source of universal motion, but he also speculated that certain "active principles" (a Neoplatonic and perhaps alchemical notion) were the secondary causes of gravity.[3] For theological reasons, Newtonians before the late eighteenth century hesitated to call gravity an inherent property of matter or to explain it by a mechanical hypothesis (despite Newton's invocation of a nonmechanical elastic "aether" after 1707). Any principle of spontaneous activity inherent in matter might give aid and comfort to the Epicurean heresy that the world could arrange itself by chance. Before the time of James Hutton and Joseph Priestley, the view that the ceaseless activity in matter was itself divine was equally unacceptable as a dangerous Spinozist or pantheist heresy. Newton himself therefore stressed that the essence of matter was unknown, while only the phenomenon of gravitational attraction could be observed. God had somehow endowed the smallest particles of matter with dynamic properties. And indeed, the Newtonian term "force," though stripped to stark mathematics, conveyed the analogy of mental activity, of divine or human will.[4] Early dis-

21

ciples of Newton, whether in England or in France (such as the two leading French advocates, the physicist Pierre-Louis Moreau de Maupertuis (1698-1759) and the philosophe Voltaire), scrupulously denied that they considered attraction essential to matter.[5]

Newtonian reluctance to assign matter inherent properties of attraction resulted in at least two far-reaching consequences —one about the notion of matter, the other about acceptable explanation. First, matter could have a property inexplicable by mechanics. All kinds of attractive forces might be involved in chemistry and physiology; and Newton's *Queries* at the end of the *Opticks* (1704) encouraged further speculation. Whether or not one assumed the necessity of an independent spiritual entity directing these forces depended upon one's beliefs about God's role in the world. The second effect of Newtonian modesty was the acceptance of nonmechanical explanations as legitimate. The "Newtonian paradigm" of explanation in the physical and life sciences justified ignorance of mechanisms because Newton had found rigorous mathematical description sufficient for useful knowledge.[6]

From the late seventeenth century until the mid-eighteenth century, philosophers turned Newton's caution into heresy. Locke argued quite safely that, given the powers of God and the forces of matter, it was not inconceivable that God could have endowed matter with thought. The deist Voltaire gleefully seized this remark out of context to defend skepticism on the soul, but more radical critics concluded that matter itself, with dynamic properties, could form the rational soul.[7]

THE GREAT CHAIN OF BEING

The followers of Newton had helped envisage a new unity of nature through the measurable yet mysterious capacities of matter. They thus unwittingly blurred the traditional divisions of the Great Chain of Being, an ancient conception of natural unity. The Great Chain was a fixed hierarchy of beings based on continuity—no gaps in forms—and plenitude—a niche for all possible creatures encompassing mineral, vegetable, and animal worlds. Physical and spiritual man was at the midpoint, while spiritual creatures occupied all links of the chain between the human and the divine. Plato and Aristotle had first expressed a notion like the Great Chain; Neoplatonists, Locke, and Leibniz perpetuated it; and eighteenth-century naturalists such as Charles Bonnet elaborately embellished it.[8] For Christian thought, the Great Chain illustrated design in Creation, enshrined the immutability of living species, and appropriately separated material and spiritual beings. Cartesians also found the radical dualism of the chain congenial, even if they did not believe in angels. Newtonians certainly did not incorporate the Great Chain as a scientific assumption, but their belief in nongravitational attractive forces, electrical or physiological, acted to link ever more tightly all beings. Yet the very Newtonian concept of universal attractive forces could lead the imprudent to ask if there might not be just one force diversely manifested and acting in one homogeneous substance. Thus, the crucial links in the chain between nonliving and living, mineral and vegetable, and vegetable and animal, animal and man, might not be inflexible barriers. The Enlightenment philosophy of metaphysical monism became plausible.

Eighteenth-century naturalists also explored the possibility that allegedly fixed species might vary or that both systematic breeding and reproductive accidents might create new species. Not until 1800, in the work of Jean-Baptiste de Lamarck (1744-1829), was there a true hypothesis of "transformism"— transformation of one species into another from common ancestry. Yet the widespread acceptance of the Chain of Being suggested to some eighteenth-century thinkers the hypothesis that each link in the chain might change over time. Thus, a dualist and fixed version of the Chain of Being could become the starting point not only for monism but for Enlightenment transformism. Both monism and transformism were essential ingredients in Cabanis's thought.[9]

There were many efforts to introduce dynamism into the Great Chain. In 1744 the Genevan naturalist Abraham Trembley (1700-1784) questioned plant-animal differences. About the same time, Maupertuis, an amateur naturalist as well as Newtonian physicist, speculated about embryo formation and, later, about "accidental" variations among organisms. In 1748 the English Catholic priest John Turbervill Needham (1713-1781) reaffirmed the once refuted hypothesis of spontaneous generation of living creatures. The next year the great naturalist Georges-Louis Leclerc de Buffon (1707-1788) published the first section of the multivolume *Histoire naturelle* questioning the fruitfulness of the idea of species. From 1749 to 1754 Denis Diderot (1713-1784) and Maupertuis both extended their hypotheses to a quasi-transformist view. Meanwhile, against clandestine and public advocates of materialism, Buffon, the Swiss naturalist Charles Bonnet (1720-1793), and the philosopher Etienne Bonnot de Condillac (1714-1780) defended the traditional dualist body-soul relationship.

The diversity of religious views among these men shows how investigation of the phenomena in itself did not lead either to orthodoxy or to heresy. Trembley and Bonnet wished to remain orthodox Calvinists, while Needham wished to remain in good standing as a Catholic cleric. Buffon was at least privately a deist, though he maintained appearances by retracting objectionable passages from his published works. And Maupertuis retained a strong conviction in divine Providence. Diderot, however, interpreted the same scientific evidence to justify a monist and transformist philosophy.[10]

Cabanis could have drawn on many works in developing his ideas on the unity of nature, but we shall discuss only works he cited or could not have ignored. Cabanis's citation practices are indeed mysterious. He mentioned Maupertuis only once, and then as a mathematician; he cited Diderot only as an art critic; and he never mentioned the baron d'Holbach (1723-1789)—even though the latter two appeared in or hosted salons that Cabanis attended. Certainly by 1802, the publication date of the full text of the *Rapports*, Bonaparte's Concordat with the Vatican had made materialism distinctly unfashionable. Cabanis simply may have wished then to avoid provocative references to notorious materialists. But this hypothesis cannot explain his silence during the freer atmosphere from 1789 to 1799—nor is any explanation as yet readily apparent.

THE NATURALISTS: NEEDHAM AND BUFFON

To Cabanis, the naturalists' investigation of special regenerative forces was a consistently fascinating project. Diderot and the physician Julien Offray de La Mettrie (1709-1751) had given special attention to Trembley's 1744 memoir on the fresh-water polyp, which challenged plant-animal division and demonstrated a regenerative force manifest in many species.[11] Cabanis himself was certainly aware of Needham's 1748 memoir to the Royal Society of London on the spontaneous generation of "animalcules" from sealed, heated beef broth. Needham thought this "vegetative force" could be the "principle of all physical or chemical metamorphosis" and that it "vivifies organized bodies, is irritated in their limbs," and "furnishes the soul material for thought." Thus, Needham speculated on the existence of a single active force without threatening the existence of God or of the independent rational soul. Despite the naturalist Lazzaro Spallanzani's refutations of spontaneous generation from 1756 to 1776, the baron d'Holbach quoted Needham for his own materialist purpose in 1770. In 1802-1805 Cabanis attempted unsuccessfully to confirm the generation of life from organic matter (heterogenesis) as well as from inorganic matter (abiogenesis).[12]

Cabanis also read closely Buffon's comments on universal forces as well as his challenges to the notion of species and fixed species. In 1749 Buffon spoke of embryo formation caused by "penetrating forces" arranging molecules, each with an appropriate imprint. In each species, these forces operated according to a characteristic "internal mold," a power analogous to gravity.[13] In 1765 Buffon speculated that the law of gravitational attraction encompassed all short-range forces among inorganic particles, including chemical affinities. This inorganic affinity was analogous to the penetrating forces of nutrition and reproduction.[14]

Clearly Buffon remained cautious about tightening crucial links in the Great Chain. He never claimed that the forces of affinity were inherent in living matter. He never surrendered the distinction between living organic molecules, for which Needham's animalcules were apparent evidence, and inanimate matter. By 1778 he admitted that organic molecules could have been spontaneously generated, though only at an earlier stage in the history of the earth.[15] While preserving boundaries between the nonliving and the living, Buffon vigorously maintained the existence of an immaterial soul to distinguish animals and men. More complex animals were not automata but had the same sensations, feelings, and "material pleasures" as human beings. Yet, like the Cartesians, he asserted, "The internal man is dual; he is composed of two principles different by nature and opposed in their action."[16]

For all his belief in universal forces, Buffon was no monist. Yet he strengthened the plausibility of variation within living species. From 1753 he recognized that cross-breeding could produce new species and that fertile hybrids might exist. He noted that variations in species might be induced by diet, climate, epidemics, and habits, and that as long as the environmental cause persisted, these variations could be transmissible to descendants. In 1766 he attributed "degeneration of animals," without a true change in species, to diet or other environmental causes. Thus, Buffon contributed several important concepts to Cabanis's thoughts on the unity of nature—the speculation that all material forces were more or less complex affinities, that the possibility of spontaneous generation did exist, and that environment could induce variation in living species. Cabanis's discussion of the influence of climate called this last opinion of Buffon "eminently philosophical."[17]

TOWARD A MONIST PHILOSOPHY OF LIFE:
MAUPERTUIS, DIDEROT, D'HOLBACH

While Buffon at the Jardin du Roi and Maupertuis at the Academy of Berlin both held prestigious positions, Maupertuis's ideas in the life sciences were the contributions of an amateur, which were more widely diffused because Buffon found them interesting.[18] Cabanis's views on the relationship between sensitivity and matter and his beliefs on change in species bear the unmistakable influence of Maupertuis. Mathematical proof of the nonrandom inheritance of physical deformity or irregularity led Maupertuis to reason that in embryo formation there may be excesses or deficiencies in the forces of affinity that arranged the particles of male and female seminal fluids.[19] By 1751 he was ready to change the traditional notion of matter to explain this phenomenon. Recalling the Newtonian explanation paradigm, Maupertuis wrote: "the more phenomena one had to explain, the more properties one had to assign to matter." Since blind attraction was not a subtle enough principle for embryology, "some principle of intelligence—something resembling what we call *desire*, aversion, memory"—might exist in the "smallest particles of matter." These principles would exist in inorganic matter as well and would not be distinct spiritual entities, like Leibnizian monads. In embryo formation, each particle would have a memory of its own original organ and its situation in the parent and would re-form the embryo on the parental model. A memory failure might result in a monstrosity or a throwback to a characteristic of previous generations. Climate and diet might influence traits of descendants (as torrid zone heat on blackness of skin) or produce deviations (albinism in blacks) that later would revert to primitive form.[20]

Dissimilar species could form from the union of two individuals because of:

> a few fortuitous productions, in which the elementary particles would not have retained the order they kept in the parent animals; each degree of error would have made a new

27

species; and the infinite diversity of animals we observe today would have occurred by repeated deviations; in time, in the course of centuries, this deviation might, by imperceptible movements, increase.[21]

Accidental changes in the elementary particles might produce inheritable defects, though positive, advantageous effects, including the transmission of talents fortified by education, were also possible.[22] Maupertuis strikingly anticipated the research of August Weismann in 1892 by suggesting an experiment to cut off rat tails to test the inheritability of acquired characteristics (though, quite typically, he never carried out the suggestion). He also anticipated Cuvier in attributing some changes in species to geological catastrophes. Though gaps might therefore occur in the Great Chain, Maupertuis was ready to recognize the existence of a single substance—matter coexisting with intelligence—in the natural portion of the chain.

Despite Diderot's malicious charges of skepticism or Spinozism in his *Pensées sur l'interprétation de la nature* (1753), Maupertuis saw no threat to divine Providence in his speculations. God was indispensable; it was God who had to grant matter psychic qualities. Unlike Spinoza, Maupertuis never merely equated God with a principle of intelligence. And unlike the Epicureans, Maupertuis invoked intelligence for continuity in species as well as chance for change.[23]

The most significant Enlightenment impetus to Cabanis's monism and transformism came from the philosophes Diderot and d'Holbach. The subtle mind of Diderot absorbed the evidence of the naturalists as well as Maupertuis's provocative insights in constructing a far-ranging philosophy of the self-sufficiency of nature. By 1749, when he wrote *Lettre sur les aveugles*, Diderot had accepted the idea that motion was inherent in matter (possibly from the English pantheist John Toland) and had explored the ancient Lucretian speculations on spontaneous generation of life and on change in species through the survival and reproduction of "monsters." In the Encyclopedia article entitled "Animal" (1751), Diderot insisted on the unity

28

of all living and thinking creatures including man. By 1753 he had become aware of Trembley's polyp experiments, which heightened the unity in the Great Chain, de Maillet's bold visions of universal germs of life, and the medical materialism of La Mettrie.[24]

In the *Pensées* of 1753, after noting similarities among quadrupeds (probably derived from Buffon's *Histoire naturelle*), Diderot asked, "Would we not naturally conclude that there is but one first animal, prototype of all animals, some of whose organs nature has only lengthened, shortened, transformed, multiplied, obliterated?" Fascinated with the chaotic world of Lucretius, Diderot developed a view of species transformation in which each species went through a life cycle of changes, but in which there was no direct link between one species and another. As he later wrote, the "worm is working its way up to be a man . . . perhaps man is working his way down to be a worm."[25] Diderot's Great Chain was certainly less orderly than that of Maupertuis, even with due allowance for "accidents" in Maupertuis's hypothesis. Yet Diderot's notion of species change was quite similar to the subsequently expressed opinions of Cabanis.

In his mature years Diderot grappled with critical questions concerning the emergence of sensitivity and consciousness from matter and of thought from sensation. Cabanis might have acquired knowledge of Diderot's private speculations from a colleague in the Institute, the classicist Jacques-André Naigeon (1738-1810), who held Diderot's manuscripts. Most likely, however, Cabanis met Diderot himself at Auteuil or at the d'Holbach salon (though the date of October 1774 recently suggested by Sergio Moravia for this meeting is improbable, since Cabanis was then in Poland).[26] The role of particular works of Diderot in influencing Cabanis is difficult to estimate. Moravia's emphasis on the role played by *Principes philosophiques sur la matière et le mouvement* (1770; published by Naigeon in the *Encyclopédie méthodique* in 1792) seems to me to be exaggerated. Diderot there criticized Cartesian mechanism with its inert image of matter. But he stressed the heterogeneity and variation of molecular forces and the varying affinities of chemical substances without explicitly discussing any emergence of the living from the nonliving.[27]

Diderot's hypotheses in *Le Rêve de d'Alembert* (written in approximately 1769, circulated in part in Grimm's manuscript *Correspondance* in 1782, published fully only in 1831) were certainly closer to Cabanis's concerns about the nature of sensitivity. Here Diderot vacillated between the view that sensitivity was a universal endowment of all particles of matter and the view that sensitivity emerged with organization. He chose neither view definitively, though in a private letter of 1765, he wrote that "sensitivity is a universal property of matter, inert in inanimate bodies [like potential energy] but activated in these bodies by their assimilation with a living animal substance."[28] In *Le Rêve de d'Alembert* there were long discussions of the activation of sensitivity in the common organic processes of nutrition and reproduction. Diderot also elaborated a theory of heredity similar to Maupertuis. He discussed malformation of "threads" in the embryo, which produced monsters, speculated on Lucretian "generation" of large animals, and argued that species might change because organs respond to needs (adaptation and selection in the terms of later theorists).[29] The physiology in the *Rêve* was also highly significant for Cabanis, but its consideration belongs amid the discussion of the related influences of Montpellier medicine in Chapter 3.

Cabanis was also inspired by the more polemical philosophy of Diderot's friend, Paul-Henri Thiry, baron d'Holbach (1723-1789). While we now know that the *coterie holbachique* was neither predominantly atheist nor socially radical, the baron himself, behind all of his pseudonyms, was a self-proclaimed materialist who disturbed Voltaire as much as he disturbed the orthodox. The coterie was an important liaison group for diverse philosophes, including abbé Morellet (a subsequent guest of Mme Helvétius) and the medical Encyclopedists G.-F. Venel and P.-J. Barthez (before their move to the Montpellier Faculty in the 1760s). Thus, d'Holbach's guests, as well as d'Holbach himself, had an intellectual, if not personal, impact on Cabanis. Destutt de Tracy claimed that Cabanis "saw the baron frequently" at Auteuil and at the d'Holbach salon for several years.[30]

In the *Système de la nature* (1770), the heaviest salvo of d'Holbach's *machine de guerre*, the baron attacked the last fortress of orthodoxy—the spirituality of the human soul. His goal was to replace allegedly pernicious morality based on theology with a sound natural ethic founded on wisely administered legislation and carefully directed education. Though the subtitle read, *Des loix du monde physique et du monde moral,* less than one-tenth of the book discussed the "system of nature." D'Holbach was primarily concerned with man—and, as a context, the natural, necessary order that enveloped him. To d'Holbach, matter and motion explained all phenomena, and empirical investigation, the only appropriate method for natural knowledge, revealed only matter. Matter had no psychic or vital properties, as with Maupertuis, but only an innate principle of motion, which, properly arranged and conditioned, produced life and thought.[31]

For the attribution of inherent motion and force to matter, d'Holbach, like Diderot, drew on varied sources, including the ancient Stoics and John Toland. Less explicitly than Buffon and Maupertuis, he developed the concept of universal attraction as the basic physical force, with increasingly complex laws of affinity ascending even to human social relationships. He wished to arrive at the most complex properties of matter by first studying the simplest. Thus, by analyzing complex into simple motions, the higher-level affinities of embryology appeared to be the same in kind as reciprocal attraction of chemical molecules. Appropriately enough, d'Holbach cited Needham's spontaneous generation experiments to argue that fermented putrefied organic matter could produce life (though like Lucretius and Diderot, he also believed in spontaneous generation of large animals). At the summit of affinities were self-love, a higher form of inertia, and sympathies and antipathies, whether in family or society.[32]

Unsurprisingly, d'Holbach adopted a physiology that main-

31

tained that physical constitution and environmental influences determined human activity. Cabanis almost literally transcribed the chief contention of d'Holbach's introduction: "The distinction so often made between the physical and the mental has been visibly abused. Man is a purely physical being; mental man is only this physical being considered from a certain viewpoint, that is, relating to some of his faculties existing because of his particular organization."[33]

Consonant with this materialist view of the Great Chain was a physiology reducing mind to matter. D'Holbach's chemical and geological erudition led him to a physicochemical theory of temperament. The most dominant element in the body, he thought, was common fire, or "phlogiston," which preserved fiber mobility and nerve tension and stimulated fluid flow so as literally to create the "fire of genius." Nerve fluid, he speculated, was "electric matter" in varying proportions, and motions or changes in the brain produced all intellectual phenomena. Since the brain could react to impressions by activating itself or other organs, there was no need to attribute its faculties to a soul. Like Diderot, d'Holbach thought that sensitivity, so evident in the organization of the brain, was merely inert in inanimate matter.[34]

D'Holbach repeated the commonplaces of eighteenth-century medical theory on temperament to illustrate the illusion of human freedom. "The habitual state of fluids and solids composing the body" influenced intelligence and character. "Tones" of the brain might determine individual variations. Moreover, external factors—air, food, and wine—could alter the internal indicators of temperament—heat and density of blood, organ arrangement, relaxation and tension of nerves and fibers. In any case, man was always a "passive instrument of necessity—a material being, organized and structured to feel, think, and be modified in special ways."[35]

Where Maupertuis appeared to dignify all matter to explain intelligence, d'Holbach seemed to enslave all human intelligence to inexorable, though complex, laws of motion. While Maupertuis flaunted reverence for divine design and Diderot in his later years often kept his iconoclastic remarks for posterity, d'Holbach, retaining his anonymity for all but a few in the loyal coterie, gleefully published a major work which left no scope for God or design.

Though the chemical terminology was obsolescent, the physicochemical basis of d'Holbach's physiology gave a new dimension to materialism. The materialization of life and thought, presented with the pamphleteer's verve, was a *succès de scandale*. Cabanis was more prudent in tone and ultimately less reductionist in his metaphysics. He adopted d'Holbach's monist view of the human body without seeming to deny the special status of life and without succumbing to a bleak view about the indifference of nature to human purpose.

In the Romantic stereotype, any materialist doctrine that denied the spiritual soul also denied eternal punishment and thereby subverted morality. But critics of materialism often failed to distinguish the hedonistic La Mettrie and amoral novelists and philosophers from d'Holbach's attack on theologically supported morality. The baron never praised idle pleasure-seeking or downgraded virtuous actions. He held that man's struggle for self-preservation and his pursuit of happiness were merely submission to the most powerful human motivations rather than free choices. Yet d'Holbach thought that virtue—making others happy or being useful to society— was consonant with, indeed was the only means of achieving, happiness. "Merit and Virtue," he claimed, "are founded on the nature of man, and on his needs."[36] Such a facile solution of moral dilemmas might have been unsatisfactory, but it did retain the distinction between vice and virtue.

In fact, d'Holbach's views on altering a naturally inherited temperament or perfecting intelligence could have been held by many physicians who were neither materialist nor determinist. For d'Holbach, moral responsibility was precisely the effort to use climate and diet to "correct the defects of a vicious organization and temperament as harmful to society as to the individual possessing it." Thus, each of us could "in a way create" our own temperament; "if one consulted experience rather than prejudice, medicine would provide moral philosophy with the key to the human heart, and in healing the body it would sometimes be assured of healing the mind."[37] Not even Cartesian dualists maintained the independence of the soul from the body, though they might prefer to consider the soul immutable. Physical explanations of mental illness and body-soul relationships were the standard fare of contemporary medicine. Many moralists also raised questions about free will and rational control of the passions. D'Holbach's views were scandalous only because he collapsed body and soul into one. His formulation of the role of medicine otherwise could have been shared by the orthodox, though it furnished a convenient blueprint, after refinement of the physiology, for Cabanis's monist science of man.

Even on the question of determinism, d'Holbach's belief that all human action was motivated and that free will was a delusion did not lead him to deny the individual's capacity to improve temperament and benefit from experience. D'Holbach hoped that education, the "agriculture of the mind," would plant virtuous habits. "The heart of man," he added, "is a terrain which can produce poison or fruit" according to its cultivation.[38]

ORTHODOX MENTAL MECHANISM: BONNET

Avant-garde irreligion was not a necessary condition for conceptions about necessity in the human condition, or for conceptions about the unity of nature, however. The Swiss Protestant naturalist Charles Bonnet (1720-1793), despite his own claim to orthodoxy, also developed hypotheses about the physical basis of the human mind and the links of man and nature. Bonnet, who was praised by Cabanis as a "great naturalist as well as a great metaphysician," had performed experiments in natural history, including the parthenogenesis of the aphid, or plant louse, before turning to more speculative works on the Great Chain of Being and on the human mind—notably *Contemplation de la nature* (1764), *Essai de psychologie* (1754), and *Essai analytique sur les facultés de l'âme* (1760).[39] Indebted to Réaumur and Haller as a naturalist, and to Leibniz and Locke as a philosopher, Bonnet, despite some unorthodox speculations on animal souls, remained a reverent believer in Providence and the human soul.

As a naturalist, Bonnet combined the traditional belief in fixed species with the new concept of change in species as a result of environmental catastrophes. His final version of the Great Chain allowed for improvements in vegetable and animal species (not minerals), though each living species would remain in a constant relationship to all others. After the Revolution conservative philosophers in France were attracted to a theory of progress such as this, which retained the old hierarchy in new form.[40] Bonnet also stressed the continuity between animals and men. He saw a physical basis in the brain for intellectual faculties, accepted the empiricist view that knowledge came from the senses, and even accepted the belief that all human actions were predetermined. Yet he shunned the perils of materialist heresy and remained confident that his own hypotheses gave no aid and comfort to skeptics.[41]

The Newtonian explanation paradigm gave Bonnet a license to formulate hypotheses that did not deal with the essence of mind. Bonnet believed that the soul was a simple, active, immaterial principle, but he also maintained that we could not know its essence or its form of union with the body. He assumed that the brain ministered to the soul not by the motion of particles, but by an interaction of forces. While he sometimes used mechanistic metaphors, such as the musician-soul playing the harpsichord-brain, he would not locate the soul in the brain. With Newtonian agnosticism, he noted that the observable relationships between forces of soul and sensitive fibers did not vary in the hypotheses of physical interaction, occasionalism, or preestablished harmony. And in a phrase worthy of Galileo, Bonnet said that man was no less perfect even if he was material.[42]

Bonnet's dualist commitment and avoidance of materializing the soul thus freed him to speculate about mechanisms of

35

physical-mental interaction. In the 1760 *Essai* he independently conceived a Condillac-like statue to describe the awakening of the sense of smell, the development of attention, memory, and other faculties. An elaborate hypothesis asserted that sensations resulted in changes in molecular arrangement of nerve fibers, so that there were dispositions in each fiber to reproduce certain movements. Association of ideas and habits arose from the supple nature of the fibers and the reproduction of movements that had already impressed ideas on the brain. The dimensions of fibers and the facility of motion of their molecules would relate to temperament, or the ability to yield to impressions. There were specific nerve fibers for each kind of sensation, even "moral" and "intellectual" fibers. In a note added in 1781, Bonnet even speculated that the subtle fluid in the nerves was analogous in effect to the electric fluid, though the fire in the electric fluid might be different when combined in the nerves than elsewhere.[43]

Bonnet thus unhesitatingly offered a physical hypothesis of sensitivity, though he carefully denied that it concerned anything but the nervous system and the brain. In 1781 he specifically stated that an explanation in terms of nerve fiber molecules only expressed an effect, like Newtonian attraction, with an unknown cause and even an unknown inner mechanism.[44] Thus, heresy was not implicit in his speculation on the mode of operation of sensitivity.

Like Locke and d'Holbach, Bonnet did not hesitate to conclude that a sensitive being must follow the Law of Pleasure. The body was subject to this necessity, he agreed, but such a necessity preserved liberty since the freedom of the will was only its executive power to do as it pleased. The will did not passively accept pleasurable sensations, but actively chose them.[45] Clearly, Bonnet's uplifting liberty was not far removed from d'Holbach's sobering necessity.

Cabanis absorbed a rich intellectual heritage from naturalists and philosophers of diverse religious views who collectively represented Enlightenment notions concerning the unity of nature. Certainly the idea of a Great Chain of Being was still a commanding concept. Yet all thinkers faced the problem of how organization, feeling, and intelligence could arise from ordinary matter. The ancient idea of souls at various functional levels was unsatisfactory after Cartesian mechanism radically separated mechanical matter and the rational soul. A range of phenomena such as spontaneous generation, regenerating polyps, or the well-known human physical-mental interaction could be accommodated in the dualist metaphysic, but at a price—strange, inexplicable forces that tightened the unity of the Chain and were legitimized by the precedent of Newtonian attraction. Thus, the nearly orthodox Needham and Bonnet or the prudent deist Buffon could avoid heresy by leaving a realm of mystery surrounding the action of these forces.

Similarly, variation in species and the idea of a common prototype accepted by Maupertuis and Diderot made the concept of inexplicable natural forces more plausible. Only those already inclined to deism, atheism, or criticism of Revelation, however, would therefore stress the self-sufficiency of nature in perfecting mankind, adopt metaphysical monism, or approach transformist ideas on change of species. Even the more daring philosophes had to concede qualities of a psychic nature (Maupertuis) or emergence of sensitivity from a latent state (Diderot and d'Holbach) that might suggest some purpose in the simplest movements of matter. The choice between dualism and the curiously similar monist extremes of panpsychism or materialism might thus be determined by beliefs about God and the soul and their relationship to the Great Chain of Being.

Condillac's "Analysis" and the Unity of the Sciences

Neither monism nor transformism was an opinion prerequisite to belief in the unity of human knowledge. Like many dualists, d'Alembert expressed the essential Encyclopedist spirit when he wrote of the "chain that binds together" the sciences.[46] Monism might mean a greater willingness to export methods of the physical sciences to the study of man and society, but the quest for unity in the sciences was first a quest for method. Inevitably, the search for valid methods led to discussion of the abilities and limitations of the human mind. Whether or not this discussion had monist or dualist preconceptions, it did legitimize questions that might challenge Revelation.

New canons of scientific method did not spring fullblown from the minds of Bacon, Galileo, and Descartes. Late medieval and Renaissance physicians and philosophers distinguished inductive from deductive procedures in reasoning, and by the late sixteenth century Galileo's predecessor Giacomo Zabarella (1533-1589) had spoken of combining "analysis," or "resolution" (inductive), with "synthesis," or "composition" (deductive).[47]

In the early seventeenth century, amid an atmosphere of excitement about practical navigation and useful craft knowledge, Francis Bacon demanded a new inductive logic that would rise gradually from "senses and particulars" to "general axioms." His incomplete legacy in the Novum Organum (1620) was a search for a universal method that would compile tables of particular instances of presence, absence, and variation of a particular "form," such as heat. After all the necessary exclusions and comparisons, one could arrive by sound reasoning at an expression of the "simple nature" of heat.[48] Despite the completion of only the portion of the Novum Organum dealing with metaphysics, and not physics, Baconian method became a widely hailed model for the French Idéologue circle.

Because Bacon had stressed the "analytic" empirical step of the double method, French epistemologists found it convenient to look to René Descartes for a model of the "synthetic" deductive procedure.[49] In the Regulae ad Directionem Ingenii (c. 1628, published 1684) and in the Rules of Reasoning in the Discours de la méthode (1637), Descartes spoke of a heuristic step of dividing each "difficulty" into parts; a second step was the intuitive apprehension of a simple nature as the simplest term in a series; and a final step was the deduction of its necessary relationships. One might, for example, intuitively determine that the essence of matter was extension and then by deduction arrive at its other properties of shape and impenetrability.[50] By the mid-eighteenth century, however, these procedures were placed in a context of sense observation, which made obsolete the mere intuition of a simple nature.

Newtonian scientific method, as expressed by the astronomer Roger Cotes, insisted on combining Baconian induction with Cartesian deduction: "From some select phenomena they deduce by analysis the forces of Nature and the more simple laws of forces, and from thence by synthesis show the constitution of the rest."[51] This empirical-rational Newtonian method complemented the study of the mind by Newton's contemporary John Locke. Locke had not systematically used procedures of analysis or synthesis, but he steadfastly denied the Cartesian assumption of innate ideas and refused to postulate an essence of mind. Rather, he studied only the operations of the mind and concluded that all human knowledge of the corporeal world derived from sensation, which furnished simple ideas, and from reflection, which was the awareness of the operations of the cognitive self and the source of complex ideas.

The mid-eighteenth-century schoolmaster of Ideology, Etienne Bonnot, abbé de Condillac (1714-1780), was still a "geometric spirit" owing much to Descartes's procedures for deduction,[52] yet his entire effort to study the mind was permeated with Locke's empirical assumptions and Newton's method of combining reason and experience. Condillac banished metaphysics, seeking to "penetrate all mystery . . . to discover the nature and essence of things," and redefined "metaphysics" as the study of mental operations.[53] He proposed a universally valid method of analysis that would increase the degree of certainty in metaphysics and morals. Cabanis and his colleague Tracy considered their task as Ideologists to be that of critical revision of Condillac's treatises. Hence, for our discussion, Condillac's definition of the method of analysis merits full consideration.

To Condillac, analysis was not only the inductive step of reasoning but the general name for the two component stages of "decomposition" and "composition."[54] The first step, decomposition, "distinguishes all the ideas belonging to a subject; and examines them until discovering the idea which generates all the others." The distinction of a single fact from a mixture, or the focus on one sensation from an indistinct bundle of impressions, would "decompose" a confused picture. In nature striking objects naturally became predominant, so decomposition was effortless, and invalid reasoning resulted from prejudices and mistakes rather than from a natural process. A glance through a château window, with each area perceived separately, would thus arrange its confused simultaneous perceptions into successive orders of dominance and relationship.[55] As with Descartes, the simplest, most striking ideas or facts were logically and temporally prior "principles," but they came from the world of the particulars of sense-experience rather than from innate ideas.[56] Composition followed more closely the deduction of Descartes's *Regulae*, for it was a reasoning by identity, or successive transformations of the primary fact to restore the simultaneous order of perception. The proper classification by resemblances and differences would enable a systematic arrangement of facts or ideas "in order of their gradation."[57]

Condillac saw the analytic method as the key to both the formation of language and the construction of philosophical systems. Natural analysis in early man fixed dominant sensations by easily ordered signs (cries, gestures, and ultimately words). In primitive languages, signs began to denote subjects of primary and urgent interest, but the meaning of words lost clarity as words began to denote objects unrelated to immediate needs. Thus, to gain clarity in a science, its language, distinct and characteristic in each science, had to reflect the analytic method. Analysis would produce a useful philosophical system, a "body of knowledge with mutually dependent parts, which is derived from a single principle; so that a good system is simply a successfully expanded principle."[58]

Condillac realized the difficulty of constructing perfect languages, however. The unity of the sciences was thus an elusive goal, and analytic method had to be appropriate to the subject. Complete analyses were possible only with the "evidence of reason," the deductive certitude of arithmetic, geometry, and some portions of metaphysics. In physics, as in demonstration of the Newtonian world-system, the "evidence of fact" had to support the evidence of reason. In physics, "principles" were empirical phenomena, not unknowable essences. Indeed the essence of a physical substance such as gold was unknowable; one could only enumerate the properties that collectively identified it, such as heaviness, malleability, and ductility.[59] Often conjecture and analogy were necessary in the observational sciences, and experimental confirmation was decisive.

In the study of man, metaphysics was between mathematical certainty and physical probability. Condillac argued that the "analysis of the faculties of the soul" was "complete if we wish to return to simple sensations" but "incomplete if we wish to penetrate the nature of the thinking being." The faculty of sensation was indeed a "principle," a primary physiological phenomenon, generating all other mental operations, but it was at best a "secondary essence" of mind. The true essence of mind, material or spiritual, remained unknowable, since one could observe only a change in the soul—feeling occasioned by a corresponding motion in the body.[60]

Thus, Condillac's pursuit of unity in the sciences, tempered by a realization that each science had a characteristic method and characteristic degree of certainty, was an important forerunner of Idéologue thought. The entire notion of analytic method and the importance of clear language was an equally significant legacy to the Idéologues. But perhaps most important of all was the content of Condillac's psychology.

Forerunners of Psychology: Condillac and Helvétius

Condillac's deductive manner of presentation was thoroughly different in style from the medically trained Locke's rich description of chaotic experience. Yet Condillac did reaffirm Locke's empiricism, and for Cabanis, this reaffirmation established the primacy of sensations, and by implication, of physical sensitivity, in the formation of thoughts as well as desires. In

41

addition, Cabanis was drawn to the questions that Condillac answered inadequately concerning the corporeal influences on sensations. Condillac avoided troublesome problems of physiology. Whether sensation occurred by movement of animal spirits or by stirring of brain fibers was of no importance to Condillac. He vaguely equated the "physical and occasional principle of sensitivity" with "determinations of the vegetative movement" and that of memory with these "determinations become habits."[61] For Condillac, empiricism and dualism were perfectly compatible.

Condillac's first major work, the *Essai sur les origines de la connaissance humaine* (1746), discussed the basic problem of how thoughts derived from sensations. Sensation was the raw material of knowledge, a kind of gravitational principle of the mind. Striking sensations generated the second faculty of attention, and attention, in the absence of the object, or reminiscence, formed memory and imagination. Unlike Locke, Condillac denied the mind any distinct active power of "reflection"; he explained the higher faculties of comparison, judgment, and reasoning by the medium of the habitual use of signs. According to Condillac, language was an efficient means of associating ideas.

In his *Traité des sensations* (1754) Condillac modified his system by analytically deriving all the faculties of the mind from simple sensation without the intervention of language. For this purpose, he used the well-worn device of a statue-man awakening, one sense at a time, to awareness of itself and the world. He showed that signs were indispensable only for theoretical knowledge and abstract reasoning.

At the same time, Condillac correlatively derived all of the faculties of the will, as well as all of the faculties of understanding, from primitive sensations. Each sensation was pleasurable as well as painful, affective as well as cognitive; and desires arose from comparison of sensations. By a kind of automatic reaction "as a result of its organization" the statue-man sought the beneficial and avoided the harmful even before its full consciousness of motion.[62]

42

Condillac recognized in passing that temperament, physical condition, and passions might influence attention and might therefore influence reaction to sensations. The conformation of organs, or even the inscrutable nature of the soul, might affect the facility of association of ideas. He asserted that such influences might even be salutary for the mind, for in periods of illness or in the transports of pleasure, the imagination often reacted upon the senses to produce images livelier than those produced by external objects.[63]

Yet Condillac never allowed such arguments or his general empiricist view to lead him into simplistic determinism. He never concluded that either external or internal impulses of the moment exercised absolute control over man. Beneficial habits came from experience, and the power of habit could counteract impulses of immediate pleasure and pain. Indeed, man's superiority over animals stemmed precisely from his ability to fix sensations through language and to make rational choices on the basis of experience. Man might then realize that previous false judgments were not conducive to his true happiness, while animals would be trapped in the circle of rudimentary reflections appropriate to their limited needs.[64]

Human freedom, for Condillac, meant the ability to cultivate good habits, uproot harmful ones, and educate and enlighten self-interest by the experiences of sorrow and shame, which were the consequences of intemperance. Condillac did not see man as a helpless swimmer against the current, except in fits of passion. He wrote, "Confide the conduct of a vessel to a man who knows nothing of navigation, and the vessel will be the plaything of the waves. But a skillful pilot will know how to suspend or halt its course; with the same wind he will know how to change direction; and only in a tempest will the helm disobey his hand. Such is the image of man."[65] If this was determinism, it was qualified and flexible. Language and experience, awesome burdens to some modern philosophers, were claimed by Condillac as essential to human liberation.

As a cleric and tutor of princes, Condillac respected dualist orthodoxy and defended human freedom. There have been too many misleading interpretations of Condillac that see logical, if unrecognized, implications of materialism and determinism in his philosophy. But these implications are largely invented by the critics. Condillac would never admit that sensations were merely physical, or that we could know the essence of mind. The empiricism of Condillac in itself threatened belief in the soul only for those whose faith was already vanishing.

If Condillac was a prudent empiricist, Helvétius was the *enfant terrible* among Locke's disciples. Yet Cabanis explicitly named Helvétius with Condillac among those who had proven empiricism beyond a doubt.[66] Cabanis's intimate association with Mme Helvétius and with the abbé Lefebvre de La Roche, editor of Helvétius's works, increases the probability that he carefully considered the issues raised in the ill-fated *De L'Esprit* (1758) and posthumously published *De L'Homme* (1772). In these, Helvétius's principal concern was with the now traditional issues of psychology, learning, and motivation, but also with moral and social relationships.

The foundation of Helvétius's philosophy was the belief that physical sensitivity was the sole principle of mental and moral activity, so that the basic law of human behavior was the search for pleasurable sensations. Unlike the physicians, he attempted to show that the effect of temperament, sense organs, climate, food, and physical causes in general was insignificant in determining either intelligence or passion. His unsophisticated approach to physiology appeared in such contentions as the irrelevance of nerve mobility to intelligence because women, with more mobile nerves, were less intelligent than men. Men of genius, he claimed, were of all proportions, strengths, and temperaments, and they inhabited all climates. Never had people of any particular region enjoyed constant intellectual superiority, either.[67]

Helvétius therefore took the extreme position that only mental factors influenced intelligence; he defined "experience" in the broadest sense as the totality of external sensations. Talents and virtues were the effect of education rather than the gift of nature, since "commonly well-organized" men had equal aptitudes for reason. Ultimately, contended Helvétius, "education is capable of everything." Differences in experience thus explained inequalities in intelligence. Some men might also have stronger passions, or a greater capacity for attention, than others. The distinguishing factors were not physical temperaments, however, but unequal motivations—the varying degrees of interest that men had in given situations. "The mental universe," argued Helvétius, "is ruled by the laws of interest no less than the physical universe by the laws of motion." All pleasures and passions could then be considered variations of agreeable physical sensations. Devoted love, loyal friendship, benevolent aid to the poor, and single-minded scholarship were all manifestations of the pursuit of physical pleasure. It is on such explanatory principles that Helvétius proposed to establish the science of man.[68]

Cabanis was just as much a critical disciple of Helvétius as of Condillac, and the opinions he would have challenged are well illustrated in Diderot's unpublished assessment of Helvétius's works. There Diderot defended the conventional view that internal physiology and climate at least partially determined character against Helvétius's extreme environmental empiricism. Diderot could not understand Helvétius's disregard of natural aptitudes. Though he agreed that education was important, he did not believe that it could erase the influence of temperament. Writing in ignorance of anatomy, physiology, and medicine, Helvétius had nowhere mentioned differences in strength of organic fibers or quality of humors. The state of the brain, Diderot maintained, might affect judgment, and the sensitivity of the diaphragm, seat of pleasures and pains, might make men compassionate or stern. In common experience, physical afflictions affected intelligence, and physical remedies helped cure mental disturbances. Age also influenced mental acuity, and climate, as Montesquieu had argued, differentiated the effects of the same form of government in two locations. Temperament, then, could not be ignored, and Helvétius was mouthing an absurdity if he thought his servant as potentially great as he.[69]

45

The social implications of this controversy were fewer than might be expected. Strict environmentalists might call attention to the need for education and the possibility of cultural deprivation. Yet Helvétius was no more a thoroughgoing democrat than Diderot, despite the egalitarian implications of his postulation of equal intelligence at birth. Moreover, the temperament theorists did not usually correlate temperament to social and economic class. The dissolute noble or tax-farmer might be as incorrigible as the greedy peasant or the shiftless laborer, while proper education could still alter the dispositions of the lowly as well as the great.[70]

Diderot also vehemently objected to Helvétius's simplistic assumption that self-interest, interpreted as the pursuit of physical pleasure, was the paramount human motivation. Diderot considered the pleasures of anticipation and imagination uniquely human, while physical sensitivity alone moved animals. Diderot appeared offended by Helvétius's far-fetched illustrations. Does a man give alms to the poor, he asked, all the while secretly contemplating the prospect of a good bed and a fine supper and coveting his neighbor's wife? By this reasoning, Helvétius abused otherwise sound principles.[71]

Diderot also accused Helvétius of inadequately discussing the relationship of physical sensitivity to matter, sensation, and thought. In fact, Helvétius did state the view that the faculty of sensation, like attraction, was a property of bodies and that it arose from animal organization. Though sensitivity might be the "essence of the soul," it disappeared with the death of the body, as magnetism did with the disintegration of iron. Nevertheless, despite Helvétius's mechanistic metaphors (physical sensitivity as the wheel of the human machine) and his presumed atheism, he was no more logically impelled to embrace materialism than was Condillac. We can discount Helvétius's wry invocation of theological aid in attaining knowledge of the "principle of life" within us. But we can accept his claim that discussion of sensitivity and memory as modifications of either spiritual or material substance "does not enter the plan of my

46

work. What I have to say about the mind agrees as well with either of these hypotheses."[72] Despite Helvétius's unorthodoxy, even he could take refuge in the now conventional retreat from exploring the essence of mind or matter.

Moreover, despite Helvétius's glorification of physical sensitivity, his ethic of reason and calculation was meant to lead to social harmony. Moral science would "enable men to live among themselves as happily as possible" by achieving the "felicity of the greatest number" (the phrase that inspired Bentham). The wise legislator would use just laws to link personal and public interests and would manipulate passions and the universal pursuit of pleasure to produce virtue. Only evil or incompetent governments allowed the pursuit of self-interest to lead to injustice.[73]

Thus, the psychology of Helvétius and Condillac led to no moral consequences that were unacceptable to Cabanis. Indeed, Cabanis looked favorably on the idea that physical sensitivity was the key to behavior. But, like Diderot, he stressed the need to bring the knowledge of a physician to correct the extravagant or incomplete statements of both Condillac and Helvétius.

Condillac had succeeded in highlighting the ideal of the logical unity of the sciences with their shared analytic method. Applied to the operations of the mind and will, analysis resulted in the selection of sensation as the generative principle of all mental faculties, and pleasure and pain as the concomitants of all sensations and the immediate, though not irrevocable, determinants of the will. Self-love enlightened by experience became the keystone of morality, and the inculcation of socially useful habits, the aim of ethics. During the Revolution some moralists would even justify natural rights without reference to God, by merely reasoning that all men have similar faculties and therefore similar needs.

Neither an empiricist epistemology nor a utilitarian ethic implied a rigid materialism. Condillac could believe that knowledge arrived through the senses but was integrated by a spiritual soul. And Helvétius could claim that men always sought physical pleasure without troubling about whether sensitivity existed in the body or in the mind.

Cabanis's association with the philosophes, especially with Diderot, d'Holbach, and the Auteuil circle, predisposed him toward monism as well as empiricism. His inner motivations for irreverence toward orthodox religion, aside from a distaste for abuses and a rebellious temperament, remain an unsolved question, as in the case of the young Diderot. But his specialized training as a physician definitely changed his view of the kind of uniformity existing both in nature and in method applied to all the sciences.

CHAPTER II

The Body as Mechanism

Ancient Temperament Theory

n the medical literature that Cabanis studied, the mind-body problem was as ancient as the temperament theory in the Hippocratic *Corpus* and the physiology of Galen. Yet the medical legacy left to Cabanis involved a complex change in the idea of temperament—from the Greco-Roman theory of humors to a concept focused on the physical sensitivity of the nervous system. Seventeenth-century concepts of mechanism and Newtonian concepts of force began to displace the ancient concern with bodily fluids. These notions developed in two distinct conceptual models, or paradigms, defined as follows: "mechanism," which stressed the analogy of the body to a machine, and "vitalism," which stressed the nonmechanical, teleological functioning of distinctive living "principles," or forces. We can understand Cabanis only by realizing that these two paradigms gradually and unforeseeably converged as they began to describe the same phenomena in increasingly similar manner. Cabanis ended up with a bias for Montpellier vitalism, which in its view of life and medicine provided a strong antidote to the dose of materialism that he absorbed from Diderot and d'Holbach. From all schools of medical thought—ancient, mechanist, and vitalist—Cabanis appropriated the goal of improving physical health in order to strengthen the mind. Physicians of diverse metaphysical and religious viewpoints could agree on the importance of preventive hygiene and treatment of disease in developing intelligence and character.

Our interpretation of Cabanis therefore requires study of the ancient temperament theory as well as of the more recent convergence of mechanism and vitalism. French physicians had rarely abandoned their loyalty to the ancients. Galenism had remained dominant in the schools, even when challenged by Paracelsian chemotherapists, and the observational, "Neo-Hippocratic" revival at Montpellier in the sixteenth century further enhanced the prestige of the ancients.[1] The Hippocratic *Corpus* became the most pervasive medical influence. Faculties of medicine commonly required commentaries on the "Aphorisms" or another Hippocratic work in degree examinations. In the reformed Paris School of Medicine in 1798 Cabanis himself prepared lectures on texts from Hippocrates as part of the course in "advanced clinical" observation.[2]

In his homage to Hippocrates (c. 460-377 B.C.), Cabanis recognized the distinction between authentic and apocryphal works. He read the *Corpus* with an eighteenth-century bias and sifted from it whatever seemed consistent with empiricism and clinical medicine. The following aspects of Hippocratic theory had the greatest appeal to Cabanis: (1) a method of observation and reasoning that retained the independence of medicine while also establishing its link to other theoretical disciplines, (2) a full consciousness of human diversity, as expressed by the idea of individual physical equilibrium (*krasis*) among the four humors corresponding to appearance, intelligence, and character, and as affected by inherent factors such as age and sex as well as external influences such as air, season, climate, topography, diet, and physical habits, (3) a therapy based on the healing power of nature, a struggle to restore individual constitution to its natural equilibrium, and (4) the specific unity of the living organism and interdependence of its parts. Cabanis held Hippocrates' philosophy in such high regard that he used a phrase from the "Decorum" as the epigraph to his own essay on medicine, *Coup d'oeil*: "The physician who is also a philosopher is the equal of a god."[3] Hippocrates scorned false systems yet insisted on "ordered experience" (*expérience raisonnée*). Hippocrates' goal was thus to "introduce philosophy into medicine and medicine into philosophy."[4]

50

The following paragraphs will summarize, in excerpts from translations of the Hippocratic *Corpus*, those observations and theories that seem to have been most significant to Cabanis. Cabanis saw Hippocrates as a forerunner of Locke, Helvétius, Bonnet, and Condillac in his insistence on the primacy of sense observation. Thus, in observing disease, Hippocrates would "perceive and fix the general relationships of all these scattered facts."[5] Yet in the treatise "The Art" (or "The Science of Medicine"), he warned against dogmatic physical hypotheses that suggested a single principle as the cause of disease. The physician must observe all he can—appearance, breathing, excretions of the patient—and perhaps even induce identifying symptoms to reveal the disease. Pondering these signs, the physician can then complete his diagnosis of the disease, prognosticate its future course, and prescribe therapy according to records of similar past cases and cures.[6] Cabanis felt Hippocrates' terse, precise, unemotional descriptions of phenomena in the "Epidemics" and his rules for medical reasoning in "Prognostic" and "Aphorisms" made him a superior model for modern physicians despite his obsolete *materia medica*.

Cabanis was also comfortable with the primary theoretical assumption in the *Corpus*, the definition of health as an appropriate mixture of humors. The author of the lecture "On the Nature of Man" named the four humors—"blood, phlegm, yellow bile, and black bile"— and asserted that the "correct proportion in strength and quantity" of these substances would assure well-being.[7] An excess, separation, dilution, or thickening of a humor might bring on disease.[8] Meanwhile, in characteristic reaction to disease, the body naturally struggled to restore lost balance by "coction," or digestion, of the disturbed humor. The result was either favorable resolution of the crisis (evacuation of the humor or abscess formation) or inability to restore equilibrium, which would be a cause of death. The characteristic periods of crisis in each disease could also become a significant diagnostic tool.[9]

Hippocratic therapy thus had to reinforce, not hinder, the healing force of nature in order to restore natural equilibrium.

51

"Nature," wrote the author, "is the healer of disease. Nature finds by itself, without intelligence, the way and means; nature, with neither instruction nor wisdom, performs what is suitable; tears, humidity of the nostrils, sneezing, yawning, coughing. . . ."[10] Lest the physician remain passive, however, there was a warning that a "spontaneous cure" was a "false and meaningless idea" in acute diseases and poisonings. The physician must guide the progress of disease, "so that it develops according to its natural tendency." Salutary crises must be neither premature nor delayed. The therapist must do everything possible to oppose the cause of disease.[11]

This principle of balancing medical caution with intervention would become not only an important ingredient in Cabanis's warnings about overactive medicine but also a striking parallel to his political philosophy based on the beneficence of natural law. Neither his medical therapy nor his political thought was deduced from the other, but they had structural similarities. Cabanis did not mean to imply that assisting free operation of natural law, either in medicine or in politics, implied passivity. He recognized that eighteenth-century medical therapy had progressed far beyond simply allowing nature to take its course. Remedies were more plentiful than in the era of Hippocrates. And in any case, physicians had to plan their treatment rationally since they could not rely on natural restorative powers in civilized society. In some cases, Cabanis counseled, "nature's misguided efforts must be stopped or channeled in another direction."[12] Similarly, natural laws of human behavior, such as the prevalence of self-interest or sympathy, had to be actively assisted if the achievement of a harmonious society were to be possible.

What was later called the temperament theory also gave Cabanis his fundamental parameters for internal and external idiosyncratic influences affecting body-mind relationships. In the Hippocratic *Corpus*, therapy had to allow for variation in humors due to age, sex, and specific physical constitution. But external environmental factors were equally important. Seasonal or short-term weather changes affected predominance of particular humors; thus the physician also had to record atmospheric conditions ("Epidemics"). "Morbid secretions in the air" as well as harmful regimen might induce certain ailments.[13] The author of the treatise "Airs, Waters, Places" provided a comprehensive geophysical account of endemic illness and characteristic health of natives of certain localities. The seasons, wind exposure, and qualities of water and soil as well as habits of eating, drinking, and work were shown to affect puberty, fertility, characteristic mental and physical traits, and susceptibility to disease. The argument, stated simply, says that "climates differ and cause differences in character, the greater variations in climate, so much the greater will be differences in character." An unstable climate would produce diverse characters; a mild climate, cowardly and mediocre minds; and an extreme climate, bold and agile minds.[14]

Despite the intervening revisions of these ideas by more modern physicians, the Hippocratic principles were still recognizable in Cabanis's list of influences on "ideas and passions"—age, sex, individual equilibrium, or temperament, disease, climate, and regimen. Temperament, in the broad sense, was metaphysically neutral—acceptable to Diderot and d'Holbach as well as to dualists. Helvétius, for his part, disputed the importance of internal factors, but the medical tradition was already so strong in Diderot that he had to acknowledge that nuanced efforts to perfect intelligence and character would be necessary in view of the diversity of temperaments. For Cabanis, Hippocrates provided the ideal compromise between the cultural environmentalism of Helvétius and the climatic theory of Montesquieu. In the *Corpus*, Hippocrates spoke of the significance of the tyrannical government as well as the mild, temperate climate in shaping the "docile and cowardly" temperament of Asians. Habits of life, such as the continual horseback riding of the Scythians, were at least as important as climate in affecting their flabby constitutions and the infertility of their women.[15]

While the Hippocratic writings provided precepts for therapy and raw materials for the art of human perfectibility, they also stressed the physiological unity and interdependence of parts within the body. Cabanis's discussion of internal and external sensations cited a Hippocratic maxim on organic unity: "Tout y concourt, tout y conspire, tout y consent" (Everything cooperates with, conspires toward, and consents to seek that purpose). Expressed differently, "Life is a circle, where we can find neither beginning nor end, since in a circle, each point of the circumference can be beginning or end."[16] This conception of unity provided the blueprint for modern vitalism and for emphasis on organic vehicles of unity such as the nervous system.

While Galen of Pergamum (c. A.D. 130-200) systematically developed Hippocratic equilibrium into the temperament theory, Cabanis devoted only one and one-half pages of his medical history to Galen compared to the eleven pages given Hippocrates. To Cabanis, Galen was a systematizer, a weaver of hypotheses who betrayed the prudence of Hippocratic observation. Yet because Galen was unhampered by Christian scruples concerning materiality of the soul, he could set certain precedents for physical-mental correlations, and did so, especially in his treatise showing that the "habits of the soul are the consequence of the temperaments of the body."[17] As in Platonic theories of a hierarchy of souls, Galen believed that a "psychic pneuma" (later called "animal spirits") in the brain and nervous system controlled sensation, muscular motion, and reasoning, and that "vital pneuma" in the heart enriched the blood, assisted ebb and flow of blood, and controlled complex passions such as ambition. Later Galenists added a "natural pneuma" in the liver to control vegetative processes, nutrition, and simple appetites for physical pleasure.[18]

Galen also established nine classes of temperaments: four simple classes, with the dominance of each of the four qualities—warm, cold, dry, and moist; four composite classes—sanguine (warm and moist), phlegmatic (cold and moist), bilious (warm and dry), and melancholic (cold and dry); and one ideal "temperate" state. Arabic commentaries on Galen emphasized the importance he placed on the "non-naturals" in shaping the soul. He defined non-naturals as being things neither natural to the body, nor against nature, yet indispensable: (1) air, (2) motion and rest, (3) sleep and wakefulness, (4) *ingesta* (food, beverages, drugs), (5) *excreta* and *retenta* (things excreted or retained), and (6) emotions or passions. Even in the original Galenic view, changes in non-naturals through diet, habits, or exposure to a different climate were thought capable of altering temperaments sufficiently to make citizens more virtuous.[19]

Iatrochemistry and Iatrophysics

While Cabanis supported critics of Galenism, he had only faint praise for Paracelsus (c. 1490-1541) and little sympathy for the Iatrochemical school of Franciscus Sylvius of Leyden (1614-1672) or the English physician Thomas Willis (1621-1675) who reduced temperament to an acid-alkaline balance. Yet Cabanis did see a reaffirmation of Hippocratic principles in the antihumoral physiology of an heir of the Paracelsians, the Flemish alchemist and physician Johannes Baptista van Helmont (1577-1644).[20] For the Hippocratic "healing force of nature," van Helmont substituted a spiritual guiding principle, or *archeus*, immanent in material ferments. The *archeus* controlling the stomach and diaphragm, with their "system of epigastric forces," could affect the mortal, sensitive soul and therefore mind-body relations. Moreover, van Helmont believed that a principal *archeus* supervised a subordinate hierarchy of organic *archei*. The entire body was thus a federation of organs, each with its inherent dynamic principle. When Cabanis studied eighteenth-century Montpellier physiology, he recognized that van Helmont's *archaeus*, stripped of mystical trappings, could be converted into the peculiar physical sensitivity of each organ. Therefore, van Helmont was a valuable progenitor of Cabanis's ideas.

The Iatrophysical school of the seventeenth century presented a more formidable challenge to concepts of the uniqueness of life and the autonomy of medicine. Inspired by Descartes's mechanical philosophy and by the statics and kinematics of Galileo and Torricelli, a number of physicians who flourished in Italy, England, France, and the Netherlands adopted the image of the body as a hydraulic machine.[21]

DESCARTES

Descartes's portrait of man in the posthumously published *De L'Homme* and in the more subtle *Traité sur les passions de l'âme* borrowed much from Galen as well as from medical contemporaries to produce the paradigm of dualist mechanism. Cabanis certainly respected Descartes's attempts to localize the area of body-soul interaction and to study the cerebral and nervous systems. He took issue, however, with Descartes's fundamental premise in *De L'Homme*—that the body is like a "statue or machine composed of earth," acting according to the laws and mechanisms of ordinary, passive matter.[22] For Descartes, all corporeal phenomena, sensory awareness, memory, "passions of the soul," and the substrate of ideas occurred physically and corresponded with the abundance, flow, activity, and homogeneity of animal spirits. Only thought and will were the province of the rational soul. In animals, consequently, all motion was corporeal and mechanical. The unsolved problem for Cartesian physiology was how inert matter could move itself unless it contained an active material principle. And if such existed, what was the role of the human soul? Still, the mechanistic approach could produce striking physiological insights. For example, some involuntary muscular motion, such as withdrawal of the hand from flame or blinking of the eye before an approaching object, was seen as strictly mechanical. To a limited extent such a notion anticipated the modern reflex concept, in which involuntary motion requires no conscious intervention.[23]

The body-soul interaction in man was complicated because of the inviolable Cartesian barrier between laws of matter and laws of mind. Descartes searched for a middle term between "the ghost" and "the machine" and found the position and alignment of the pineal gland. According to Descartes, both external senses and internal senses (hunger, thirst, joy, sadness, love, anger) or the will of the soul moved the gland, which affected animal-spirit flow and therefore affected feeling and movement. If the mechanism was vague, the interaction was undeniable. Descartes himself maintained that "even the mind is so dependent on temperament, and on the dispositions of the organs of the body, that if it is possible to find some way to make men wiser and more clever than they have been thus far, I think it must be sought in medicine."[24] Descartes agreed that the physician was the prime auxiliary in the struggle to control passions by reason.

DUALIST MECHANIST PHYSIOLOGY: BOERHAAVE AND GAUB

Though the Iatrophysical school was not all Cartesian, all of its members proceeded to relate body to soul without surrendering the dualist idea of active soul and passive, or mechanical, body. The renowned Dutch clinician, chemist, and botanist Hermann Boerhaave (1668-1738) was a pious Calvinist who in his youth wrote dissertations against Epicurean, Hobbist, or Spinozist heresy. Fascinated by the Italian mechanist physicians Giovanni-Alfonso Borelli (1608-1679) and the contemporary Giorgio Baglivi (1669-1706), Boerhaave unhesitatingly accepted a mechanical view of the body. In his *Institutiones Medicae* (1708) and his *Aphorismi* (1709), Boerhaave helped establish the distinctive eighteenth-century mechanist notion of temperament as an equilibrium between solids (membranes, vessels, and fibers) and fluids, or humors. Boerhaave realized that physicians could contribute to healing mental disturbance by healing physical disease, including disturbances in solid-fluid equilibrium. Body-soul interaction was phenomenally observable, while study of the soul itself was beyond the ability of the physiologist.[25]

Despite Boerhaave's praise of Newtonian caution on ultimate causes, his elaborate medical theories impressed Cabanis as more oversystematic betrayal of Hippocratic empiricism. Boerhaave used the evidence of mechanics, microscopy, and vascular injections to postulate ever smaller vessels and ever more subtle fluids—in short, a series of invisible mechanical agents—to explain all major bodily functions. Cabanis was particularly critical of Boerhaave's concern with vessel diameter, fluid impulsion, and digestive chemical "acrimony." Yet Boerhaave's observation of mental and emotional phenomena could not avoid recording apparently nonmechanical upsets. By 1731 he used a Hippocratic term *enormon* to denote a mental principle of arousal that acted in some unknowable way to influence bodily movements as well as ideas. He had no fear of localizing this principle in the "sensorium commune"—"all the places where the union of the cerebral cortex and spinal medulla gives off the origins of the elementary . . . nerve fibers."[26] The sensorium commune played a role above and beyond the merely corporeal cerebral cortex, which was, to Boerhaave (as to Baglivi), a kind of gland that secreted very fine nerve fluid. Because it was neither wholly physical nor wholly mental, the sensorium commune was a safe, neutral term that disguised the difficulty concerning the essential mystery of mind-body interaction.[27]

Boerhaave's temperament theory and mind-body phenomenalism were thus components of the classic dualist mechanist paradigm. In principle, mechanists were committed to explaining as much as possible by treating the corporeal as mere matter and extending the explanations of physics into physiology. Even if the soul remained unknowable and matter remained passive and inert, a science of man dedicated to improving intelligence and character would be, for Boerhaave as for Galen, theoretically possible.

One dualist pupil of Boerhaave in Leyden, Jerome Gaub (1708-1780) explicitly studied mind-body relationships and illustrated the flexibility in the mechanist tradition. At the same time, an erudite member of the Paris Faculty of Medicine, the Cartesian dualist Antoine Le Camus (1722-1772), showed how far a mechanist could develop a "hygiene of the soul." Neither yet took account of new physiological experiments that

58

could potentially undermine the dualist aspect of mechanism.

In two closely reasoned lectures delivered in 1747 and 1763, *De Regimine Mentis Quod Medicorum est . . . (On the Duty and Office of Physicians in the Management of the Mind)*, Gaub developed Boerhaave's suggestions concerning the *enormon* and introduced the idea of mutually responsive active powers in body and soul.[28] Cabanis was probably familiar with lectures so closely related to his own themes in the *Rapports*, though he directly cited only Gaub's esteemed pathology textbook. To Cabanis, Gaub was more a "semi-animist" than a mechanist—someone who, like certain physicians of Montpellier and Edinburgh, believed in active principles of motion within the body.[29]

In his first lecture Gaub provided a sharply focused restatement of the traditional temperament theory and of its effect on the mind. He maintained that age, sex, disease, and mode of life (including the non-naturals) would obviously affect mental clarity. The mental effects of fever, intoxication, and pregnancy were commonplaces of daily experience, and physical disturbance might even be detrimental to moral character. Gaub remained faithful to phenomenalism, believing that one could know only the "kind and degree of . . . reciprocal power" of mind and body, not their ultimate nature.[30] The soul and body coexisted, and the existence of the soul without the body was not verifiable by the physician.

Yet Gaub departed from Cartesian mechanism in the way he perceived mind-body interaction. Rather than focusing on detailed analysis of the nervous system or brain structures, Gaub postulated three principles of spontaneous arousal—one in the mind and two in the body (an adaptation, in fact, of the Galenic pneumas). The unlocalizable *enormon* of the mind, active in sensation and motion, violently shook and agitated the mind in response to desire or aversion. The *enormon* of the body, contained in the nervous system, or what Gaub called "neural man," had two parts—the mentally activated principle of sensation and voluntary motion (the cerebrospinal system) and the *enormon* of the vital and natural functions, including movements of excised organs. Otherwise, the body was inert and mechanical.[31]

Once again the principle of therapy was to use the nonnaturals to affect the *enormon* of the body and thereby improve mental acuteness and moral dispositions. Variations in temperament were thought to be responsible for diversities in mind and character. No amount of sermonizing would cure the drunkard if he were allowed to consume wine. Gaub wrote, "The root deeply seated in the body must be torn out . . . in the case of Alcibiades, not even the teachings of Socrates would prevail." Physicians ought to make men "as superior in character and behavior as possible." In order to do so, they need to search for "special regimens, universal therapeutic methods, and particular remedies with which we can awaken, sharpen, or strengthen any faculty of the mind whatsoever, and moderate, arouse, or repress its paroxysms, instincts, and propensities as needed."[32] These suggestions had great potential in the approach to nervous disease. Treatment of the body, in Gaub as in Descartes, was the key to treatment of the soul.

Clearly, the pious Gaub was sensitive to the potentially heretical implications of introducing an active principle into the body. He devoted a second lecture to stressing the power of the mind over the body. In addition, in its introduction he publicly denounced "a little Frenchman" and "a repulsive offspring, to wit, his mechanical man" published "not long after sitting before this chair and hearing me speak, and in such a way that it seemed to many people that I had furnished him with, if not sparks for his flame, at least matter for embellishing his monstrosity." Gaub was clearly referring to Julien Offray de La Mettrie and to his book *L'Homme machine* (1747). The charge was only partially true, however. La Mettrie borrowed anecdotes easily available elsewhere and did not owe his initial inspiration to Gaub.[33]

Unlike La Mettrie, Gaub demanded equal status for the mind. In his second lecture, he once more appealed to common experience to show that anger, fear, envy, hatred, and even great joy might corrupt the humors or cause digestive upsets. Repressed passions, whether anger, grief, or love, might also have dangerous physical effects. The physician, "more effective and specific than moral preachments, must act on the body to restrain, moderate, and bring to order the principle of arousal, the *enormon*, whose vehemence leads the thwarted mind of man astray to the detriment of the body." Gaub cautioned, however, that only in extreme cases, such as attempted cures of paralysis, might violent emotional shocks be salutary.[34]

CORRELATION OF MIND AND BODY: LE CAMUS

While Gaub refined the mechanist paradigm, Antoine Le Camus developed its premises more systematically in a study of correlations between mind and body. The three books of *Médecine de l'esprit* (1753; revised ed. 1769) offered a complete analysis, in the fashion of Condillac, of intellectual and moral faculties (the understanding and the will), their correspondence with the physical, and a therapy to maintain desirable, and correct harmful, influences. Because the treatise anticipated the goals of Cabanis's unfinished projects, one modern critic has claimed that Le Camus was a forerunner of Cabanis.[35] We have already shown, however, that internal and external influences on temperament were so integral a feature of eighteenth-century medicine that no one work could have been Cabanis's major inspiration. While Cabanis himself never cited Le Camus, Diderot named him in a manuscript note as a source for his *Eléments de physiologie*.[36] In any case, Le Camus is an important control for this discussion. His optimistic objective of human perfectibility and his adherence to the empiricist psychology of Locke and Condillac illustrated how acceptable and ordinary a medically based science of man was, so long as there was no assumption of activity in the body.

Le Camus clearly stated that the soul was neither material nor mechanical, but a "contingent, rational, spiritual, and immortal substance." Yet he assumed it could be "constrained in its own operations by truly mechanical operations . . . often . . .

against its will." In his analysis of the understanding and the will, he acknowledged the primacy of sense-knowledge while insisting that this view did not threaten the truths of religion. Like Descartes, Boerhaave, and Gaub, Le Camus classified thirst, hunger, and sexual appetite as "internal sensations" and dreams and hallucinations as "reflected" sensations. Only the 1769 edition devoted a chapter to "Sensitivity and Sensations," to acknowledge the research of Haller and Encyclopedist physicians. Still, Le Camus envisaged sensitivity not as a special active property of matter, but rather as a mechanical "tonic force," or "muscular force," in animal fibers.[37]

In the second book of *Médecine de l'esprit*, Le Camus listed eight physical causes affecting the mind and will: generation and heredity, sex, climate and seasons, education of the mind and body, temperaments, regimen, age, and health and illness. This list is clearly derived from ancient tradition and from the notion of the non-naturals. But Le Camus followed Boerhaave and other mechanists in asserting the correspondence of size of vessels, elasticity of solids, and state of fibers—not just humors—on mental aptitude, character, complexion, and hair color. Since climate, manner of life, and physical exercise all influenced the blood, and therefore, temperament, "by these mechanical causes . . . one can procure a particular kind of character or genius; one can transmute (*permuter*) sterile, unrewarding terrain into an abundant and fertile one: thus temperaments are a physical means of acquiring intelligence, or correcting its defects."[38]

In the final book of the treatise, Le Camus synthesized empiricist psychology with mechanist physiology. He proposed to adjust climate, mental and physical education, and regimen (duly proportioned to age, sex, and individual temperament) in order to remedy assorted excesses or deficiencies in sensitivity, memory, imagination, judgment, virtues, and passions. From his tedious catalogue, two therapeutic prescriptions will suffice as illustration: for overly relaxed nerve fibers due to a wet climate, watery blood, or the natural temperament of women and children, move to a hot, dry climate, exercise frequently, sleep less, and eat hearty foods to strengthen the stomach; and stiff fibers need humidity, baths, rest, a vegetarian regimen, and perhaps some bleeding. What greater powers, Le Camus wondered, would one need to engage for each person to become intelligent?[39]

Despite these remarkable anticipations of psychosomatic medicine, Le Camus could not be an ideal model for Diderot, d'Holbach, or Cabanis, for without inherent activity in the fiber, the physical body could never generate thought. Le Camus marked a milestone in a typical eighteenth-century approach to hygiene. In addition to the philosophical postulate of dualism, Le Camus's prescriptions were limited by an individualistic approach—personal self-improvement rather than a social commitment to public health. Insofar as this private approach characterized all such medical works from the time of Galen to that of the Idéologues, they were, as a recent article argues, elitist. Only those who were literate, leisured, and wealthy could afford travel to a different climate, the luxury of a varied diet, or the opportunity to change work habits or life styles. Publicizing precepts of hygiene was no doubt a way of overcoming the secrecy of the medical guild. But more important for the social commitment of Cabanis and his colleagues, the physicians active in politics during the French Revolution did not rest their hopes on private hygiene alone but also on a thoroughgoing medical and hospital reform that implied a right to health through public measures.[40]

In the theoretical medical legacy left to Cabanis, the dualist soul-body polarity had to be broken by a new idea—a nonmechanical, but corporeal, force—before there could be convergence of the mechanist and vitalist paradigms. To escape the Cartesian impasse, in which animal motion could not be satisfactorily explained either by body or soul, physiologists turned to what Thomas Steele Hall has called the "physiological unknown," an "inexplicable explicative device" that was the counterpart of Newtonian gravity in physics.

HALLER AND THE PRINCIPLE OF IRRITABILITY

The renowned Swiss experimental physiologist, physician, poet, and polymath Albrecht von Haller (1708-1777) used such a device to explain the peculiar behavior of nerve and muscle fibers. He made muscle fiber the bearer of an active, irreducible property of "irritability." Unwittingly, he became a crucial link between vitalists, who celebrated the uniqueness of life, and materialists, who celebrated the dynamic properties of matter. Vitalists and mechanists were confronted with the same phenomenon, and to explain it, they continued to patch and repair anomalies in their respective paradigms. Gradually their labels described phenomena so similar that the difference in terms seemed a purely metaphysical choice.

In the seventeenth century, several physicians had questioned the traditional Galenic explanations of muscular contraction as the flow of animal spirits through the nerves. The English physician Francis Glisson (1597-1677) had first used the term "irritability" as a general property of living matter in his *Tractatus de Ventriculo et Intestinis* (1677). Glisson's work brimmed with obscure scholastic and Helmontian terminology, but among other insights, he saw the importance of the nerve fiber as an element in "natural perception," which did not always produce conscious sensation.[41]

As a commentator on Boerhaave's lectures, with full awareness of the work of Glisson and Stahl on muscle tone, Haller developed the notion that some organs, such as the stomach and heart, "do not sense distinctly" and that these "obtuse" sensations were independent of the nerves.[42] Moreover, Haller's pupil J.-G. Zimmermann began animal experiments in the 1740s (described in an inaugural dissertation of 1751) that pursued the subject of non-nervous contractions.

Haller offered his theory in a dissertation presented to the Royal Society of Sciences of Göttingen in April and May 1752, "De Partibus Corporis Humani Sensilibus et Irritabilibus."[43] In this paper, he reported, "I call that part of the human body irritable, which becomes shorter upon being touched." Irritability was an inherent tendency of the muscle to contract. Haller then continued, "I call that a sensible part of the human body, which upon being touched transmits the impressions of it to the soul, and in brutes . . . which occasions evident signs of pain and disquiet in the animal." Sensitivity, then, depended on transmission by nerve fibers of sense impressions to the brain, though in animals, pain, or later convulsions, was the only observable phenomenon. Sensitivity was inseparable from consciousness and a unified (presumably central) nervous system. Nerve ligatures always affected sensitivity but they did not remove irritability. In a sectioned nerve of a dog, there could be movement with no apparent sensation. Furthermore, there was no proportional relationship between sensitivity and irritability in particular organs. The force of irritability was a muscular property, while the force of sensitivity was a nervous property. Though sensitivity was normally present in voluntary muscular motion, involuntary motion, or residual motion in excised muscle, was due to irritability alone.[44]

Throughout the discussion, Haller kept his agnostic Newtonian reserve—the sources of irritability and sensitivity, he maintained, "lie beyond the reach of the knife and microscope, beyond which I do not choose to hazard many conjectures." He appealed explicitly to Newton's caution:

> What therefore should hinder us in asking why irritability should not be that property of muscular fiber to contract itself when touched and provoked, without it being necessary to assign a cause, just as no probable cause of attraction or gravity has been assigned to matter? The cause of irritability is physical, hidden in the intimate fabric, and revealed by experiments sufficient to show its existence but too gross to trace its nature.[45]

Haller was aware that a metaphysical storm would break over the notion of irritability, an active force in excised muscle tissue. Yet this *vis insita* (inherent force), he insisted, was no mere arrangement of matter but a divine power. No corporeal

forces could produce motion. His own dualist mechanist outlook rejected the contention that physical phenomena *caused*
mental phenomena. As the hands of a watch at noon corresponded to the sun at the meridian, so did body and soul correspond; yet the sun did not move the hands.[46]

The semi-animist physician of Edinburgh, Robert Whytt
(1714-1766), launched a bitter attack against the materialist implications of the idea of motion that was neither strictly mechanical nor initiated by the soul. Whytt argued that there
must be sensitivity and a sentient principle that was the instrument of the soul wherever there was motion.[47] Meanwhile, as
early as 1747, the scandalous La Mettrie used the concept of an
active force in living matter to question the existence of the
soul. In 1752 Haller felt compelled to reject both animism and
materialism. He argued that there was no part of the soul or
consciousness in flesh cut off from the body. Irritability was
therefore independent of the soul, which was neither extended
nor divisible, and also independent of the nerves. Haller astutely warned that "those who, like Stahl, attribute irritability
to the soul, and make both things inseparable, give Demetrius
[La Mettrie] more plausibility. If both are inseparable, and one
invisible while the other is evident to the senses, one has nearly
excluded the first."[48]

Both Haller and semi-animists could now accuse each other
of materialism. To Whytt, any active force in the body would
assign to mere matter a capacity to move that should be assigned to the soul. Self-sufficient matter threatened the whole
idea of Creation and Providence. To Haller, a single force of
sensitivity would involve the soul in all kinds of merely bodily
motions that needed no conscious or mental direction. In this,
there would be a risk of equating spiritual activity with the
merely physical.

Subsequent eighteenth-century nerve physiologists quoted
or contested Haller's experiments to their own purposes. Many
debated the existence of animal spirits, nerve fluid, or vibratory
aethers. But most tended to accept the existence of nonmechanical forces, either nervous or muscular, over the image of pas-

THE BODY AS MECHANISM

sive, inert, living matter.[49] The pious physicians of Edinburgh could be confident that their sentient principle would avoid the theological dangers of mechanism. And students of libertine tracts and clandestine manuscripts could use Haller's experiments as a catalyst to promote materialism. To Diderot and Cabanis, Haller's experimental physiology was a great repository of reliable information in need of interpretation.

The Activation of Matter: La Mettrie

When the notorious physician La Mettrie dedicated his *L'Homme machine* to an outraged Haller, it was a stroke of malicious humor and ironic justice. After receiving his M.D. at Reims in 1733, La Mettrie studied with Boerhaave in Leyden in 1735-1736 and translated an abridgment of Boerhaave's *Institutiones Medicae* into French. In 1747, when he heard Gaub in Leyden, he became aware of the experiments of Haller's circle in Göttingen. Haller himself complained La Mettrie "learnt all he knew about [irritability] of a young Swiss with whom I am not acquainted; who never was my pupil, nor is he a physician, but he had read my works, and seen some of the famous Albinus's experiments [Bernhard Siegfried Albinus, professor of medicine at Leyden] and upon these La Mettrie founded his impious system, which my experiments totally refute."[50] (A medical historian has identified the "young Swiss" as a minor philosopher and economist, Georg Ludwig Schmid (1720-1805) of Avenstein, a correspondent of Haller and later tutor to Duke Ernst-August of Weimar.[51])

While La Mettrie amply praised the dualist mechanists Descartes and Boerhaave, his own mechanism followed more closely still another paradigm—that of Newtonian inexplicable forces. Lester Snow King summarizes a conventional interpretation of La Mettrie's role: "While Descartes had regarded animals as machines, the dualistic philosophy gave to man a soul which the animals lacked, and which differentiated a human from a machine. It was only a small step, but a mightily important one, to say that the mind of man was not a separate substance."[52] Certainly La Mettrie showed great respect for Descartes and even speculated that Descartes might have been a materialist had he not feared theological censorship. But Vartanian's critical edition of *L'Homme machine* has gone far to balance La Mettrie's loyalty to Iatrophysics with his original conception of motion in the body.[53] Descartes's living body was an automaton with a mainspring continually running down; La Mettrie's was a perpetual motion machine with an inherent active principle. A self-winding machine was neither ordinary mechanism nor Cartesian automaton. Certainly La Mettrie's intention, like Diderot's and d'Holbach's after him, was to assimilate the human species to the animal kingdom and to support the idea of a corporeal Chain of Being with one substance of varying complexity. Yet unlike Maupertuis, he never attributed inherent activity or intelligence to all matter, only to living matter.

In developing the man-machine image, La Mettrie listed irritability in his catalogue of phenomena of involuntary motion. In this catalogue, he also cited ordinary reflex phenomena (pupillary contraction in increased light, vomiting, and excretory processes) as well as residual reflexes after death (contraction of excised muscles, palpitation in dead animals, persistent intestinal peristalsis, heart and muscle revival after injection of hot water into blood vessels, and persistent movement of a frog's heart, previously noted by Boyle and Steno). These empirical observations led La Mettrie to the hypothesis that "each little fiber," independent of the nerves, had an "innate force." The structure of the nervous system led to certain other properties of sensitivity. By analogy to the "small subordinate springs" in many organs, La Mettrie argued that the brain had, at the origins of the nerves, an "inciting and vigorous (*impétueux*) principle that Hippocrates called enormon (the soul)." By this elementary principle of motion, "animate bodies will have all needed to move, feel, think, repent, and behave; in a word, for all physical and mental behavior."[54]

Refusing to accept nonempirical metaphysical entities, La Mettrie asserted that the soul was not separate but "only a principle of motion, or a sensitive material part of the brain . . . a principal spring of the entire machine." Organization of the body was paramount. No one could know how movement and feeling reciprocally excited each other. Somehow movement produced sensation, and by Locke's empiricist philosophy, sensation produced thought. La Mettrie speculated, "I think thought so little incompatible with organized matter, that it seems to be a property of it, as is electricity, the motive faculty, impenetrability, extension." Like Newtonian gravitation, thought was an inexplicable property of matter. For all his fascination with ancient Epicureanism, La Mettrie required neither Epicurean chance nor the God of the orthodox for an explanation—only the awesome power of Nature.[55]

All the familiar body-soul correspondences detailed by Gaub and Le Camus or by contemporary speculative psychologists like David Hartley and Charles Bonnet could now assume a new significance. The influences of age, sex, temperament, disease, and the non-naturals (including diet and climate) on mind and character could now be interpreted as the interactions of portions of a single uniform substance. With no spiritual soul, there was no difference in kind, only in degree (primarily in use of language) between apes and men. Consequently, an image of the universe including Final Causes or divine Providence seemed inappropriate. Yet in *this* treatise, La Mettrie chose to mute his much-vaunted mockery of conventional morality and natural law (as he did not in *Discours sur le bonheur*, 1st ed., 1748). Like d'Holbach later, he here argued that a natural law controlled both animals and men and, at least in the human species, assured that virtuous acts would bring pleasure, except to the depraved. Thus, criminals might be malformed individuals needing medical treatment. Man composed of material substance would still act in moral fashion, and the merely natural and material was therefore so much more extraordinary.[56]

La Mettrie's own irreverent satires on the medical profession, his alleged gluttony, insolence, and personal hedonism only confirmed the conviction that metaphysical materialism threatened morality as well as religion. Even the atheist d'Hol-

69

bach labeled La Mettrie "insane," while Diderot described him as "frenetic" and was clearly disgusted with his ethical views. And while no one ever doubted La Mettrie's influence on Cabanis, there were no references to La Mettrie in Cabanis's works. Whether this remarkable silence was due to La Mettrie's overly mechanistic metaphors remains a moot point.[57]

To be sure, La Mettrie was more impressionistic in *L'Homme machine* than either Le Camus or Cabanis were in their methodical treatises. Like the works of dualist mechanists, La Mettrie's considerations on the human body tended to stress the similarities in the corporeal Chain of Being and the legitimacy of a single scientific method for physics and physiology. With elimination of the spiritual soul, there was an even more decisive unity in nature and in the sciences. Yet La Mettrie certainly illustrated how Haller's experiments could modify the mechanist paradigm. After the postulation of the inexplicable force of irritability, life was not *merely* mechanical. Surely La Mettrie himself did not hesitate to use the term "materialism."[58] But living matter was no longer inert and passive. The irritability of muscle fibers was a property of matter, as incomprehensible as gravity. If the soul was a motive principle, it could be a corporeal motive principle, a kind of complex cerebral muscle.

For Cabanis, the oversystematic mechanists had attempted to reduce the human body to dynamics and hydraulics against all the canons of Hippocratic empiricism. At the same time, mechanists like Boerhaave had used a Hippocratic term *enormon* to indicate a nonmechanical principle of arousal. Gaub had developed this notion to interpret the phenomena of mental-physical correspondence, and Le Camus had shown the limits of dualist mechanism without such a notion. Now the solid-fluid balance theory of temperament was ripe for revision to account for the forces of irritability and sensitivity. La Mettrie had stood Haller on his head to arrive at a monism that was not entirely mechanical. The animist and vitalist physicians would also use inexplicable principles allowing degrees of spiritual activity sometimes scarcely distinguishable from corporeal activity. If they ultimately appealed more to Cabanis, it was their precise analysis of degrees of nervous activity that seemed to him to best refine the notion of temperament. Then, too, the vitalists, or philosophers inspired by them, especially preserved the respect for the uniqueness of the living body that was the foundation of Cabanis's physiology.

★ CHAPTER III ★

The Soul and the Vital Principle in Physiology

The Omnipotent Soul: Stahl

hile the mechanists were assigning strange active forces to living matter, the vitalists, like Descartes, were confining the soul to reason and inventing special "principles" to perform seemingly purposive bodily functions. Just as Descartes had insisted that everything corporeal was mechanical, so the forerunners of vitalism insisted that the soul or its spiritual agents directed all corporeal activities. The late seventeenth-century medical world was filled with concerns of the Iatrophysical school, such as measurement of fluid forces and vessel diameters, and with concerns of the Iatrochemical school, such as acrimony of humors. Against this background, the cantankerous chemist and physician of Halle, Georg Ernst Stahl (1659-1734), demanded a return to Hippocratic empiricism and a useful sifting of the theories of Paracelsus and van Helmont.[1] Stahl believed that nature could not be understood by use of the chemical balance and that only clinical observation would reveal the incalculable properties of life. He had both a pietistic and scientific sense of the limitations of the intellect and thus rejected the overweening effort of mechanists to explain what he felt had to remain mysterious. At the same time, he helped create the distinctiveness of the term "physiology" as a subject apart from physics. While his medicine was based on external observation, his physiology was peculiarly life-oriented. Its testimony alone should make historians skeptical of Michel Foucault's contention that the idea of life could not be developed in an era when

72

the study of animals was dominated by natural history classification.[2]

Although a renowned theoretical chemist himself, Stahl thought chemistry and other "accessory sciences" to be useless in medical theory. In a characteristically entitled dissertation, *Paraenesis, or the Necessity to Remove from Medical Teaching All Foreign Objects* (1706), Stahl chided anatomists for being more concerned with counting torn fibers than healing a wound.[3] Anatomy ignored the nonmechanical, purposive, directing principle of life. While Cabanis believed in linking scientific and medical knowledge, he approvingly quoted Stahl's strictures on the "most serious efforts" of applying doctrines from other sciences to the "sciences seeking to know and to regulate the animal economy."[4]

Stahl based his disdain for medical systems on the radical discontinuity between medical subject matter and the inanimate objects of the physical sciences. Anticipating Bichat, Stahl believed life to be the force that prevented the decay of the inherently corruptible and heterogeneous elements of "organic aggregates." Harmonious organization was neither mechanical nor chemical. In physiology, the soul held corporeal activities under absolute control, though "the soul does not perform its actions or achieve its goals *immediately*, but in mediate fashion and for the most part entirely by means *corporeal* and infinite in number." The soul was the directing agent of the corporeal instruments. It lent cohesion to material constituents that would otherwise disintegrate.[5]

Though Stahl insisted on divine purpose and the powers of the soul, he refused to postuate a hierarchy of souls or spiritual agents. While he distinguished *logismos*—the conscious intellectual faculty—from *logos*—the "instinct of reason" supervising voluntary motion, conscious sensation, and involuntary vital processes—he never distinguished two or more souls. The soul as *logos* controlled circulation, heartbeat, and muscle tone in an intelligent and rational way. No mechanism could explain the specific capacities of each structure. As Cabanis noted, Stahl believed that the soul "digests in the stomach, breathes in the

lungs, filters bile in the liver, and thinks in the head. . . ."[6]
Stahl thought that neither the quality nor the heat of the
humors could be chemically or mechanically maintained. By
circulation, secretion, excretion, and variation of tonic motion
the soul refreshed the body and expelled corrupted matter. In
pathology, the "substantial motive force" of life was identifiable with the Hippocratic healing force of nature, needing only
assistance by the physician to overcome disease. Medical
therapy would most profitably stimulate the appropriate secretions and excretions to rectify errors of the soul.[7]

Stahl particularly stressed the activity of the soul in impress-
ing tonic motion on nerves to convert sense-stimuli into conscious useful perceptions. Sensation served a specific purpose—
that of preventing bodily harm. While Haller later acknowledged the importance of brain response in perception, Stahl's
imagery more clearly stressed the freedom of the soul to direct
attention at will. A weary soldier would sleep through a can-
nonade, while a mother would hear a child's cry. The soul was
no more passive in sensation than a man is in hunting birds.
Even in assimilation of nutritive substances, the separation of
appropriate "corpuscles" was a "truly elective act."[8]

While Stahl emphasized the sovereignty of the spiritual principle, especially in the physical effects of powerful emotions, he
adopted the common dualist doctrine of temperament and the
non-naturals. He did not hesitate to correlate qualities of mind
and character with density, velocity, and chemical composition
of the humors, or with hardness, compactness, and diameter of
the solid vessels.[9] The insistence on the dominion of the soul
ran all the dangers later noted by Haller. In Stahl's own lifetime, the philosopher Leibniz, in a bitter correspondence (published in 1720 under the appropriate title of *Negotium
Otiosum*) argued that only a corporeal substance could have direct action on the body. Stahl weakly replied that the soul could
move living matter because there had to be an "immaterial
cause" for motion, an "incorporeal thing."[10] Stahl repeated so
often and with such conviction that the body was only the instrument of the soul that we must dismiss Leibniz's accusation

of materialism as a characteristic ploy against philosphical adversaries (as in the famous exchange with Newton's spokesman Samuel Clarke). But Cabanis himself deliberately ignored the "animist" aspect of Stahl's physiology (rational control of all bodily functions by the single soul). He claimed, rather incredibly, that Stahl used the term "soul" to please the orthodox but meant by it a synonym for terms such as *enormon*, sensitivity (the explanatory term of the Montpellier school), living solid (used by Friedrich Hoffmann of Halle, Gaub, and William Cullen of Edinburgh), or vital principle (Barthez of Montpellier).

This disingenuous interpretation precisely reflected Cabanis's desire to purge Stahlian thought of its animism while retaining its vitalist aspects (in this case, the belief in a nonphysicochemical conserving principle that would function as the inexplicable forces of mechanists did). Cabanis valued Stahl's image of the self-conserving, unified living organism as a legitimate revival of ancient clinical observation. Indeed, Cabanis lavishly praised Stahl as the "greatest physician to appear since Hippocrates," primarily because of his detailed observation—as of hemorrhages and chronic abdominal infections.[11]

"Semi-Animism": Whytt

While Stahl had several disciples at German universities, the most significant revisionists were active at Edinburgh and Montpellier. At the Medical Faculty in Edinburgh, the renowned experimental physiologist and clinician Robert Whytt (1714-1766) studied with Alexander Monro *primus* and, before his return, also with Boerhaave and Albinus at Leyden and with the neuroanatomist James Winslow in Paris. Several times Cabanis cited Whytt's justly admired treatise on nerve disease, published in 1764 (translated into French in 1767 and 1777).[12] Like Stahl, Whytt contested Cartesian mechanism but he denied charges that he was a Stahlian.

In an *Essay on the Vital and other Involuntary Motions of Animals* (1751; rev. ed. 1763) as well as in the treatise on nervous disorder (1764), Whytt painstakingly refuted explanations of reflex phenomena and muscular contraction by mechanisms, chemical reactions of nerve fluid and aether, or electrical effluvia.[13] From experimental evidence—oscillatory, diminishing responses of muscles to stimuli and contraction of the membranes, rather than of the internal fibers of muscles—Whytt arrived at the hypothesis of a purposive "sentient" principle governing muscular contraction. Similarly, he attributed pupillary contraction to a sentient principle in the brain that, excited by unpleasant light stimuli, determined nerve action. He attempted to show mathematically that the heart could not produce sufficient mechanical force for circulation, or the nerve fluid, for muscular contraction. Involuntary responses also might follow imagined rather than actual stimuli, "as when salivation follows the sight, or even the recalled idea of *grateful* food." In modern terms, Whytt described an integrated functional response, with a conditioned reflex as a special case. In his own terms, Whytt described "feelings" of the sentient principle rather than properties of matter. The human body was so constructed that "the whole is a system far above the power of mechanics."[14]

Whytt's twelve-year debate (1752-1764) with Haller on irritability focused on his refusal to admit nonnervous contraction. For Whytt, irritability was merely a special case of sensitivity. He maintained that Haller's experiments were inaccurate because the shock to already injured animals had masked the additional pain they felt on stimulation of "insensitive" organs. For Whytt, sensitivity was present in every organ, not merely in nerves; even tendons had "obtuse" sensation. Various animal experiments performed after decapitation as well as the contraction of irritated excised muscle fibers showed "traces" of the sentient principle. Any dissociation of sensitive phenomena into two forces was unjustifiable on grounds of simplicity of explanation and was also potentially materialistic in attributing active motions to the body.[15] Conversely, critics charged that Whytt made the soul physically extended. To Haller, activity of the soul in excised muscles was itself potentially materialistic.

For his part, Whytt carefully refined his notion of degrees of activity of the sentient principle. The principle explained, for example, organic "sympathies" where no nerve connections were observable or where mental phenomena played an inhibiting role. Sympathies between stomach and brain or between uterus and mammary glands were commonplaces of medical experience. They were no more mechanical than was thought "a motion of the particles of the animal spirits, or other subtile matter in the brain." At the same time, sympathies were preeminently attributable to the brain itself and to "spinal marrow."[16] The role of the spinal cord, effectively established by Whytt, could be illustrated by the residual sympathies in decapitated animals. In an experiment performed by his friend, the physiologist Stephen Hales, Whytt discovered that such sympathies could be inhibited by pithing the spinal cord of a decapitated frog.[17] Consequently, the spinal cord was part of the sensorium commune, and "reflexes," whether of the cord or pupillary contraction, were special cases of sympathies.

Like Stahl, Whytt insisted on the unity of the soul that supervised involuntary motion. But he explicitly defended himself against Haller's charges of Stahlianism by differentiating rationality and consciousness in the soul (absent in "infants, idiots, and brutes") from the feeling of the sentient principle.

> The mind, therefore, in producing the vital and other involuntary motions, does not act as a rational, but rather as a sentient principle; which, without reasoning upon the matter, is as necessarily determined by an ungrateful sensation or *stimulus* affecting the organs, to exert its power, in bringing about these motions, as is a balance, while, from mechanical laws, it preponderates to that side where the greatest weight prevails.[18]

At one point, Whytt even used the term "quasi-mechanism" for involuntary motions, despite his principles of "semi-animism." While he believed that spiritual activity endowed the body with peculiar properties, he also acknowledged that it was a strangely enslaved spiritual principle that was "necessarily determined" in vital phenomena. Whytt even admitted that animals have sentient principles differing only in degree from men.[19]

Semi-animism could thus be the mirror image of La Mettrie's addition of an unexplainable active property to the Cartesian beast-machine. Whytt, no less than Haller and La Mettrie, was using a "physiological unknown." Vitalists could maintain their orthodoxy by stressing the purposeful activity of the sentient principle, and mechanists could stress the determined response of merely inert and insensitive matter. But the convergence of paradigms facilitated the tasks of Diderot and Cabanis. Activated matter or unfree sentient principle—either interpretation might threaten belief in the soul and lead to heretical monism.

An interesting corollary to Whytt's nerve sympathy doctrine might have suggested to Cabanis his cherished analogy between physical and moral sympathies. Whytt first noted that if, as Scottish philosophers claimed, we instinctively approved or disapproved of moral phenomena, then the involuntary physiological reaction of stimuli to organs might seem more plausible. No reasoning was involved in either realm. The next year (1764) Whytt reversed the argument to give a new wrinkle to the ancient "body politic" metaphor. Organic sympathy, he suggested, was a model for the cooperation observable in social sympathies.[20] In the individual, nature had illustrated desirable harmony, and healthy societies followed the same premise.

Montpellier Medicine

More influential than Edinburgh in the development of the thought of Diderot and Cabanis was the doctrine of the venerable University of Medicine in Montpellier—vitalism in theoretical medicine and cautious Hippocratic clinical observation in practical medicine. Endowed by Pope Honorius III in 1220 and placed in a medieval commercial crossroads, the Montpellier Faculty had retained its preeminence long after the economic decline of the city. In several ways Montpellier medicine played a significant role in the late Enlightenment.[21] Its emphasis on sensitivity in physiology reinforced Condillac's empiricist theory of sensation as the basis of knowledge and motivation. Several Montpellier physicians were Encyclopedists, close friends of Diderot or members of the *coterie holbachique*. In fact, one may argue that Montpellier physiology shaped Diderot's materialist world-view as much as did his fascination with the naturalists, with Lucretius, and with clandestine materialist manuscripts. For both Diderot and Cabanis Montpellier medicine was an antidote to mechanical reductionism and a stimulant to interest in the dynamic philosophy of life of Buffon and Maupertuis. When Cabanis reviewed modern medical developments, he asserted that the doctrine of Montpellier, perfected by the "application of philosophical methods" and by the "progress of collateral sciences" more and more "approaches the truth," which would not be the property of a school but of all.[22]

BOISSIER DE SAUVAGES

The first Montpellier professor to leaven Iatrophysics with "vital principles" and "physiological unknowns" was François Boissier de Sauvages (1706-1767). Known as the "physician of love" for his dissertation on simple remedies to "cure" love, Sauvages was a Montpellier graduate (1726) reared in the mechanist tradition. He translated the Iatrophysical classic *Haemastaticks* by Stephen Hales (as *Statique des animaux* [1744]) and attempted quantitative measurement of heart force, arterial pulse, blood circulation, and organ density. A confirmed Newtonian, he saw the basis of medical theory in experimental physics, "mathematical philosophy," and precise anatomical knowledge.[23] Yet in his later works, after study of Stahl, he came to recognize "a principle of vital movements, superior to ordinary mechanism." Sauvages himself legitimized, in Newtonian fashion, use of inexplicable principles: "One sees, however, mathematicians who use the letters x and y to designate unknown quantities, and with so much greater success, that they discover by such means truths inaccessible to other philosophers." To control pulse, respiration, secretion, assimilation, and other involuntary motions, there was need of an "intelligent force," for all the hydraulic structure of the body. Everyday experience showed that the mind, or "soul," could accelerate the heartbeat, and one must assume that other faculties of the soul direct other motions.[24]

The physiology of Sauvages represented a curious transition between animism and mechanism. His pathology brought into France the methods of "nosology," or classification of disease, of the English physician Thomas Sydenham (1624-1689).[25] While Sauvages was a botanist and corresponded with Linnaeus, the first French sketch of the *Nosologie* appeared in 1731, even before Linnaeus's *Systema Naturae* (1735). Sauvages followed Sydenham in describing a two-stage classification—first, a history, or "graphic and natural description," and second, "philosophical nosology," or reduction of all diseases to "definite and certain species."[26] Sauvages would observe only evident symptoms in the attempt to differentiate the idiosyncratic effects of age and temperament from the "peculiar and constant phenomena" of the disease. In this respect, Foucault has correctly argued that eighteenth-century classifiers emphasized the external rather than the internal location of a disease. While Cabanis clearly considered Sauvages's nosologies artificial and inadequate, the Baconian-style observation and classification was later at the heart of Cabanis's "analytical" method in medical theory.[27]

BORDEU AND SENSITIVITY: RESTRICTION OF THE SOUL

For Cabanis, the most significant Montpellier physician was the Gascon, Théophile de Bordeu (1722-1776, D.M. Montpellier 1743), staunch advocate of inoculation, personal physician to Madame du Barry, and principal character in Diderot's dialogue *Le Rêve de d'Alembert*.[28] Cabanis not only cited Bordeu's original works, but often followed Bordeu's history of medicine in his *Coup d'oeil*. He also claimed that his own mentor Dubreuil had medical theories related to views of Bordeu.[29]

From fragmemts of the dogmatic structures of Iatrophysicists and Stahlians, Bordeu constructed an original conception of life and physiological function. For Bordeu, life consisted of the "faculty of the animal fiber to feel (*sentir*) and to move itself . . . inherent in the primary elements of the living body [like] the gravity, attraction, and mobility of various bodies."[30] The primary living structure was the nervous system, which controlled the equilibrium of two inversely proportional forces—sensitivity and muscular mobility. All nervous activity was sensitive, and Haller's irritability and Whytt's sympathies were special cases of nervous sensitivity.[31] As early as 1742, in his baccalaureate dissertation *De Sensu Generice Considerato*, Bordeu had divided functions into those of "evident motion and occult sensation," such as circulation and respiration, and those of "evident sensation and occult motion," such as internal and external sensation.[32] Thus, Boerhaave's notion of obscure sensation could reappear in a different context, a context in which a kind of feeling could remain subconscious. In a later treatise, Bordeu refined the idea of sensitivity to include not merely the "fiber," but the arrangement, cohesion, and composition of the sheaths of fibers, the nonsensitive mucous "cellular tissue" (Haller's *tela cellulosa*, the modern areolar connective tissue).[33]

Bordeu always carefully allowed for the active influence of the spiritual soul and he recognized its primary role in conscious functions and emotions. But he subsumed all vital activity under the guidance of a distinct animal being, namely the force of nervous sensitivity. As his thought matured, sensitivity overshadowed the soul in nearly all discussion of corporeal activity.[34]

Bordeu's "federative" concept of the body (as Moravia has called it) shaped the medical presuppositions of Cabanis's science of man. Unwilling to limit sensitivity to the brain and spinal cord, yet unsure of the precise relationships of central and sympathetic nervous systems, Bordeu revived van Helmont's hierarchical *archei* in the form of three centers of sensitivity. The brain was the primary center, but there were two subordinate centers—the heart, or precordial region, and the stomach and diaphragm, or epigastric region.[35] The relative strength of each center, and of the sphere over which it presided, could account for the diversities observed according to age, sex, and temperament. Internal organs also had nerve connections with a corresponding "department" in the brain. Tension changes in these connecting fibers could explain the physical effects of emotional reactions (nausea, salivation, tears). All individual characteristics were thus a function of equilibrium of centers of sensitivity or relative activity of these nerve networks.[36] Bordeu now transformed the Hippocratic "unbroken circle" metaphor into the image that fascinated Diderot:

> A swarm of bees, gathered in clusters and suspended from a tree as a vine; each part is, so to speak, not an animal, but a kind of self-contained machine, which in its fashion concurs in the general life of the body.[37]

For therapy, the inferior centers might even be more important, since the brain was not an autocrat, and each "partial life" interacted with the "general life."[38]

If the federative concept was essential for Cabanis's physiology, so was the model of active sensitivity. Bordeu's description of gland functioning was at once a pioneering work of endocrinology and a model for the active sensitive response. To Bordeu, glandular secretion was no mechanical compression or separation, as in Iatrophysical theory, but a response to an irritating body or other stimulus from nerves linking the gland and brain. After a preparatory spasmodic state, or "erection" (the genital and mammary models were appropriate), there was extension of glandular ducts, activation of blood vessels, and nerve convulsions that contracted and emptied the reservoir of the gland. Secretion was a "kind of sensation," even a kind of "taste," without consciousness in which the nerves would "retain and choose" substances in the blood. The nerves of external sense-organs, like the nerves of glands, reacted, after preliminary arousal, to extend toward pleasurable sensations and withdraw from unpleasant ones.[39] Although Bordeu associated sensitivity with nerve structure, he believed sensitivity to be a basic force in all living matter and dared to speculate that it might be either essential to matter or a necessary attribute of organization.[40]

The vitalist Bordeu was thus prepared to make statements on the fuzzy borderline of materialism. Yet he would make no concessions at all on the autonomy of medicine. Despite a lively interest in chemical explanation of respiration, Bordeu warned that chemists would never unravel the complexities of digestion. He decried the use of physical instruments, such as a thermometer to measure fever, a meter to record pulse beat, or a microscope to examine fluids, and he used "experimenter" as a derogatory epithet.[41] Like Stahl, he saw the key to prognosis and therapy in careful clinical journal-keeping that correlated individual temperaments, atmospheric conditions ("constitutions"), and the progress of disease.[42]

LACAZE, FOUQUET, AND DE SÈZE

Several lesser-known Montpellier physicians amplified Bordeu's views and gave Cabanis a specific legacy. Bordeu himself and G.-F. Venel, Dubreuil's mentor, contributed to a work (*Idée de l'homme physique et moral* [1755; Latin ed. 1749]) ostensibly authored by Bordeu's "rich uncle," the physician to the duc d'Orléans Louis Lacaze (1703-1765; D. M. Montpellier 1723). Extravagantly conceived and tortuously written, the physiological sections elaborated ideas concerning sensitive-motor equilibrium and ideas on the "phrenic center" (Bordeu's epigastric region) as the regulator of vital forces. Lacaze followed Haller's addition to temperament theory by dividing men into "sensitive" and "motive" categories. The largely nonempirical corollary held that society developed moral sensitivity and reflection while savagery promoted muscular activity.[43] Later, Cabanis would have a prime goal of promoting physical temperaments with socially desirable moral correlates.

Moreover, Lacaze's schema permitted the argument that histor-ical development changed human nature itself—a fruitful view for partisans of human perfectibility.

Lacaze was even more hostile than Bordeu to physiological experimentation and dissection. His idea of sound medical method was good clinical observation, free from the "laws of experimental physics." This deep-seated antagonism toward exportation of the methods of the physical sciences was evident in Cabanis's conception of the autonomy of medicine.[44]

The Montpellier graduate and later professor Henri Fouquet (1727-1806) provided an easily accessible summary of the ideas of Bordeu and Lacaze, among others, in his *Encyclopédie* article "Sensibilité, sentiment." Cabanis placed him among the great physiologists from Montpellier who were responsible for the striking advances in medical theory since the age of Galen. Fouquet's main purpose was to extend the range of the vital or sensitive principle to include Haller's observations of irritability and all other muscular motion. He supported Whytt in reiterat-ing all the arguments of the debate with Haller. His vigorous opposition to "even the best-conducted experiments" on living organisms once again showed the clinicians' fear of distorting the delicate phenomenon of life. Finally, Fouquet indulged in the fascinating Neo-platonic or neo-Stoic speculation that sen-sitivity was an emanation of a universal intelligence. This latter reflection anticipated the private metaphysical musings of the mature Cabanis.[45]

Still another graduate of Montpellier, a professor at Bor-deaux, Victor de Sèze (1760-1830), was Cabanis's colleague after 1796 in the "analysis of sensations and ideas" section of the Second Class of the National Institute. In *Recherches physiologiques et philosophiques sur la sensibilité* (written 1778; published 1786) de Sèze developed even more fully the ramifications of the key concept of sensitivity. Cabanis never cited this volume but presumably he was aware of a work dedi-cated to President Dupaty of the Parlement of Bordeaux, the godfather of his wife, who was also the intended heiress of Du-paty's papers. Like Lacaze and Fouquet, de Sèze castigated "cruel animal experiments," denigrated the "optical illusions" of microscopy as an aid to pathology, and even questioned the medical value of Harvey's discovery of blood circulation. Attacking the basic spirit of the *Encyclopédie*, de Sèze doubted that "all sciences are a branch of a common trunk" and questioned the common physiological belief that animal life was governed by mechanical, hydraulic, and chemical laws.[46]

Despite these barriers between the sciences, de Sèze expressed a vision of the unity of nature by means of a hierarchy of affinity-force laws. As a vitalist, he reversed Buffon's order and began at the highest level—the free choice and conscious sensation of the spiritual soul—and descended through subconscious "sensations," irritability, tonic motion (evident in some vegetables), chemical affinity, and attraction. In physiology, de Sèze, like Bordeu, allowed for sensations unrelated to external sense-organs such as hunger, thirst, and sex drive—a view of sensation later stressed by Cabanis. Moreover, he followed Bordeu's notion of sensitive response as an erection, or *érétisme*, of fibers which in the brain, if excessive, could produce a "frenzy." De Sèze thus explicitly developed a new idea of sensitivity in explaining physical-mental correspondence.

Given the hierarchy of forces, de Sèze solved the problem of the emergence of life and feeling by postulating that life was latent everywhere—sensitivity was a "faculty that the true state of organization permits an active principle to display." As Fouquet had already argued, the vital principle might conceivably be an emanation of the "spirit of life circulating in all bodies." For de Sèze, then, the continuities and correspondences in nature posed no threat to a vitalist viewpoint or religious orthodoxy. But like his Montpellier colleagues, he refused to extend methods of study from the inorganic to the organic realm.[47]

BARTHEZ, THE VITAL PRINCIPLE, AND THE CONVERGENCE OF MECHANISM AND VITALISM

Montpellier vitalism reached its culmination in the prerevolutionary era in the works of the vain, ill-tempered Paul-Joseph Barthez (1734-1806), who publicly vilified the "sect" of Stahl and Bordeu. Barthez was first physician to the duc d'Orléans (1781), later consulting physician to Louis XVI, Chancellor of the University of Medicine in Montpellier, an eminent jurist, contributor to Diderot's *Encyclopédie*, and occasional guest of d'Holbach. After the political passions of the Revolution cooled somewhat in 1798, the young physicians and medical students at the Paris School of Medicine insisted that the former royalist and partisan of noble privilege Barthez be permitted to become a corresponding member of their Société médicale d'émulation, a highly significant research circle. After preliminary expositions of his physiology in Latin orations of 1772 and 1774, his principal work was *Nouveax Elémens de la science de l'homme* (1778). Cabanis was convinced that this treatise was "filled with great medical insights as well as philosophy and erudition" and that it "merits a more striking success."[48] Despite the high reputation of Barthez's work, the greatly expanded second edition (1806) seemed rather quaint in its continued opposition to the new chemical theory of respiration and its preference for vague vitalistic explanations of animal heat.

While Barthez narrowly defined the "science of man" as physiology, he shared Cabanis's view that physiology was indispensable to broader theories of mind and character. The "Preliminary Discourse" to the physiological discussion was also a veritable discourse on method for the life sciences, far more precise than Buffon's remarks in the *Histoire naturelle*. Enshrining the Newtonian explanation paradigm and anticipating the positivist credo, Barthez rejected the search for essences and recommended the quest for laws showing "succession of the phenomena." Observation, said Barthez, would reveal "experimental causes," acting in a fashion as seemingly occult as electricity or magnetism, but in a fashion admissible if effects were empirically evident. The much-maligned "occult causes" were useless only if they transcended the phenomena. In physiology, mechanists erred in expecting the "occult faculty" of impulse to explain all, while animists erroneously explained corporeal motion as the work of a "spiritual being." Both ignored the "most general experimental cause" in man—the "vital principle" causing feeling and motion in the body.[49]

86

In practice Barthez found it difficult to adhere to his lofty standards. In a treatise entirely concerned with the vital principle, Barthez never could define it unambiguously. It was neither body nor organization nor soul nor any body-soul intermediary. It was purposive, though not conscious; multiform, but not extended. In the "Preliminary Discourse," he insisted that it was not a "distinct being," but rather a "simple vital faculty of the human body." It was determined, not free, and mortal, unlike the soul. Though Barthez scorned Newtonian caution by ascribing to all matter an "activity residing essentially in matter," he refused to admit that living matter *produced* the activity or moved itself. In a supplement of 1806 he warned that organic structure was "absolutely passive."[50] Like de Sèze, he envisaged a hierarchy of principles of motion, from impulse, attraction, chemical affinity, and electricity to "living forces" with "laws of a transcendent order compared to the laws of physics and mechanics." Barthez could not accept any implication, whether from Haller or the vitalists, that fiber activity was of, as well as in, living matter itself. This ambiguity produced scarcely compatible accounts of the vital principle. On the one hand, Barthez had reduced its physiological force to Sauvages's algebraic unknown—an epistemological riddle that was not an explanation, only a name and a "theoretical abstraction." On the other hand, Barthez wrote a lyrical echo of Fouquet's conjectures that the vital principle might be an emanation of a universal principle created by God to animate the universe.[51] At the same time, Barthez could account for the regularity of vital phenomena without surrendering the uniqueness of life or the free, spiritual activity of the rational soul. Cabanis absorbed both the methodological caution and the metaphysical interest in the emanations of a universal intelligence.

Barthez's physiology discussed the activities of the vital principle in sensitive and motive forces, as well as in sympathies and in "modifications" due to age, sex, temperament, disease, and the non-naturals. Against Haller, he argued for the primacy of a "sensitive principle" in irritated excised muscles. Against Whytt and the vitalists, he contended that some sensitivity can

be independent of nerves, as in pathologically inflamed liga-
ments and tendons and the response to stimuli of nerveless
zoophytes.[52]

Unlike his Montpellier colleagues, Barthez insisted that motive forces had "characteristic primordial laws" and were therefore as significant for the vital principle as nerve structure and
sensitivity were. A paralyzed patient, asserted Barthez, might
recover movement without feeling; hence no nerve movement
or animal spirit flow could in itself be necessary to move muscles and internal organs. The motive forces regularly controlled
imperceptible "tonic movement" in muscle fiber molecules and
spasmodic, perceptible tonic movements in reactions to cold or
fever.[53]

Similarly, Barthez refused to attribute to nerve connections
alone the sympathies (transfer of disturbance) or "synergies"
(cooperation of organs) occurring in organs with functional relations but no direct nerve connections. Barthez thought that
even Whytt had considered sympathies "too materially." Sympathies such as that between the brain and epigastric regions
were sometimes products of immediate activity of the vital
principle.[54]

While Cabanis followed more closely the Montpellier physicians who encompassed all such phenomena under the heading
of "sensitivity," he was very much indebted to Barthez for placing in fresh perspective the concept of temperament. Moving
beyond the solid-fluid balance theory, Barthez redefined temperament as the "ensemble of constant affections which specify
in each man the system of forces of each individual." Traditional, indirect methods of determining temperament required
either external observation of appearance and behavior or medical analysis of the elasticity, dryness, and strength of fibers (solids) and abundance and density of humors (fluids). The ancient
classes of temperament were a valuable guide, but Barthez preferred a direct determination. The crucial factor was the "total
energy of the radical [potential] forces of the vital principle in
the entire body" and its "respective energy in various organs."
Indicators of this energy might be convulsive movements or

weakness or uncommon liveliness in sensations and appetites. These movements and sensations might in turn suggest chronic organic disturbance that would influence temperament classification. One also had to observe modifications produced by habits or use of the non-naturals in the forces of the vital principle. Changes in air, climate, diet, and exercise would all affect sensitivity and mobility. Temperament classification was important, because any therapy had to adjust these environmental agents to restore natural equilibrium.[55] The concept of temperament was thus for Montpellier physicians either associated with an all-encompassing nervous sensitivity itself or with an indefinable vital principle that controlled both sensitive and motive forces in the body.

In Montpellier medicine, the active forces performed more and more corporeal functions while Stahl's omnipresent soul was confined to thought, its Cartesian essence. This refinement in views of purposiveness in the body was not entirely regressive in the history of the life sciences. Montpellier caution curtailed the mania for physical and chemical hypotheses and increased respect for factual observation. At the same time, Montpellier physicians no doubt discouraged physiological research and experimental medicine. Their epistemology involved importing Newton's concept of unknowable forces into an area where its usefulness was doubtful. Barthez thought that his vital principle was as valuable an experimental cause as gravitation was; yet Newton could assign mathematical relationships to the forces observed and, for all his piety, encouraged hypotheses and experiments without suggesting that the human intellect was all-powerful. To the Montpellier school, measuring life like brute matter was a kind of sacrilege. Yet they certainly had a well-developed concept of life before the age of biology, and their clinical approach to medicine anticipated the marked advances of the early nineteenth century.

In forming Cabanis's thought, the mechanist-vitalist convergence was crucial. To Descartes and Le Camus, matter was passive and mechanical. Mental feelings and passions could be correlated with the merely mechanical strength of fibers or flow of animal spirits. Nowhere in the body was there the activity of thought and will. To Stahl, a spiritual soul was responsible for direct supervision of all true activity in its corporeal instruments. The Montpellier vitalists suggested that corporeal forces were indeed active, though not spiritual. As sensitivity or the vital principle explained more and more physiology, the spiritual soul was crowded out of all but rational activity. Since nervous sensitivity was not mechanical, merely corporeal forces could account for mental phenomena—sensation and feeling. While there was no satisfactory solution to the age-old dilemma of how the physical becomes the mental, Condillac's psychology deduced thought from sensitivity, and therefore an active force of sensitivity could plausibly generate the active function of thought. Thus, for those with sufficiently unorthodox inclinations, Montpellier vitalism could be as provocative as the modified mechanism of Haller. La Mettrie could claim that irritability was the single active physical principle necessary to produce feeling and thought. Diderot could claim that the active sensitivity of Bordeu could explain the emergence of feeling from material organization. To be sure, neither Haller nor Bordeu could be accused of dangerous heresy. But just as the materialist La Mettrie could transmute mechanism, so could the materialist Diderot turn Montpellier vitalism to his own purpose.

The convergence of vitalism and mechanism certainly did not dictate the choice of monism or dualism. Bonnet could have a sophisticated view of nervous sensitivity while remaining a dualist. D'Holbach would choose a monism filled with physical and chemical terminology, speculate on a hierarchy of forces of affinity, and yet be little influenced by the vitalist-mechanist convergence. Nor would all those influenced by physiology become monists. The Montpellier physicians carefully reserved a place for the rational soul. But those with unorthodox inclinations, such as Diderot or Cabanis, were deeply affected by the vitalist-mechanist convergence. Their monism had a distinctly vitalist tinge in which the forces accounting for nervous sensitivity could also account for intelligence. For them, a simplistic mechanist materialism was now untenable.

DIDEROT AND MONTPELLIER PHYSIOLOGY

Diderot's hypotheses on spontaneous generation, species change, and the awakening of sensitivity might have been inspired by Buffon, Needham, and Maupertuis. But he gleaned from Montpellier physicians the physiological vocabulary that enabled him to place so much faith in the capacities of organized matter. In a letter of 1765, he had explicitly maintained that "sensitivity is a universal property of matter, inert in inanimate bodies . . . but activated by assimilation with a living animal substance."[56] But Diderot exercised none of the caution of de Sèze or Bordeu in speaking of latent sensitivity. In private letters or reading notes, he left no room for the soul or for free will in psychophysical correlations. Diderot's influence on Cabanis's physiology seems definite, but no easier to substantiate than in the case of transformism. Grimm published fragments of the *Rêve de d'Alembert* in 1782, and the Committee on Public Education of the National Convention allegedly received a copy in 1794 (accessible to Cabanis's friends Garat and Ginguené). Cabanis's acquaintance with Diderot's literary executor J.-A. Naigeon would also suggest access to the *Rêve* and possibly to Diderot's voluminous reading notes.

From about 1765 to his death (1784), Diderot gathered materials for a collection later entitled *Eléments de physiologie*. In a manuscript note dated 1778, he proposed to consult many of the same authors who influenced Cabanis—Stahl, Whytt, Bordeu, Barthez, William Cullen (Whytt's colleague at Edinburgh), and Pierre Roussel of Montpellier among the animist, semi-animist, and vitalist physicians; Le Camus, Haller, and La Mettrie of the mechanist or modified mechanist tradition; and Bonnet and Helvétius among the naturalists and philosophers.[57] The order of presentation and sometimes the substance of entire sections followed Haller's *Elementa Physiologiae Corporis Humani* (8 vols., 1757-1766). But Diderot was undeniably radical in his views on mind-body interactions. He relentlessly attempted to show how the soul depended on health, age, fatigue, and diet and asserted that life in excised organs undermined belief in unity of the soul. Like d'Holbach, he argued that the soul was merely a portion of the body correlated to other portions—merely a name for the "organization of life." Sensation, memory, affection, and the will were merely corporeal functions of the brain and nervous system, organs with no special distinction in status. The human body was certainly not reducible to a traditional image of mechanism but it was still a passive machine. Voluntary motions were not "free," but "necessary," either because of the needs of our organs and passions or because of our habits.[58] Once again, what Bonnet and Condillac would call "liberty" became "necessity" in the terminology of Diderot and d'Holbach.

Diderot continued to insist on the unity and interdependence of the organism. He found the "vibrant sensitive cord" of the fiber the key to the active force of sensitivity. Moreover, he adopted Bordeu's swarm-of-bees image in which each organ was like a "distinct animal" having its "particular kind of touch," its particular manner of sensing.[59] As in Montpellier medical works, the diaphragm had a particular sensitivity important in emotional expression, and fits of sensitivity meant spasms in nerve tension, which, in their extreme state, were, as Bordeu might have said, an *éréthisme violent*. The brain was the seat of consciousness and dominated subordinate centers of sensitivity except in sleep, illness, or violent passions. Diderot also repeated the common conception (from the time of Malpighi, adopted by Baglivi, Boerhaave, Cullen, and Buffon) that the brain was a secretory organ and that the variable composition of the nerve fluid it secreted could affect minds and characters. This glandular image of the brain was specifically rejected by Bordeu, and though Cabanis notoriously adopted it, he hardly used it in a gross materialistic fashion.[60]

Thoroughly consistent with his views in *Le Rêve de d'Alembert*, his refutation of Helvétius, and his letter to Hemsterhuis, Diderot combined a monistic metaphysics with an unmistakably vitalist physiology in his *Eléments*. He tried to reconcile the model of sensitivity as active with his conviction that sensitive response was determined rather than free. Yet assimilating man to nature did not mean denying the distinctiveness of life or denigrating human stature, as his refutation of Helvétius clearly illustrated. Diverse human temperaments prevented treatment of men as if they were all from the same mold, and human pleasures of memory and anticipation were far different from animal pleasures. In Diderot's ethical thought, far too complex for thorough discussion here, human beings were neither inexorably fated nor mere automata. As with d'Holbach, there was ample room for improvement even in a refractory temperament. Men were modifiable, and they could strive for self-realization.[61] Diderot had synthesized the Encyclopedic aspirations for unity in nature and the sciences with the medical experience of diversity.

Since Cabanis had a similar intellectual heritage, it was hardly surprising to find his thought to be an amalgam of insights from the philosophes and theories from the physicians. Before beginning his major work on psychophysiology, he would arrive at definite opinions concerning method in medicine and the need to apply the clinical approach to hospital reform. These early essays illustrated his commitment to the unity of the sciences as well as to the special status of medicine. Within a year of completion of his early essays, he was caught up in the whirlwind of revolutionary politics. Practice had to precede fully elaborated theory. Assumptions about human nature had implications for social policy, and method in medicine could be applied in reorganized hospitals and amid new professional standards.

CHAPTER IV

Methodical Medicine in the Service of Humanity

Cabanis's Medical Education

abanis became a full-fledged physician before he aspired to found a science of man. Relating medicine to the other sciences was thus a more immediate problem in his early philosophical writings than the metaphysical issue raised by psycho-physical relationships. His search for a valid medical method could not begin before he had considered existing medical institutions and public health policies. The obstacles to any truly observational medicine were partly the legacy of bookish medical education and partly the ill-defined role of hospitals. After writing about the degree of certainty of medicine, Cabanis became concerned with reforms in medical education and later with questions about the general purpose of education. From criticism of inadequate clinical training, he moved squarely into the lively debate over both the medical and charitable functions of hospitals. Throughout his subsequent political career, Cabanis focused his attention on issues of public education and public assistance. As an early enthusiast for the Revolution of 1789, his first publications highlighted his political convictions and encouraged his well-placed friends to promote him to administrative responsibilities, such as the Paris Hospitals Committee in 1791. In politics, Cabanis faced the dilemma of deciding at what point the natural order needed the corrective hand of government, just as in science he had to decide when the natural order of facts needed the rational rules of method.

Though Cabanis entered the ancien régime medical world and profited from its abuses, his training was not entirely orthodox.

94

Probably some time in 1777, he began following his much-revered mentor J.-B. Léon Dubreuil on his rounds at Charité hospital in Saint-Germain-en-Laye. Certainly it was Dubreuil (himself a student of Venel, the Montpellier physician and friend of Bordeu) who was responsible for Cabanis's initial inclination toward Hippocratic, observational medicine.[1] But while we have only Cabanis's reminiscences about his apprenticeship with Dubreuil, there is other documentary evidence of his enrollment in the Faculty of Medicine of Paris. The following list, taken from Cabanis's certificates of course attendance, indicates the subjects he studied and his teachers during the period from October 1780 to June 1783:

October 1780- June 1781	pharmacy	Jean-Jacques Leroux des Tillets (1749-1832)
1781-1782	pharmacy	Jean-Baptiste Eugène de Mangin
1782-1783	physiology	J.-B. Langlois
1782-1783	surgery (Latin)	Jean-Augustin Coutavoz
1782-1783	pathology	Benjamin-Michel Solier de la Romillais
1782-1783	*materia medica*	Edouard-François-Marie Bosquillon (1744-1814)[2]

Though there was a profusion of mediocre medical schools in France during this period, Cabanis's professors in Paris did not offer inferior training. In 1785 Bosquillon published translations of William Cullen's *Physiology* (2nd ed. [1784]) and *First Lines of the Practice of Physick* and corresponded with the Edinburgh Society of Medicine. Of course, these activities might not have affected the content of Cabanis's *materia medica* course, but Bosquillon's preliminary discourse to Cullen's *Practical Medicine* did align Hippocrates with modern believers in a vital principle. Bosquillon was best known as an erudite bibliophile and Greek scholar. He annotated a Latin translation of Hippocrates's *Aphorisms* and, since 1774, had lectured in Greek language and philosophy at the Collège

Royal. De Mangin was an editor of the *Journal de médecine*, which appeared from 1776-1790. And Le Roux was a progressive advocate of the union of medicine and surgery in 1783, wrote a memoir on British and Dutch hospitals for the Academy of Sciences commission on hospitals in 1786, administered hospitals for the Paris Commune in 1790-1791, and became a professor at the reorganized Paris School of Medicine in 1799. (Paradoxically, Cabanis and Le Roux competed against each other in 1795 for a teaching post, which neither received.) During the Consulate and Empire, Le Roux was an editor of Corvisart's new *Journal de médecine* (1801-1811) and became dean of the Faculty of Medicine.[3] Thus, Cabanis's teachers included eminent men, though not necessarily avid reformers.

Had Cabanis taken the usual route toward a medical degree, his flurry of course registrations in the third year after passing two desultory years would have been unorthodox. The guildlike regulations of the Paris Faculty of Medicine, last revised in 1751, were rigid and demanding. At entrance, the student had to be at least 22 (Cabanis was 23), Catholic, and the holder of an M.A. For a medical baccalaureate, the student normally took twelve courses in three years and prepared four oral examinations—in physiology and anatomy (things natural), pathology and therapy (things against nature), hygiene and diet (the non-naturals), and the aphorisms of Hippocrates. There were practical exams in anatomy, and in botany and *materia medica* as well. The candidate also presented two Latin theses—one in physiology or pathology and therapeutics and one in hygiene. Although Cabanis's writings showed his erudition in hygiene and in Hippocrates, his dossier is silent on course preparation in these subjects. Each examination and thesis presentation required payment of high fees and refreshment expenses. While the baccalaureate entitled the student to comment on medical texts, for the next two years he assisted his younger colleagues and diligently attended thesis disputations and anatomical dissections. Only at this stage could he accompany a doctor on house calls if he desired and, occasionally, to hospitals. For the licentiate, or license to practice, the candidate, after two more years, had to present at least two more theses and pass two more practical examinations—one in anatomy and one in medical practice. The latter exam lasted a week and involved questioning by professors at their homes, with refreshments again provided by the student. After formal presentation to university, church, municipal, and royal officials, the candidate received his letters of licentiate. Since the Faculty held a guild monopoly on medical practice in Paris and the suburbs, the candidate needed to become a Faculty member. Royal decrees stipulated two more years of apprenticeship with a hospital physician and a further ceremony at which the candidate defended contradictory theses. The clinical requirement was usually waived or minimized, but the rhetorical display invariably took place. At an expensive banquet, the student received the doctor's bonnet and swore the Hippocratic oath as well as fidelity to the statutes of the Faculty. With one further step—chairmanship of a thesis examination—the doctor earned the privilege of teaching, if selected by his peers, at the Faculty. The total cost to the physician of examinations, theses, and ceremonies could well have been over 5000 livres—a tidy sum for those not independently wealthy and more than the annual income of some country doctors.[4]

In November 1783, rather than prepare for examinations, Cabanis chose to sign a contract with Franz Anton Mesmer, the notorious purveyor of "animal magnetism." This episode might suggest a still unsettled, rebellious temperament or a longing for the mystical, unfulfilled by membership in the Masonic Loge des Neuf Soeurs. The likelihood is more simple—Cabanis never became an adept or an enthusiast for the popular fad of Mesmerism. He was probably as curious as other more distinguished savants. The chemist Berthollet also signed with Mesmer before leaving the sessions in disgust. And Cabanis's own pathology professor, Solier, had practiced animal magnetism in 1779. Yet all but the diehard converts recanted their infatuation in the summer of 1784 when the Faculty of

Medicine solemnly approved the condemnation of Mesmer by the Royal Commission and threatened expulsion of any Faculty member continuing to vaunt the virtues of animal magnetism.[5]

Cabanis was certainly still in good standing as a student in December 1783 when the dean signed the letters prerequisite to baccalaureate examinations. Yet, perhaps disturbed by Dubreuil's death that year, he decided to leave Paris. Quite possibly, he simply lacked the fees required to obtain degrees in Paris and was unwilling to borrow the funds. In May 1784 the respected pediatrician J.-Ch. Desessartz, cited by Rousseau in *Emile*, provided Cabanis with letters of recommendation to the dean of the Reims Faculty. Desessartz, who held degrees from both Reims (1757) and Paris (1768), described Cabanis as a shy, though worthy student.[6] Cabanis might have found attractive the lax standards in Reims for students who did not intend to practice in the city. Such students could openly plagiarize theses, with satisfactory disputation responses deemed sufficient for thesis acceptance. In rapid succession Cabanis received the baccalaureate (15 June—Thesis: "An Datur Etiam Vitalium Organorum Somnus?" affirmed by Pascasius Borie, Paris, 1746), the licentiate (21 September—*An a Pastu Quies?* affirmed by Antoine Gardane, Paris, 1765), and the doctorate (22 September—"An Quinque Medicinae Partes Medico Necessariae?"—an invariable thesis required of all candidates).[7]

This cavalier scholarship seemed incongruous with Cabanis's emotionally fervent poetic version of the Hippocratic oath, composed for his doctorate reception. Published in a Limoges periodical in April 1785, the "Serment d'un médecin" evoked Dubreuil's wisdom and pledged to consider medicine a holy ministry to God and the poor. While Cabanis later adopted a less impassioned theism and discarded the conventional piety of these verses, he never abandoned his exalted conception of the dedicated, almost saintly medical fraternity, who should wish their names "blessed rather than famous."[8] Contemporary testimony also confirmed that Cabanis took the oath to aid the poor in their humble dwellings as a first priority. There are few documents relating to Cabanis's life from 1784-1789, but his biographers cite his sympathy and generosity for the poor of Auteuil, where he apparently practiced medicine.[9] The antityrannical apostrophes in the "Serment" certainly corresponded to Auteuil sympathies for the American Revolution.

The Profession of Medicine

Cabanis's early essays certainly showed awareness of the lively debates in the medical profession. Newer medical trends sometimes bypassed the Faculties, steeped in their jurisdictional prerogatives. For one thing, the Paris Faculty demanded loyalty from the supposedly less literate corps of surgeons, who had until 1743 been ignominiously associated with the barbers. Since the late medieval period, physicians alone could examine patients, prescribe remedies, and supervise treatment, though in rural areas there were too few physicians to enforce this monopoly. Surgeons, in turn, had the exclusive right to perform operations. In 1751 Paris Faculty statutes even required from all bachelors of medicine an oath before a notary that they renounce the practice of surgery and pharmacy to "preserve pure and intact the dignity of the medical corporation."[10] In practice, the legal barriers did not absolutely preclude several well-known eighteenth-century French physicians from teaching or writing about surgery. Moreover, Louis XV had consistently favored surgeons—first by founding a Royal Academy of Surgery in 1731 and then by endowing positions for demonstrators at the College of Surgery, by requiring the M.A. (and thus the prestige of Latin literacy) of all surgeons in 1743, and by planning sumptuous new buildings for the College, while the Faculty of Medicine remained in inadequate quarters. Like other concerned members of both professions, Cabanis hoped to end the jurisdictional controversy, which persisted into the Revolutionary era.[11]

Cabanis was also aware of other royal encroachments on the Faculty monopoly. The teaching of the medical subjects of anatomy, natural history, chemistry, and practical medicine took place in free public lectures at the Collège Royal. Industrious students could also hear the lectures of the distinguished anatomist Félix Vicq d'Azyr and of the brothers Rouelle, brilliant chemists, at the Jardin royal des plantes.[12] In addition, the hierarchy of royal physicians and surgeons who performed public health services in hospitals and prisons was exempted from the requirement of Faculty membership and thus those in the capital could hold degrees from jurisdictions outside Paris. Their superior officers, the *premier médecin du roi* and the *premier chirurgien du roi* superintended medicine in the households of the King, Queen, and royal family and thus controlled lucrative appointments at all levels.[13] Dubreuil himself had been a royal physician at Saint-Germain hospital in the Paris region.

The emergence of a rival scientific and administrative body, the Royal Society of Medicine, was a far more important challenge to the Faculty. The society fostered a spirit of medical reform that would leave its mark during the Revolution and help shape Cabanis's notions on medical standards. The cattle plague of 1770-1776, bringing high costs of meat, milk, and draught animals, led the dynamic Controller-General Turgot to appoint a commission in 1776 to gather information on the causes of epidemics and epizootics and to recommend measures for their prevention and control. Under Necker's administration in 1778, the commission obtained revision of its original mandate to form a Royal Society of Medicine, with thirty Parisian members, sixty provincial associates, sixty foreign associates, twelve nonmedical associates, and an unlimited number of correspondents. The Society undertook to aid intendants in compiling a "medical topography" of France. They sent elaborate questionnaires to physicians throughout the kingdom to attempt to relate weather conditions, soil, terrain, minerals in water, crops, and past epidemics to current epidemics and endemic disease.[14] The replies concerning climate, geography, and modes of life have recently proven an invaluable resource of quantifiable information for the history of climate, medicine, and public health near the end of the ancien régime.[15] The exclusive right to license patent medicines and to inspect mineral water content and distribution gave the society a substantial income to carry on its projects. By 1779 it was virtually an academy, with an annual history and memoirs edited by Vicq d'Azyr as well as prize competitions. Of course, the Faculty of Medicine was insulted by the implication that it could not control epidemics and at the authorization to nonphysicians (such as the chemist Lavoisier and the philanthropist La Rochefoucauld) to comment on medical subjects. When it could not sufficiently infiltrate or supersede the society, the faculty expelled its own members who became Society* affiliates and intrigued against their students. After the Royal Council annulled such decisions, the faculty even went on strike for a month in the winter of 1778-1779. But neither the King nor the Parlement of Paris supported the faculty, and it was constrained to tolerate grudgingly its successful competitor.

While the dispute shows a classic conflict of corporate spirit and encroaching royal bureaucracy, it also involved key issues in medicine. The active naturalists, chemists, and anatomists in the society enthusiastically promoted collaboration between physicians and other scientists. Vicq d'Azyr encouraged publication of experimental as well as clinical memoirs and fostered the observational approach to medicine. Like Cabanis later, he wished to safeguard the special character of medicine but he also foresaw that in the long run the "accessory sciences tend to approach medicine ever more closely, and that works of physicists, anatomists, and chemists continually hasten such unification."[16] Vicq was also an adherent of Condillac's empiricism, with its stress on observation, precise language, and analysis.[17] He ultimately wrote one of the most significant documents of medical reform, the "Nouveau Plan de constitution pour la médecine en France," submitted through his own political maneuvering to the comité de salubrité of the Constituent Assembly in 1790.[18] This plan insisted on the union of medicine and surgery, the association of both medicine and surgery professors with hospitals, public competition for teaching posts, abolition of mediocre medical schools to reduce the total from twenty-three to five, instruction in French rather than Latin,

101

and abolition of examination fees. Thus the society was capable of placing the medical world in ferment with a plan completed in the early phase of the Revolution. Coupled with the increased emphasis on the clinical approach in the military and naval medical corps and the foundation of a model clinical teaching hospital in 1774 at the Hospice of the College of Surgery, the trends fostered by the society showed that the old bookish approach to medicine was clearly obsolete.[19]

When Cabanis enrolled in the Paris Faculty of Medicine in 1780, his training with Dubreuil would have already alerted him to the pitfalls of the formalized curriculum. Yet while he sympathized with most of the reforms advocated by the society, he was skeptical about the immediate contributions to medicine of the other sciences. To understand Cabanis's attitudes in perspective, one need only briefly examine the viewpoint of a protégé of Vicq d'Azyr and active member of the society, the physician-chemist Antoine-François de Fourcroy (1755-1809). Throughout his career, Fourcroy concerned himself with the utility of chemistry for medicine.[20] He insisted that the chemical composition of bodily fluids and solids, in illness and in health, as well as of drugs and their affinity to the body *were* relevant for the practitioner. In the society memoirs, Fourcroy developed a chemical theory of aging, an index of "animalization" (later partially adopted by Cabanis), based on the nitrogen content and galvanic properties of fibers.[21] In 1791 Fourcroy, his pharmacist assistant Vauqelin, the surgeon Jacques Tenon, and the physicians Philippe Pinel and Jean-Noël Hallé founded a short-lived periodical literature digest called *La Médecine éclairée par les sciences physiques*. Fourcroy recommended active cooperation between medicine and the other sciences and condemned narrow observation which would reduce medicine to "systematic empiricism." Later, despite conventional acknowledgment of the uniqueness of life, Fourcroy would urge Paris medical students to discern the "mechanism of life," the nature of disease, organic injury, and the composition of drugs.[22]

To Cabanis and to the Neo-Hippocratic clinicians of Montpellier, human knowledge was both more limited and more potent. On the one hand, they warned that no chemical experiment could reveal the secret of life; Barthez had clearly argued that the vital principle transcended laws of ordinary matter. And on the other hand, the clinicians, as well as Cabanis, were sanguine about the need for such knowledge in physiology and pathology. To them, life might remain unknowable, but unaided observation was powerful enough for successful medical practice.

Du Degré de certitude de la médecine:
Explanation and Classification

Cabanis's first essay in the philosophy of medicine, *Du Degré de certitude de la médecine*, thus had an ambivalent relationship to the attitudes of some members of the society. He certainly sought to establish medicine as an observational science as valid as other natural sciences. Yet he claimed medical knowledge could not penetrate ultimate secrets and he thus stressed the clinical at the expense of the experimental. The Newtonian explanation paradigm—Newton's caution in explaining gravity—and the metaphysical skepticism of Locke and Condillac became the foundation of Cabanis's attitude to medicine. *Du Degré de certitude de la médecine*, completed in 1788, published only in 1798, was a reasoned defense of the status of medicine and a call to rouse the enthusiasm of medical students. The preface reminded the reader that the political excitement of 1789 had delayed publication, and Cabanis insisted on the approval of his colleagues at the new School of Medicine before final submission to the publisher.[23] The essay attempted to respond to seven traditional objections to the validity of medicine—ignorance of the source of life, or the "principle animating us," and its means of action; ignorance of the nature and cause of disease; variation and complexity of disease according to the patient's age, sex, temperament, climate, regimen, and so forth; mysterious nature of drugs and of their action on the body; difficulty of interpreting the reason for cures or the outcome of experiments in medicine; contradictions in medical theory through the centuries; and difficulty of absorbing enough knowledge for effective medical practice.[24] Rather than stressing the need to probe further, as did Fourcroy, Cabanis asserted that medicine already had effective means of preventing and curing disease.

The very title of the essay suggests acquaintance with the eighteenth-century arguments that the observational sciences could not have deductive certainty. By 1788 Cabanis knew the marquis de Condorcet, who had written on observational error in the sciences and who had adopted arguments like those of Hume on "degrees of belief and assurance" in knowledge. Condorcet was eager to extend the rapidly developing probability calculus to the "moral and political sciences." In his reception speech at the Académie française in 1782, Condorcet had already written, "in meditating on the nature of the moral sciences, one cannot indeed help seeing that, based like the physical sciences upon the observation of facts, they must follow the same method, acquire an equally exact and precise language, attain the same degree of certainty." Condorcet reasoned that the results of some sciences are more certain than results of others but that the probable truth of any given result could be expressed with the same certainty. Though all observational knowledge was probable, it was sufficiently valid for everyday life.[25]

Cabanis had a similar concept of observational certainty but he remained skeptical of mathematical applications in medicine. At the end of Degré de certitude, he added a note on the observation of a "very enlightened friend" (almost certainly Condorcet) on the value of probability calculus in the moral sciences. Reinforcing sound metaphysics (the analytical method of Condillac), the probability calculus would hasten progress in philosophy. Yet Cabanis warned that, despite the need for calculation of muscular strength or the need to know mathematical optics and acoustics, applications of mathematics to medicine had "far from hastening its progress, infected it with the most false and dangerous plans of treatment."[26] With this statement, he was probably referring to the misguided efforts to calculate the mechanical force of muscles in digestion or the force of the heart in circulation, or to theories of "critical days" for drugs in intermittent fevers. Like Locke, Condillac, and Buffon, Cabanis knew that the sciences of observation could not claim deductive certainty; yet he feared the distraction of mathematical demonstrations of probability values, even though his whole subsequent approach had statistical implications.

The introduction to the *Degré de certitude* stressed both empirical and rational components of the origins of medicine. Primitive peoples observed the power of the healing force of nature in spontaneous recoveries. Despite his inferiority to animals in instinct, early man had inclinations to rest and eat less during illness. In Rousseauist fashion, Cabanis argued that these instinctive talents declined inversely with the development of sensitive and intellectual faculties. Stahl might have suggested the view that man was, of all creatures, the most sensitive and most susceptible to disease.[27] Early physicians were skilled observers of the appetites, desires, and salutary evacuations of those who recovered. They aided their memories by classification of disease by symptoms, duration, and crises, and of patients by temperament, regimen, and habits. Then they had to relate and compare the facts, make analogies to new cases, and systematically order the conclusions. With experience, treatments became increasingly assured of success; and after long experience, successful treatments, according to Cabanis, would be "practical certainties." When medical method was fully mature, it still could never lead to the certainty of demonstration, but only to "more or less precise approximations"—all that men could hope for in the "practice or the application of reasoning to positive facts."[28] Here, then, was a kind of "large numbers" rule for medicine—the more often a treatment worked, the more likely one thought it would work in the future. Although Cabanis makes no explicit references here to probability theory, or to theories of inductive reasoning, his confidence in medicine rested on the high statistical probability that empirically proven relationships would hold true.

Cabanis maintained that medical progress was an example of the "indefinite perfectibility" of man (the term used by Rousseau in the Second Discourse and made famous in the posthumously published *Sketch* by Condorcet) accomplished by transmission of experience. Any objection to medical knowledge on the basis of complexity of disease could be overcome by proper method—attentive observation, due regard for the peculiarities of each case, classification of the disease, and treatment on the basis of experience. Here, too, was the reply to the critique based on contradictions of medical theorists. These variations in dogma actually masked the agreement of talented observers since Hippocrates—their rules of diagnosis, prognosis, and therapy were quite similar since they were based on experience.[29]

Amid this optimism, Cabanis recognized the pitfalls of overzealous nosology, or classification of disease. The grand schemas of Sydenham, Sauvages, and Cullen were as necessary as botanists' charts of plant species. But the futile multiplication of species, the mania for systematic categories, the conspicuous gaps and exceptions clearly showed the artificiality of all such tables. Rather than abolish all rules, however, one had to notice the frequent agreement of empirics and avid classifiers on symptoms. Cabanis hoped to create a new nosology that would correlate therapy with each category. By the time Cabanis published the more elaborate medical methodology *Coup d'oeil* in 1804, however, he had to admit that this project had already been partially accomplished. Philippe Pinel's *Nosographie philosophique: Méthode d'analyse appliquée à la médecine* (1798) was the "happiest contemporary effort at classification." In 1788 Cabanis was content to stress the need for verbal "signs" (as Condillac had)—a language to fix fleeting phenomena. He thought that observation would reveal a small number of repetitive phenomena in disease (pains and fevers, for instance) that varied in intensity, duration, order, and relationship. Observation would thus furnish the letters of a pathological alphabet. Accurate description, rather than mere nomenclature, would improve any reformed nosology. Whatever the disadvantages, classification in as natural a way as possible would be invaluable for the practitioner.[30]

Aside from answering objections to the practical feasibility of medical knowledge, Cabanis discussed the inability to understand fully the object studied. Here Cabanis claimed that ordered empirical knowledge of life, disease, and drugs was sufficient to produce cures and achieve the same degree of certainty possible in other observational sciences. Reasoning like Newton and Locke, he affirmed that man could not discern the essence of matter, the "hidden principle" vivifying it, or any of the "first causes" of things. A causal explanation was nothing more than an ordering of facts or a determination of resemblances among them: "Two facts are connected in an order of succession; one calls the first fact the cause of the second." The only true cause, unknowable to us, was the "general principle of motion" or "spontaneous force" moving the world and all its parts. Cabanis obviously adhered to the antimetaphysical tradition of Voltaire and Condillac and to some extent anticipated the positivist views of Auguste Comte. Like Hume and Condorcet, he was confident that, even if cause did not imply logical necessity, it was a notion sufficient for scientific knowledge.

After all, Cabanis continued, men performed physical and chemical operations without understanding the "cause of the affinity, elasticity, cohesion of bodies." Similarly, they improved agriculture without knowing the "secret of vegetable life," and they formulated rules of diet for diverse ages, temperaments, and climates without knowing the mechanism or cause of digestion or assimilation. Sense observation of effects, or facts, and presumably appropriate reasoning upon them were sufficient for the formulation of scientific principles, the rules of cultivation, or the rules of nutritional hygiene.

The same radical empiricist approach applied to knowledge of disease and drugs. The physician observed the history of a disease or a "concourse of accidents," not an essence or cause. Yet deductions drawn from observation of, touching, and listening to the patient could lead to classification and treatment of disease. More remote causes, according to Cabanis, were probably

107

less important to know.[31] This attitude contrasted nicely with Fourcroy's later observation of the difficulty of determining the function of oxygen in physiology: "As the object is more difficult and more important, so is Nature's veil covering this operation more tightly drawn and folded."[32] Cabanis seemed to be saying that medical knowledge was at the fingertips of the skilled observer. Unlike the chemists, Cabanis thought that knowing the "intimate nature" of quinine would not affect the decision of whether or not to prescribe it for "intermittent fever" (malaria) and would certainly not improve its effectiveness. Observation of its effects under varied conditions was important. In fact, rather than a search for new drugs, the need in medical therapy was for a better ordering of the relationship of observed effects of the already ample existing pharmacopoeia.[33]

Like Francis Bacon, Cabanis wished to substitute method for talent. The clinical empiricists saw disdain for speculative systems and for the search for ultimate causes as a legitimate latter-day Newtonianism. Yet the precise description of effects of disease or drugs and the correlations of symptoms and therapy could never match the mathematical sophistication of Newton's laws of gravitation. Moreover, with the mere tabulation of symptoms one risked avoiding a search for meaningful relations; even for the secondary efficient causes of disease—the true pathogenic agents. Just as overzealous vitalism could conceivably inhibit experimental physiology, overzealous clinical empiricism could inhibit experimental pathology. Only later would Cabanis respond to the surgeons' concern for anatomical localization of disease and correlation of autopsy reports, in case of death, by drawing up clinical charts. Foucault is in this instance correct in claiming that the "old" clinical school was preoccupied with the external.

In *Degré de certitude*, Cabanis spent little time warning against the encroachments of the other sciences upon medicine. But even here, he was skeptical of the utility of chemistry. He did see the need to search in the collateral sciences for "what relates to our art, what can be transported into it without hypothesis." That theme would become one of the major arguments seven years later in *Coup d'oeil*.

Finally, having established the validity and feasibility of medicine as a science of observation, Cabanis concluded the essay with a ringing declaration on the mission of the physician: consoler of the suffering and the weak, the conscientious physician should be indifferent to fame and wealth, subservient only to his conscience and patriotic duty. Before publication in 1798, the conclusion was strengthened (some notes indicate revision) to a systematic expression of social responsibility. By the exemplary search for truth, the physician should combat the terror of superstition, emancipate the public from quackery, and publish his discoveries to serve all humanity. He must selflessly combat epidemics and offer his talents to his own country, not to its enemies. Thus, servant of his patients, his country, and all humanity, the physician would be one of the shock troops of enlightenment and virtue, one of a corps of "mandarins," a term Cabanis expunged from the 1803 edition.[34]

Cabanis's idea of the methods and mission of medicine would be applied in a broader context to the role of a science of man. Armed with analytical method, the physician actively intervened to restore natural powers of recovery. In the future, practitioners of the science of man would restore physical-mental equilibrium. Yet how could one even hope for a sound clinical medicine with such conspicuous gaps in medical education and such poor cooperation between Faculties and hospitals? Moreover, how could a clinical medicine emerge if its field of observation, the hospital, was a chaotic institution fulfilling many other nonmedical functions? Valid knowledge of a truly observational, scientific medicine was inseparable from a change in institutions. In the fervor and excitement of the first year of the Revolution, Cabanis turned from medical philosophy to hospital reform.

Hospitals in the Ancien Régime

While some hoped the new regime would bring an end to hospitals, Cabanis clearly thought they were essential for medicine as well as for patients. In the ancien régime, the polyglot nature and innumerable abuses of hospitals inspired vocal criticism.

There were indigent sick in the institutions of Paris known as the "Hôpital Général" (founded in 1656); but these buildings were primarily places of confinement, not treatment, for the aged and feeble, the orphans, the insane, and the social deviants (vagrants, prostitutes, common criminals, and the temporarily unemployed). For physicians, the housing of the ill and insane together with prisonlike control of criminals and paupers meant a fundamental confusion of social responsibilities, even in the small parish hospice. For government officials and economists, hospices and hospitals would foster idleness and squander public funds unless the able-bodied were removed and put to work in "charitable workshops" or the more repressive "depots of mendicity." Louis XVI himself had adopted the policy, "Work for the able-bodied, hospitals for the sick."[35] Both Physiocrats and neo-mercantilists could agree on the importance of increasing productivity by eliminating unemployment or underemployment. In the context of the new liberal economic theory, hospitals seemed "unnatural," arbitrary creations, especially to statesmen like Turgot. Private or church hospital endowments fixed capital in a necessarily unproductive, sometimes inequitable way. The testament of a benefactor could tie the hands of administrators to narrowly confessional charity that might exclude those unable to meet tests of piety or good character. Moreover, hospital boards had to consume valuable time in administration of inalienable hospital property, on which, as corporate institutions, they collected seigneurial dues. Such an archaic, feudal structure seemed anachronistic to some in an enlightened age. The entire framework of Christian charity also could lead to placing more importance on saving souls than rehabilitating bodies or facilitating return to work.

Enlightenment humanitarianism was just as powerful a motive for hospital reform as economic doctrine or the bureaucratic dream of efficiency. Despite disdain for the "people," philosophes such as Montesquieu as well as more radical writers like Rousseau or the philanthropist Claude-Humbert Piarron de Chamousset agreed that the poor had a right to subsistence. Both humanitarianism and financial problems led to criticism of the appalling conditions at the Paris institutions that were designed solely for the sick poor—the Hôtel-Dieu on the Ile de la Cité (founded allegedly in A.D. 660) and its affiliated houses. A disastrous fire in 1772 destroyed one wing of the Hôtel-Dieu and led to a plethora of reform proposals. In any case, the years 1774-1789 were a boom period for hospital construction, with seven small parish hospices founded—as many institutions as had been established in the previous 130 years. Aside from the College of Surgery hospice, Jean Colombier, a physician in Necker's civil hospitals department, and Mme Necker herself had helped establish a model Hospice de Charité in Saint-Sulpice parish in 1779. But Necker himself favored expansion and renovation of the Hôtel-Dieu rather than a new network of small hospices.[36]

THE ACADEMY OF SCIENCES COMMISSION

The head of the Maison du roi and a minister for Paris, Louis-Auguste le Tonnelier, baron de Breteuil convened a special commission of the Academy of Sciences in 1785 to examine the proposal by a Paris municipal architect for a new 5,400-bed hospital. With the full patronage of Breteuil and diplomatic support for a fact-finding tour by two members (the distinguished surgeon, pathologist, and ophthalmologist to the royal family Jacques Tenon [1724-1816] and the physicist Charles Coulomb) to English hospitals in 1787, the commission produced three reports (November 1786-March 1788) with a telling critique of the Hôtel-Dieu and a proposal to establish four new hospitals. The commission included the author of the reports, the astronomer Jean-Sylvain Bailly (1736-1793) and such illustrious savants as Lavoisier, Laplace, Daubenton, and the first physician to the King, Lassone. Tenon, the principal researcher, produced the fruit of twenty years' work on hospitals, a veritable summa, published separately as *Mémoires sur les hôpitaux de Paris* (1788).[37]

The commission found the Hôtel-Dieu in every respect insufficient, uncomfortable, and unhealthful. Housing an average

111

of 2,500 patients on 1,200 beds, the Hôtel-Dieu was infamous for overcrowding, favoritism (some patients were four and six to a bed while others had private beds), and failure to isolate contagious cases or to separate convalescents from the critically ill. The Augustinian nuns who performed essential services placed highest priority on spiritual welfare rather than on scrupulous adherence to medical prescriptions. The size of the hospital led to routine, uniformly scheduled administration of food and drugs which made a mockery of individualized therapy. The poorly heated, ill-ventilated wards, short on clean linen and woefully understaffed, resulted in longer recovery times or dangerous secondary or new infections. Physicians complained that illnesses became so complicated that proper diagnosis was nearly impossible. Surgery, performed in the wards rather than in special rooms, was less successful than elsewhere, and typhus, puerperal fever, hospital gangrene, and scabies raged inside the wards and sometimes in the densely populated surrounding neighborhoods. With a nearly twenty-five percent general mortality rate and a high, but unknown, mortality rate in childbirth, little wonder that the administration was secretive. High per-patient costs made accounting practices suspect.

In 1787 the Royal Council adopted the commission proposal to abolish the Hôtel-Dieu and construct four new 1,200-bed hospitals on the outskirts of Paris. These would constitute a compromise between those favoring many small hospices and the one large hospital proposed by the architect. Each would be both a general hospital and a specialized institution—for surgery, obstetrics, contagious cases, "fetid" fevers, or the insane. Ten separate pavilions with 120 beds each would enable isolation and differentiation of disease, as in the best English hospitals. Chemical theory on respiration would determine room size and ventilation, while scientific principles would be applied to drainage, sewage disposal, and interior organization. Each patient would be assured a single bed, and most important, medical control would be paramount.[38]

When Cabanis entered the debate, Breteuil had resigned, the

112

commission had ceased to function, and Necker was once again the Controller-General. But the establishment early in 1790 of a National Assembly Committee on Exterminating Mendicity (hereafter called the comité de mendicité) reopened the issue of public assistance in general and that of hospital reform in particular. Cabanis fully agreed with the commission that large hospitals were fundamentally vicious, that physicians had to have complete medical jurisdiction, and that hygienic principles were essential in hospital reform. But he had several disagreements with the commission, many of which stemmed from memoirs that they had rejected.

DU PONT

One of the most significant among these rejected memoirs was *Idées sur les secours à donner aux pauvres dans une grande ville* (1786), written by the physiocratic collaborator with Turgot and friend of Lavoisier, Pierre-Samuel Du Pont de Nemours (1739-1814). In this work, Du Pont carried the critique of bigness to its logical conclusion. His premise was that the most salutary, the most natural, the most humane, and the most economical care for the sick would always be at home. Specially assigned physicians and surgeons could visit at least 3,000 patients at home. With general revenues from the Hôtel-Dieu and the free services of the hospital order of the Sisters of Charity (all the more dedicated because of their annual renewable vows), each patient would receive a daily subsidy for food, drugs, and fuel, carefully supervised by parish officials. Domestic care would be one-third cheaper than a bed at the Hôtel-Dieu while bringing material and psychological benefits to the family. In an image possibly already in Turgot's manuscripts and used in 1784 by the novelist Bernardin de Saint-Pierre, Du Pont noted that the bouillon for the patient would bring meat and warmth to the home. Personal care would bring the family closer, facilitate return to work, and boost the morale of all involved.[39] In sum, self-help, as far as possible, was best.

Du Pont still had to admit that many sick poor lacked families or suitable housing for health care, so he recommended, on the basis of the success of the Hospice de Charité of Saint-Sulpice, a system of parish hospices of about one hundred beds each for about 3,000 more patients. Here, there would be fewer complications in disease, fewer secondary infections, and more rapid recovery from surgery. The hospices could treat one-quarter more patients than the Hôtel-Dieu for five-eighths the cost and with one-half the mortality rate. Rather than expensive new constructions, existing religious establishments would be converted into hospices. Finally, Du Pont proposed separation of the aged or feeble in twenty 100-bed nursing homes run by private contractors at a guaranteed rate of return. Competition among them, he naively added, would insure good patient care.[40]

The commission rejected the arguments of Du Pont and others on several grounds. First, they believed that domestic assistance would be medically ineffective—the patient would be in cold, unsanitary, overcrowded rooms with unprofessional administration of food and drugs. Second, the saving in public expenditure would be borne by the poor, who, while losing the income of the sick person, could not meet their expenses even with the calculated subsidy. Nor could working relatives lose *their* income to act as nurses. Domestic assistance might mean maldistribution by parish and might dry up the sources of private charity. Moreover, parish hospices might be in poorly equipped buildings rather than in the scientifically designed structures envisaged by Tenon. Each hospice would end up a miniature Hôtel-Dieu, with an overworked parish clergy and the added inconvenience of residency or piety tests, which the Hôtel-Dieu never demanded. Unwed mothers could not retain anonymity, there would be no space for contagious cases, and there would be a lack of competent staff to treat rare diseases and the insane and to perform difficult surgery.[41]

Observations sur les hôpitaux

Cabanis's *Observations sur les hôpitaux* appeared early in 1790. A former official of the civil hospitals department, Michel-

Augustin Thouret, reviewed it favorably in June 1790 in his capacity as adviser to the comité de mendicité.[42] While Cabanis later made clear his sympathy with Du Pont's ideal of domestic assistance, here he agreed that hospitals were a necessary evil for the ill-housed poor, if only because medical and surgical treatment often required cumbersome apparatus. He therefore supported a plan for small hospices—where better ventilation, cleaner beds, more sympathetic nurses would assure an environment as natural as possible. Overall size was the principal factor in overcrowding, internal epidemics, complication of disease, poor ventilation, and routinized administration of food and drugs. Only where the physician had complete control of treatment and where he could give individual attention in a favorable environment could there be effective medical practice. In a point-by-point critique of the Academy's "four hospitals" plan, Cabanis argued that in the small hospice, treatment of contagious diseases would be better, unwed mothers would have better chances of survival, a centralized list of available beds could avoid wasteful duplication, and, most important, clinical medicine could be made a reality.

The Academy of Sciences had carefully avoided mention of the needs of medical research and teaching, but Cabanis did not hesitate to link medical and hospital reform. Only in the small hospice would there be time to keep clinical journals with precise description of each illness and of the effect of remedies. Only there could the medical staff adjust doses and times of administration of food and drugs according to the medical history, age, and temperament of each patient in the given climate. With strict cooperation between physicians and surgeons, the small hospice would also provide humane conditions for a teaching ward. Cabanis relentlessly elaborated on the dangers of the large institution. "Great assemblages" of men in "enclosed places" would become corrupt. The labyrinthine bureaucracy would conceal both medical negligence and administrative peculation. Without the incentive of private gain or ease of public scrutiny, there would be no motivation for good service. Operating budgets would surely be lower in the small hospice. Renovation of existing buildings into 100- to 150-bed hospices would also save capital expenditures with respect to the Academy plan.[43] Reformed hospitals were thus indispensable for analytical medicine.

Cabanis's views on hospitals were analogous to his views on medical practice in another sense as well. Just as the physician had to maintain natural equilibrium and bolster natural healing forces, so must the legislator intervene to obtain a natural milieu for therapy. Though Du Pont and Cabanis, like others before them, proposed use of clerical staff, they insisted on secular control of hospitals. In the reports of 1791, the duc de La Rochefoucauld would articulate the concept of the citizen's right to public assistance if he were unable to assist himself.[44] Even the moderate monarchical Constitution of 1791 would specify the intention to organize a "general establishment" to "relieve the infirm poor, and furnish work for the able-bodied poor unable to procure it for themselves."[45] For the sick, this concept implied the right to health care. Yet health care was not naturally available any more than cures for illness occurred spontaneously. As the physician had to intervene to assure health itself, the legislator had to intervene to assure the availability of health care.

Cabanis's *Observations* also aspired to have broader implications for the subject of public assistance. He discussed food shortages, poverty, and unemployment as well as hospitals. The epigraph was characteristic: "Poorly distributed alms are yet another scourge for the poor; alms discerningly and charitably given are the safeguard of the rich."[46] Christian virtue aside, humanitarianism and self-interest both spurred charity for the able-bodied, as for the sick. Cabanis clearly wished to attack an inadequate clerically distributed charity and to insist on a secular public responsibility for assistance.

The Dilemmas of Public Assistance: Elimination of "Artificial" Inequality

Even in the seventeenth century, the royal government already gave short-term employment subsidies after bad harvests to maintain production and to avoid social disturbances. During the course of the eighteenth century, penalties remained harsh (branding or a term in the galleys for able-bodied men) for vagabondage, which in 1724 was defined as habitual begging, armed or in a group or on false pretenses, and redefined in 1764 as unemployment for six months without references or domicile. Yet while begging was once again prohibited in 1724 and 1764, beggars without resources were merely confined—at first to general hospitals, and later, after 1767, to special "depots of mendicity." At the same time, some intendants established "charitable workshops" for beggars and the temporarily unemployed. The rather grim depots sometimes detained migrant workers unfairly and, for all their overcrowding, still could not possibly absorb the numerous bands of beggars and brigands on the roads.[47] While critics have charged that the state was obsessed with productivity, the depots and the workshops both testified to official recognition that work, rather than punishment, was the only remedy for begging. Administrators like Turgot and Necker clearly realized that the poor needed social assistance in economic crises.

At least one depot superintendent, a canon-turned-journalist and protégé of Necker, Leclerc de Montlinot (1732-1801) had sincerely humanitarian aims. His experience at the Soissons depot gained him a considerable reputation, so that the comité de mendicité named him an adviser in 1790, the Department of Paris selected him (as well as Cabanis) for the Hospitals Committee in 1791-1792, and later the Thermidorian Convention and the Directory appointed him a hospitals administrator. In an essay on begging, Montlinot stressed the inability of the deserving poor to provide for old age or widowhood or to deal with disabilities. How could one hope to enforce the harsh laws against begging when poverty persisted and master artisans were not compelled to hire hands? While there were incorrigible vagrants who could be chastened only by transportation to a penal colony, the deserving poor needed jobs—and a comprehensive public assistance program.[48]

Thus, when Cabanis wrote his pamphlet, many philosophes

117

and officials had already concluded that individual laziness and improvidence were not solely responsible for poverty. If social and economic conditions drove more men to beg, the state had to provide jobs as a last resort. Cabanis began with the premises that both the self-interest of the rich and social justice required relief of the poor. First, to preserve their own property and status in a society in which hordes of beggars roamed the countryside, the rich had to realize that aid to the poor was a high priority. Cabanis here merely invoked the traditional motive for laws against begging—whether in the context of the punitive "great confinement" of vagrants and deviants in general hospitals in seventeenth-century France or in the earlier, more constructive Elizabethan Poor Law. Mercantilists and physiocrats had always stressed the wastefulness of begging. Cabanis added to this argument by pointing out the need for security and the hope that the benefactors of the poor through publicly administered relief would feel the nobler pleasures of virtuous action. He also argued, with the Scottish moralists and Rousseau, that sympathy was as natural a human quality as self-interest. Somewhat like d'Holbach, he contended later in the *Rapports* that love of fellow men was a higher-order manifestation of the physical attractions of the inanimate world and the sympathies of the animal world.[49] In any case, relief of the "poor beings whose lives and sufferings are sacred" was a natural development of the sympathy in any sensitive being. Charity, or beneficence, as its secular advocates preferred to call it, was thus an essentially human act, bound up with the universal forces of the cosmos.

Yet alms-giving degraded the recipient and encouraged idleness. Hence, for governments, public assistance was a question not merely of sympathy, but of social justice. In 1789 Cabanis agreed with the abbé Siéyès (an occasional guest at Mme Helvétius's salon) that the proposed Declaration of the Rights of Man should properly include the right to assistance for "anyone who cannot provide for his own needs"—a right any wealthy family would grant an aged, disabled servant or a servant's child. Even from a business standpoint, such assistance was a sound investment in the future services of the child. For the aged, it was a debt justly repaid.[50] The state was thus obligated not to aggravate the wrongs of centuries, but to redress them. Poverty, like excessive wealth, lamented Cabanis, was "generally the work of social institutions" and of "bad laws and customs." Indeed, "if legislators and governments had not favored with all their power the maldistribution of wealth, would the earth ever have been covered with this crowd of indigents, whose cries accuse both nature which brought them forth, and the powerful who despoiled them before birth?"[51]

With the legacy of the corrupt ancien régime, there would be no spontaneous correction of injustice. Nor could one assume that the rich would naturally understand their self-interest in poor relief or that all men would suddenly cultivate more than usual their natural feelings of sympathy. The state had to act, but act wisely. Men were equal in rights, not abilities, hence any attempt to eliminate all inequality would be disastrous. Cabanis opposed any wholesale redistribution of wealth even long before his revulsion at the radical egalitarianism of the journalist-conspirator Babeuf. He warned that Spartan communal ownership or a Roman-style "agrarian law" limiting property would be "iniquitous and contrary to the purpose of society, which is the free exercise of the faculties of each, and the peaceful enjoyment of the goods these faculties procure." Like Du Pont, he thought that the English Poor Law unjustly burdened and impoverished the middle-income ratepayer while failing to solve the problem of poverty.[52]

A wise public assistance policy would seek to eliminate only "artificial" inequality, not "natural," inevitable inequality. State action would thus not harm individual self-reliance or the freedom of proprietors. Cabanis subsequently made clear what he meant by artificial inequality. Like the Physiocrats and Adam Smith (whom Cabanis had read by at least 1791), Cabanis hoped that the state would eliminate the relics of feudalism—the monopolies, burdensome industrial regulations, inequitable inheritance laws, obstacles to labor mobility, and, most of all, hereditary privilege. Only then could one

119

break up artificially created concentrations of wealth while encouraging new economic activity to provide jobs for beggars.[53] Here Cabanis sounded like the archetypical liberal visionary—in modern terms, he would remove all hindrances to the free market in goods and labor and to free capital accumulation. Unproductive privileges distorted the natural flow of wealth earned on the basis of productivity and talent. Hence, inequalities in wealth would inevitably diminish in this liberal utopia since gross inequalities were impossible after the abolition of privilege.

In concrete terms, Cabanis hoped in 1789 for a public assistance program that, while not guaranteeing any minimum income, would assure public workshops for the unemployed. Work, not alms, would discourage troublemakers, defray the costs of assistance, and develop the self-respect of the unemployed—a sentiment conducive to social stability. While opposed to an obligatory minimum wage, Cabanis noted in 1789 that charitable workshops would help maintain the general wage level, "a factor of greatest importance for the class that lives by its hands."[54]

The therapy of work would also make prisons more humane. Inmates were generally "unfortunate victims of society," but already so corrupted that they must be isolated to prevent mutually harmful influence. But in line with Beccaria's philosophy of punishment, prisons should be not mere detention houses, but "infirmaries of crime." If inmates were to be cured of their antisocial tendencies, they must be given work to prepare for return to society and to defray institutional costs.[55]

Thus, from considerations on the need to reform hospitals, Cabanis advanced to reflections on public assistance to the able-bodied. The right to a job was as important a public consideration as the right to health care. In the same way, his concern with medical method had brought him to general notions on knowledge in the observational sciences. In both areas, his early writings were sketches to be completed by more detailed works. Throughout his early writings, there was the aforementioned analogy between scientific and political concepts. The physician supplemented clinical observation with classification and reasoning and actively intervened to calm physiological disturbance. In society, too, there was a "natural" equilibrium to be established by legislative intervention. Public assistance would help eliminate "artificial" inequality while preserving "natural" inequality. Enough work for all would mean human dignity for all. Meanwhile, reformed, smaller hospitals would allow a more nearly "natural" environment for the treatment of illness. Institutional change would place medicine in service of humanity.

Cabanis's experience as a hospital administrator as well as his observation of Revolutionary turbulence led to modified views on public assistance, particularly to the able-bodied. His horror of large assemblages of men increased with the evidence that these groups often disturbed the peace. But though Cabanis was driven to antidemocratic attitudes by Revolutionary politics, he never surrendered the goal of reducing the suffering of the poor. His political friendships in the early phase of the Revolution led him to a new interest in education, the most promising tool to increasing the skills of all and enabling the poor to emancipate themselves.

CHAPTER V

The Natural and Artificial in Society

The Fervor of Revolution

he outbreak of revolution heightened the enthusiasm of the Auteuil salon for political and institutional reform. Two of Cabanis's closest friends, the medical student-turned-ethnologist Volney and the mathematician Condorcet, became avid pamphleteers on the organization of provincial assemblies and on the Estates-General, the abuses of privilege, and the need for guarantees of equality before the law and individual liberties. Abbé Siéyès, an occasional guest at Auteuil, denounced aristocracy and demanded a constitutional government with real power for the Third Estate. The electoral assemblies chose Volney, Siéyès, and the lawyer Dominique-Joseph Garat to represent the Third Estate at Versailles, and Garat became the Assembly correspondent for the *Journal de Paris* until 1791. Another deputy, the military officer from Bourbonnais and future Idéologue Antoine-Louis-Claude Destutt de Tracy (1754-1836), accompanied liberal nobles who joined the Third Estate after the establishment of the National Assembly. Other future Idéologues, Pierre-Louis Ginguené, Marie-Joseph Chénier, and Pierre-Claude-François Daunou, expressed their hatred for tyranny and their hopes for the advent of liberty in essays, poetry, or plays.[1]

According to his own account, Cabanis was in Paris on 14 July when he heard the news of the fall of the Bastille. The next day he rushed to the Assembly chamber in Versailles to report the effervescent state of opinion in Paris to Garat and Volney. They seized the opportunity to introduce him to the greatest orator in the Assembly, the declassed noble, intrepid defender of the Third Estate, philanthropist, and intriguer, Honoré-Gabriel-Riqueti de Mirabeau (1749-1791).[2] The habitués of Mme Helvétius's villa soon divided their time between the Assembly debates and Mirabeau's salon, while Volney and Siéyès became residents of Auteuil.

Despite Cabanis's fears of social disorder, he revealed a fierce dedication to the patriot cause during the first year of the Revolution. In his native region of Bas-Limousin, peasant disorders continued in the winter of 1789-1790. The authorities of the Brive-Tulle region reported incidents of brigandage, burning of churches, pillaging of châteaux, and even a pitched battle between rioters and the maréchaussée, the royal mounted highway patrol. The provost courts of the maréchaussée of Tulle executed several ringleaders and ordered the detention of some Brive National Guardsmen as instigators. Meanwhile, a house guest of Mme Helvétius, abbé Morellet of the Académie française, without informing Cabanis and Martin Lefebvre de La Roche, published a pamphlet defending the restoration of law and order by the provost courts. Early in March 1790, the pro-revolutionary Brive municipality sent two friends of Cabanis, the physician Lachèze and the National Guard officer J.-B.-H. Serre to inform the Paris Commune and the National Assembly that the "executioners" of Tulle and the "seigneurs and other so-called privileged persons" were guilty of "atrocious excesses" and were making scapegoats of overzealous patriots.[3] Cabanis and La Roche snubbed Morellet so harshly that he bitterly left Mme Helvétius's hospitality.[4] On 26 March, Cabanis defended the Brive delegation before the Paris Commune and thanked the Commune for its address to the Assembly, which ultimately had the effect of suspending provost court judgments.[5] In a letter to Serre in April, Cabanis lamented that Limousin was so "retarded" in the Revolution but warned that persistent "habits of tyranny and slavery" would only be gradually changed. Around the same time, Cabanis and La Roche contributed to the "patriotic gift" given by the municipality of Auteuil.[6]

Despite these prorevolutionary views, Cabanis joined a rather moderate club, the Society of 1789, founded in late March or early April 1790 by Condorcet and Siéyès. Its objectives—to bring together the Lafayette and Mirabeau factions and thus stabilize the Revolution—were conservative in part from the outset. But Cabanis, not an active member, was more likely attracted by the intellectual goals—to develop a "social art" to increase public happiness, help establish a new constitution, and promote the Enlightenment spirit of progress and innovation. The high membership dues insured that the group was more for the literate elite than for the people in general. Its members included future Idéologues Garat, Chénier, and Roederer, as well as men of letters like Suard and experienced lawyers or administrators like Du Pont, Pastoret, and Talleyrand. Interestingly enough, a recent analysis showed that a very high proportion of the over 400 members—about twenty-five percent—were from the world of banking, finance, wholesale commerce, or tax-farming.[7] While the short-lived *Journal*, edited by Condorcet, published theoretical articles on the art of reasoning, it devoted much of its space to practical aspects of the "social art," improvements in agriculture, mining, and commerce—as well as to innovative, socially useful business ventures, such as a social insurance plan. Thus, in the first phase of the Revolution, this effort to establish a kind of social science joined both humanitarian and broad utilitarian goals with more narrow concerns of private self-interest.

While the Society of 1789 left an intellectual program that would be eagerly pursued by Condorcet and the Idéologues, the group itself faltered—primarily because the Mirabeau and Lafayette factions could not long hold together. The society's conservative members supported the repression of mutinous troops at Nancy in September 1790 a bit too zealously, and Mirabeau chose to return to the Jacobins the next month, with Condorcet, Siéyès, and Talleyrand following in May 1791. The Lafayette circle then drifted into the monarchist Feuillants club. Cabanis's name appears on an undated list of Jacobin Club members, and this affiliation may very likely parallel that of his moderate friends from late 1790 until the summer of 1792.[8]

Mirabeau's Physician and Speechwriter

At this time, too, Cabanis joined the circle of researchers and speechwriters who collaborated with Mirabeau.[9] Cabanis's effort is identifiable in the *Travail sur l'éducation publique, trouvé dans les papiers de Mirabeau l'aîné*, which he published in August 1791, some four months after the death of the great orator. No one has yet resolved the problem of authorship of the four discourses—On Public Education, or the Organization of the Teaching Corps; On Public Civil and Military Festivals; On the Establishment of a National Lycée (a public higher educational institution); and Education of the Presumptive Heir to the Crown. Cabanis modestly attributed them to Mirabeau, though his widow, and some critics, have claimed that he wrote them. Even if Mirabeau had not yet revised them for publication, he no doubt found the opinions expressed acceptable. A recent study presents manuscript evidence that indicates that the fourth discourse was probably the work of the future Girondin, abbé Antoine-Adrien Lamourette. And Mirabeau's correspondence shows that he also asked another collaborator, the Genevan pastor Etienne-Salomon Reybaz, to write a discourse on "national education," but there is no record of Reybaz's reply.[10] We cannot assume that Reybaz wrote any of the discourses. Passages in the first three, however, on the faculty of sensitivity, the relationship of physical and mental, the limited role of the state in general education, and the necessity for supervising medical education are all consistent with Cabanis's views and even with his style. If the topics of the discourses depended on Mirabeau, it seems likely that Cabanis provided the actual rough drafts and possibly the major ideas for the first three discourses.

REVOLUTIONARY FESTIVALS

The discourse on festivals, certainly completed after September 1790, had the general goal of channeling revolutionary passions to orderly, patriotic ends and of excluding priests from civic ceremonies. The political context dictated the curtailment of popular, unorganized exuberance by detailed rituals of poetry, drama, and prize ceremonies. Mirabeau and Cabanis both agreed on the need to institutionalize the Revolution. After the mutiny at Nancy, there were also motives for separating the civic festivals (applicable to the National Guard) from the festivals of military garrisons—avoiding dangerous incidents and keeping the army subservient to the Assembly. Only the Fête de la Fédération, already celebrated on 14 July 1790, would be exempted from this division.[11]

As in Cabanis's writings on public assistance, the premise of the discourse on festivals was the existence of the human faculty of sensitivity, of sharing the affections of fellow citizens. As in Cabanis's *Rapports*, the author of this discourse called sensitivity the "last fact of the study of man." Intensifying natural affections made us more human. Furthermore, while Revolutionary principles and laws were rational, the government needed to "move, not merely convince" its citizens. The Church had always known how to use "imposing objects and striking images" that directly affect the senses. The secular moral goal of the festivals should be to "make each of us feel our own happiness in public felicity—in virtues and sacrifices to the interest of our brothers." Beyond the arid texts of the laws, the festivals should call forth the wellsprings of natural sympathy. In the *Letter to F[auriel] on First Causes* (1806 or 1807), the mature Cabanis would make the same admission of the human need for impressive ritual.[12]

Cabanis himself participated in several Revolutionary fêtes. The electors of the commune of Auteuil, on 13 November 1791, chose Lefebvre de La Roche as mayor and Cabanis as municipal officer. Both led the commemoration on 5 August 1792 of the abolition of seigneurial dues three years earlier in a ceremony that included the dedication of a new municipal building. At a time of great excitement in Paris about an allegedly traitorous King and the threat of an Austro-Prussian invasion, the municipality of Auteuil duly constructed an "altar to the Patrie" and displayed the popular symbols, the revolutionary pike and the fasces. At the same time, they brought busts of Enlightenment philosophes into the city hall—Rousseau as author of the *Social*

126

Contract, Voltaire as "enemy of privilege," Franklin as the savant who met human needs with the printing press and lightning rod and who fought for American liberty, and Mirabeau, the "victim of despotism, orator of liberty."[13] This enshrinement of *lumières* on the eve of 10 August was fitting for the circle of Mme Helvétius. When secret correspondence from the Tuileries implicated Mirabeau as an intriguer with the Court, however, La Roche found the bust of the orator a reason for some to question Auteuil patriotism.

FREEDOM AND REGULATION IN EDUCATION

In a broader sense, the discourses on education aligned themselves along the central axis of Cabanis's thought—the spontaneous and natural situation, best left to itself, and the mode of intervention of external authority. At the same time, they renewed the long eighteenth-century debate on the need for a secular, patriotic, and pragmatic public education. Throughout the Revolution, the issues of state control, tolerance for religious or private schools, universal and compulsory schooling, scholarly "instruction" versus moral "education," classical versus scientific curriculum were reargued *ad infinitum*. The Revolutionary era was as critical for schools as for hospitals, given the schism in the clergy in 1791, which removed a portion of potential teachers, the abolition of clerical teaching orders in 1792, and the abolition the same year of the corporate legal status, if not the existence, of University Faculties and secondary-level collèges.[14]

The author of the first and third discourses adopted the familiar agricultural metaphor (already present in Hippocrates and in Cabanis's *Degré de certitude*) for the power of education. The outcome of good education was compared to the harvest of a skillful farmer who, with his knowledge of the terrain, planted and cultivated carefully to improve the "wise dispositions" of nature. Especially in impressionable childhood years, education had great power to cultivate necessary habits and eliminate destructive ones. Education was indeed a "science of freedom" providing knowledge of objects advantageous or harmful to us. Transmission of the cultural heritage of the ages thus assured "nearly incalculable progress" in the "physical and moral existence of man." At the current juncture, proper education would combat ancien régime prejudices and "lead human inclinations back to nature."[15]

Though the inventors of laissez-faire theory, the Physiocrats, favored universal free primary education, the author of the discourses more closely followed the views of Adam Smith.[16] He maintained that while the educator represented an external intervention in natural development, the trade of teaching should be left free to enterprising schoolmasters. The state should remain in its suitable sphere of judicial and police functions. State salaries for teachers would produce a harmful corporate spirit and would not allow an incentive to improve teaching. Competition for fees among schoolmasters could only benefit pupils, while fees for schooling would also prevent unrealistic ambitions from carrying pupils beyond their appropriate place in society.[17]

At least three principles forced compromise with this rather timid, rigorously liberal theory of schooling, however. First, the state could not remain indifferent to the "urgent need" and "profound ignorance" of the people. Therefore, the state must "protect, excite, and reward" parish schoolmasters with bonuses for recognized teaching ability, prizes for awards to excellent pupils, and subsidies for authors of elementary textbooks. While the constitutional clergy would provide most of the teachers, the state would supervise instruction with departmental and national education committees.[18]

Second, the state would recognize its obligation to certain talented, but impoverished children by endowing faculty chairs and allocating one hundred student stipends (one student from each department and seventeen from the nation at large), to be awarded on the basis of merit, for a higher-education National Lycée. This "encyclopedic" school would improve upon traditional curriculum by adding chairs in modern languages and literature, the sciences, public economy and ethics, and several modern philosophical subjects. A course in "Universal Method" would include "analysis," the decomposition and re- composition of objects, and classification by analogies and re- semblances. It would also discuss the laws separating and unit- ing the sciences, which were each like a branch attached to the common trunk of universal knowledge. In order to accomplish the Baconian goal of leveling wits, this course would be closely linked to "Universal Grammar," the study of signs in fixing ideas and of languages as analytic methods. A third subject, "Metaphysics," would study mental faculties in the fashion of Locke, Condillac, Helvétius, and Bonnet (all authors Cabanis cited in the *Rapports*), teach the art of comparing and judging, and set down rules for the "degree of certainty possible in each subject."[19] Thus, the plan for the National Lycée included a kind of Ideology *avant la lettre*—the kind of psychology, logic, and analysis that would be the subject of Idéologue treatises and that later was partially included in the curriculum of the secondary-level "central schools" created in 1795.

Third, the state would insure the regulation of those trades and professions (flour and grain merchants, bakers, goldsmiths, notaries, pharmacists, physicians) where the public needed pro- tection from fraud and quackery. Under any regime, the state would have to inspect pharmacies and to license health prac- titioners. The author embarked on a long discussion of medical reform, disclaiming his own competence (as if Mirabeau would *read* the speech), but claiming expert advice. The text certainly paralleled Cabanis's own views—unified education of physi- cians and surgeons, certificates for pharmacists and midwives, penalties for quacks, award of medical professorships only after competition, and stress on clinical observation, journals, and clinical teaching in hospitals. More unorthodox was the plea for a medical school in every department under departmental ad- ministration, though Paris would retain its Faculty and its Royal Society of Medicine, which would also devote itself to teaching.[20] Otherwise, the details did not differ much from Vicq d'Azyr's contemporary plan.

Another moderate innovation in the learned societies would

be the reorganization of existing royal academies into one unified "National Academy," with a third branch, philosophy, added to letters and science. To some extent, this proposal, though not very detailed, anticipated Condorcet's plan for a section of "Moral and Political Sciences," which became a component of the unified Institute of Sciences and Arts in 1795. The Mirabeau-Cabanis plan even developed the idea of meritocracy—all academicians would automatically become "active citizens," that is, they would have the privilege of voting in primary electoral assemblies and, by a special dispensation, be eligible to join the National Assembly.[21]

No doubt, the discourses appeared conservative when compared to the more famous Talleyrand report on education (September 1791) or to the subsequent Condorcet plan (April 1792). The Mirabeau-Cabanis plan did not envisage secularization or compulsory attendance and hardly encouraged universal primary schooling or any kind of social mobility. It gave the generally conservative departmental directories jurisdiction to inspect secondary and medical schools, and to choose pupils for the National Lycée. It repeated at length Rousseau's image (as well as Cabanis's views) of the "delicate constitution of women," which made them unsuitable for most nondomestic social roles and therefore excluded them from public education.[22] Even if Cabanis did not write these discourses, they follow his most persistent concerns on the physiology of sensitivity, the influence of age and sex, medical reform, the unity and relative independence of the sciences, and the power of education. As the Revolution progressed, Cabanis would openly confess that his views on public education were inappropriate. The "natural" competition of private schoolmasters, and the "natural" ability of pupils to pay fees, after all, could never eradicate ancien régime prejudices.

THE DEATH OF MIRABEAU AND REPUBLICANISM

Another clue to Cabanis's moderate views appeared in his apologetic *Journal de la maladie et de la mort de Mirabeau*

(April 1791). Mirabeau had called upon Cabanis to be his trusted physician during his final illness. Cabanis attributed Mirabeau's demise (now variously diagnosed as angina, rheumatic pericarditis, with gallstones as well) to poor dietary habits and speculated that the bad air of the assembly hall had hastened his end. Charged by the Jacobins Barnave and the Lameth brothers with incompetence, Cabanis tried to portray Mirabeau in the *Journal* as already marked by death when he first called a physician. (Cabanis's administration of quinine does show the feeble powers of eighteenth-century physicians to deal with serious ailments.) Aside from medical post-mortems, the importance of the *Journal* was its testimony of agreement with Mirabeau's views on the "alliance of true representative democracy and monarchical government," which combined the virtues of the single executive with the proper respect for natural liberties. In the second edition of 1803, Cabanis persisted in defending Mirabeau's sincerity in a note that claimed that Mirabeau himself assured Cabanis that if the King should decide to flee, Mirabeau would have been the first to proclaim the republic.[23] On 31 July 1798 he had offered Mirabeau's portrait to the Council of Five Hundred.

In any case, for Cabanis's circle, the flight of the King in June 1791 shook the foundation of all previous political assumptions. While Lafayette, Du Pont, and the more conservative faction of the Society of 1789 remained faithful to the monarchist ideal, a clandestine republican circle began to meet in July 1791 and to publish a short-lived periodical, *Le Républicain*.[24] The group included Condorcet, the future Girondin leader Jacques-Pierre Brissot, the military commander, resident of Auteuil, and patient of Cabanis, the Marquis Achille-François du Chastelet, and their Anglo-American associate Thomas Paine.[25] From the offices of Mirabeau's former newspaper, the *Courrier de Provence*, du Chastelet edited a number of articles on the theme that an elected executive council could succeed in a large country. In 1799, in a speech before the Council of Five Hundred, Cabanis recalled his own participation with "the most famous deputies of the Gironde: I can offer the most direct proofs; having often attended the secret committees where the means of application [of republican ideas] were discussed," including the declaration of the *patrie en danger* in July 1792 as a blow against the executive power.[26] Garat, Daunou, and Volney were all dubious of the stability of the monarchical constitution of 1791.[27]

Hospital Administration in Paris

The notoriety that Cabanis acquired as physician to Mirabeau helped catapult him into a position of administrative rather than political power. Less than a week after Mirabeau's death, Pastoret, the attorney for the Department of Paris, in the name of the Department Directory, appointed Cabanis to a five-man Hospitals Committee to assume administration of the hospitals of Paris.[28] His colleagues on the committee included the two advisers to the comité de mendicité, Thouret and Montlinot, the financial controller of the Pitié orphanage, Aubry-Dumesnil, and a member of the Academy of Sciences, J.-A.-J. Cousin. The origin of the Hospitals Committee goes back to the jurisdictional tangle after the electors of Paris assumed the power of the Commune in July 1789. Bailly himself, the mayor, refused to accept the resignations of the former administrators of the Hôtel-Dieu and the Hôpital-Général. On the other hand, the Commune retained all legal administrative power in its department of hospitals and charitable workshops until May 1790 and afterward in the department of "public institutions" headed by the botanist-physician Antoine-Laurent de Jussieu.[29] Meanwhile, in August 1790, the Assembly's comité de mendicité heard Thouret's recommendation to abolish the large hospital in favor of hospices of 250 beds in cities, and of 150 beds in the country.[30] Before the comité de mendicité had a chance to prepare its final reports, hospital finances completely collapsed. The nationalization of church property in 1790 and the definitive abolition of tithes in January 1791 dried up charitable revenues from the Church, while the abolition of seigneurial dues deprived hospitals of their own seigneurial income.

Hospitals also lost their share of the defunct municipal tariff (*octroi*) and theater taxes, while the Assembly subjected them in March 1791 to ordinary real estate property taxes. The result was a brutal entry into the liberal economic world.

Near the end of 1789, although the communes retained nominal power to administer "institutions belonging to them," the Assembly confided to the newly-established department directories the right to "inspect and ameliorate the regime of hospitals." In this bureaucratic maze, the Paris Department Directory (including La Rochefoucauld of the comité de mendicité) arranged to control policy while assigning the Commune merely routine administrative tasks. From the incomplete Hospitals Committee minutes and the report of Germain Garnier, a department official, to the full Department Council, we can reconstruct the committee's accomplishments. In the end, they dealt more with the most flagrant abuses than with issues of grand policy.[31] In his official capacity, Cabanis wrote several reports, all unfortunately lost, on Hôtel-Dieu mortality, reform of the Hôpital-Général, prison infirmaries, and the Foundlings Hospital. The committee tried to follow the spirit of the Bailly-Tenon reports, but the financial constraints did not permit new hospitals or hospices—only the reform of practices in existing institutions.

The committee first insisted, as a prerequisite to all other changes, on careful accounting, particularly in its audit of the inflated hospital employee food budget. As Garnier indignantly wrote, one might have thought that hospitals existed chiefly for the staff and that patients "only owe the care they receive to the benevolence of people on the staff." Like the Academy of Sciences commissioners, the Hospitals Committee favored external contracting for food supply, with competitive bidding if possible, rather than a full internal kitchen with its expense and its dangerous open fires. Second, the committee agreed with the Commune in reducing the nonmedical budget; they drastically cut the number of priests (particularly if "refractory") and choirboys and discouraged nonmedical charity, such as endowment of Masses. Third, the committee ordered wholesale sanitary and medical reform at the Hôtel-Dieu, including one bed per patient (700 beds added), better food, cleaner laundry, a separate terrace for convalescents, and more medically attentive nursing care.[32] Since 1788 there had been a great improvement in the teaching of clinical surgery through the efforts of Pierre-Joseph Desault (1738-1795), who obtained a large surgical amphitheater at the Hôtel-Dieu and gave free instruction to at least one hundred apprentice surgeons in 1791 and later to even more students.[33] The committee favored the inauguration of a clinical medicine course as well and arranged for anatomical dissections under the guidance of Vicq d'Azyr. They also proposed to move contagious cases and the insane away from the city center to specialized wards in the Saint-Louis branch of the Hôtel-Dieu.

While the committee could not by itself dismantle the Hôpital-Général, it at least began the separation of the sick from the chronically disabled and all the "infirm" from the merely poor. To conserve the public assistance budget, rich families were required to pay for hospitalized relatives, whether feeble, or "insane." At the Bicêtre asylum for men, the committee insisted on separating the "insane" from the "criminal," increased the bread ration, and, in the measure long identified with the supervising physician Philippe Pinel, substituted the straitjacket for chains in controlling the manic.[34] Relief of "insane" women at the Salpêtrière was also an urgent priority. The committee released some unjustly detained inmates and expelled those merely feigning insanity. Finally, the committee applied Cabanis's occupational therapy principle to able-bodied boys in the Hôpital-Général. The administrators arranged for private employers to hire apprentice woolspinners aged at least thirteen for a maximum eight-hour workday. Compared to the twelve- or thirteen-hour workday in English mills, this regimen was not ungenerous. The employers agreed to permit the inspection of food, clothing, and lodging given the apprentices. Department officials were not indifferent to the "sacred debt every society contracts to indigence and misfortune." But they hoped to save hospital expenditures while also insuring that there would be no distortion of the industrial economy and that the boys would gain enough self-respect to become productive citizens.

In 1791 the Department Directory and the comité de mendicité, with the adherence of the Royal Society of Medicine, approved a comprehensive plan for Paris hospitals that conciliated the Cabanis-Thouret small hospice policy with the Bailly-Tenon view. They favored domestic aid by parish surgeons where possible but insisted on a neighborhood network of fourteen hospices of 175 beds each, including several medically specialized institutions. Convalescents and venereal disease patients would be assured separate wards, while there would be a general separation of the acutely ill from chronic cases. Foundlings, the aged, and incorrigible vagabonds would be housed in distinct institutions. Most remarkably, the report recommended the creation of two 700- to 800-bed hospitals for "more complete" clinical instruction, because only in them could one assure all the "means of observation . . . collected in less space . . . in a greater variety of subjects." The report acknowledged that more pupils could be accommodated in the total number of small hospices but that a large hospital would insure better surgery and better use of funds.[35] The Academy of Sciences commission had advocated large hospitals on grounds of medical and administrative efficiency but never for the benefit of medical research or teaching. Interestingly enough, though Cabanis always remained hostile to large hospitals, his opinion softened in a 1798 speech to the Council of Five Hundred on medical schools. Only in the "vast hospitals" of large cities, he then admitted, would there be enough diversity of subjects—men and women from diverse climates, of diverse temperaments, following diverse regimens—to provide opportunities for adequate investigation and teaching both of medical uniformities and of rare cases.[36] Analytic method in medicine was statistical, requiring large numbers of subjects, either in large institutions or from compilations of hospice records.

The National Assembly implemented neither the Department mendicité plan nor any of the recommendations of the rival comité de salubrité. Nor did the Legislative Assembly approve any plan other than emergency hospital appropriations. The Paris Hospitals Committee remained in office until 10 August 1792, when the new, more radical Commune forcefully reasserted full administrative jurisdiction over the hospitals of the capital.[37]

A Revised Theory of Public Assistance

From his Hospitals Committee reports, Cabanis compiled notes for an essay, *Quelques Principes et quelques vues sur les secours publics*, written mostly in 1791-1793 but published only in 1803. The date of publication was thus long past the national commitment to public assistance during the radical phase of the Revolution. Yet it is interesting to note that while Cabanis's attitude to assistance was more cautious than in 1789, he retained the sense of urgency of a wisely planned program. In October 1796, Cabanis, Lacuée, and Baudin des Ardennes were members of a public assistance committee of the Second Class of the Institute that deputized Thouret and Montlinot to join it. Cabanis's thoughts were stimulated no doubt by the publication (at the initiative of François de Neufchâteau, Interior Minister) in 1798 of a series of translations and summaries of European publications on "institutions of humanity." Cabanis and his colleague Baudin des Ardennes reviewed the fourth and fifth volumes of this series (translations by John Howard) for the Institute after 2 November 1798.[38]

HOSPITALS, ASYLUMS, ORPHANAGES, PRISONS

Cabanis's experience with the Hospitals Committee did not change his basic ideas on hospital reform. In *Quelques Principes*, he was not committed to stressing hospitals to the exclusion of ideal forms of assistance, however. And consequently, he clearly stated his preference for aid at home and openly cited Du Pont's pamphlet of 1786. Family care would strengthen the ties of blood and reinforce natural sympathy, while local physicians and surgeons would be assigned to insure medical supervi-

136

sion. For those without available relatives, volunteer or subsidized nurses would be used to save as many patients as possible from the bad air and sometimes "negligent medicine" of hospitals and to save hospital beds for those truly in need. The municipality could assign these nurses to tutor the children of the family or to spin or weave to minimize the assistance budget or to use it more efficiently. If domestic aid was impossible, Cabanis still preferred small hospices.[39]

Cabanis reiterated the goals of the Hospitals Committee in medical treatment of the insane. He wished to eliminate the residue of the arbitrary ancien régime *lettre de cachet* from commitment procedures. Without a formal legal act and a medical certificate after proper observation, families must not be permitted to "put away" deviant relatives. Families who could afford to pay for private institutional care must not be permitted to benefit from a charitable public hospital. Confinement was essentially temporary—revocable on medical judgment alone without slow legal process—because the asylum was an infirmary, not a prison. Madness itself was often temporary, and confinement was thus an exceptional violation of individual liberty solely to prevent the patient from harming himself or others. As in his philosophical works, Cabanis stressed the effectiveness of physical agents on the mentally ill; here he favored the physical components of Pinel's "moral treatment"—better diet, air circulation, and occupational therapy appropriate to the strength of each. Cabanis again proclaimed a basic assumption of his philosophy, applied here to the pathological: a "sustained occupation, in providing a field for activity of all the organs, of the mind as well as the others, maintains the faculties in a state of equilibrium; this state constitutes the health of the brain, as of other parts of the living system." Physical agents and habits of life affected mind and character according to Cabanis. Even in an insane asylum, there must be a way of restoring a semblance of a natural environment.[40]

Similar considerations applied to institutions for foundlings, studied by Cabanis for the Hospitals Committee. The nearly ninety percent mortality rate before age ten and the inadequate apprenticeship training at the Paris Foundlings Hospitals horrified the committee. Montlinot had already analyzed the serious problem of child abandonment in the Soissons district; he read a memoir on foundlings to the Second Class of the Institute on 28 September 1796. Twentieth-century studies substantiate the eighteenth-century opinion that there was an enormous increase in the number of children abandoned in the provinces who were taken to the already overcrowded Paris Hospital.[41] On this subject, Cabanis agreed that each canton should be responsible for its own assistance program to end the already illegal, but still murderous transport of infants to Paris by unscrupulous traffickers. Cabanis also confidently predicted that the chief causes of abandonment—poverty and dissolute morals—would decrease under the new regime. The prediction was not empty revolutionary propaganda, since new legislation allowed the possibility of divorce, and even more important, gave more tolerance to unwed mothers.

Because Cabanis felt that any institution was worse than a domestic upbringing, he proposed that only sick foundlings be hospitalized in a special infirmary. Healthy children should be placed preferably in the country with foster parents who would receive a pension indexed to local prices until the child reached age seven. At that time, the foster parents could keep the child as an apprentice until age twenty-one or return him to public care. At twenty-one, either the parents or the state would emancipate the youth with an endowment equal to the public pension of the first seven years. Ideally, foster parents would legally adopt abandoned children. This seemingly modern approach followed the general practice of the Paris Foundlings Hospital of placing many more children in the country than it admitted. But Cabanis, of course, wished to avoid the horrors of the transport as well as the disadvantages of any large public institution.[42]

Cabanis visited prison infirmaries for the Hospitals Committee and devoted some space in *Quelques Principes* to repeating his views of the prison as a "hospice of correction." Then in the summer of 1796, Cabanis was named by the Second Class of the

Institute to report on the "unhealthfulness and poor condition of prisons and the means of a prompt remedy." In the tradition of the writings of John Howard, he argued that proper hygiene—better bedding, clothing, ventilation, and food—was indispensable to treatment. Borrowing English and American experience—most likely the Gloucester "penitentiary" and the Walnut Street prison of Philadelphia opened in 1790—Cabanis insisted that prisons become compulsory workshops where inmates would be productive (though with innocuous tools unconvertible into weapons). The skepticism of "great assemblages" of men induced him to adopt (probably after the precedent of the English Blackstone-Howard Bill presented to the House of Commons in 1779) the proposal of enforced work in isolation to minimize mutual corruption and allow sufficient time for remorseful meditation. Thus, prisoners would rehabilitate themselves. For truly refractory cases, Cabanis warily endorsed Montlinot's plan of 1797 to transport prisoners to a remote tropical penal colony, where they would become independent farmers. But reports of Australian penal colonies already made him pessimistic on prospects for success.[43]

BENEFICIAL NATURAL INEQUALITY: THE LIBERAL CREDO

The other sections of Cabanis's essay completely reviewed the premises of any public assistance program. Cabanis retained the ideal of cultivating individual sympathy as a natural development of sensitivity, and the conviction of the justice, as well as the considerable advantages to enlightened self-interest, of aid by the rich to the poor. More than before, he insisted that public assistance must be sufficiently reflective. His philosophy of economic liberalism now appeared in mature form. Its first tenet was the elimination of all social, or artificially created, inequalities and concentrations of wealth—monopolies, preferential subsidies, industrial regulation, property sale restrictions, hereditary offices, inequality of inheritance rights, privileges of birth or tax exemption—in short, all ancien régime relics of corporatism, feudalism, and state encroachment. The second tenet was encouragement of the beneficent aspects of natural inequality, stemming from the free exercise of human faculties, skill, diligence, and prudence. Thus, property acquired from honest labor was the untouchable foundation of society.[44]

In some passages, Cabanis echoed Adam Smith's confidence in the ability of the free market to enrich everyone. Any useful industry that enabled an entrepreneur to increase his wealth also contributed to public prosperity and the resulting economic inequalities were only beneficial and self-correcting. Indeed, the "middle class," active in commerce and industry, had been chiefly responsible for the "more equitable" property distribution of the last two to three centuries. The poor could only gain by the accumulation of wealth in "great commercial and industrial enterprises . . . which spread life and abundance around them."[45] Here, Cabanis sounded most like the fabled bourgeois "idéologue" of Marxists—the ideal spokesman for rampant entrepreneurial capitalism. We must point out that Cabanis wrote in the generation before economics became, in Carlyle's words, the "dismal science," before Ricardo had punctured the visions of Adam Smith on economic growth bringing a universal increase in living standards. Then, too, the dehumanizing rigors of industrialization were less evident in France in 1803 (or in England in 1776) than they are to historical hindsight. But the Marxist interpretation is still apparently untouched—whatever Cabanis's humanitarianism, he was an enthusiastic proponent of liberalism, and therefore, of the "false consciousness" masking the true consequences of the economic doctrine.

PITFALLS OF THE POOR LAW AND PUBLIC WORKS

We can support this Marxist interpretation by piling up Cabanis's repeated warnings on how not to give assistance to the poor. The Revolution, for Cabanis, had offered too many lessons of inappropriate economic policy in an atmosphere of political instability, which stifled commerce and produced increases in begging and crime. The precipitate property transfers, confiscations, price and wage regulations, forced requisitions, unemployment in the luxury trades, and depreciation of paper currency all aggravated the plight of the poor. Nor did Cabanis spare the Montagnards and, by implication, the Babouvists and neo-Jacobins: he called them "senseless demagogues frightening property by doctrines subversive of all order" and advocates of an "agrarian law" limiting property holdings.[46] Diffusion of wealth was certainly a goal for Cabanis, but economic equality certainly was not.

Inappropriate public assistance was not a benefit for the poor. The English Poor Law was based on the misguided principle that each parish should care for its own poor, who needed a minimum residence certificate to qualify for the rolls. The result, according to Cabanis and English critics, was to discourage the unemployed from seeking work outside the parish and to place inequitable burdens on impoverished parishes where the taxpayers themselves could hardly afford to subsidize the least fortunate. The operation of the system also showed that wherever the most funds were distributed, the number of paupers invariably increased the most.[47] Thus, the English were caught in a never-ending cycle of supporting steadily increasing poor rolls.

In addition to Cabanis's study of documents from the Interior Ministry series, he chose to review elsewhere in 1798 the massive three-volume *State of the Poor* by a disciple of Adam Smith, Frederick Morton Eden.[48] Here he vigorously opposed the Poor Law modifications of 1795 in the southern (Speenhamland) counties that provided wage supplements, related to bread prices, to give each worker a minimum real income. Cabanis thought these "indiscriminate" supplements rewarded the less productive and established the bad precedent of aiding the able-bodied, employed poor from public funds that should have been reserved for the unemployed or infirm. In 1795 Samuel Whitbread presented another bill to the House of Commons proposing that local magistrates be allowed to fix a minimum wage. To Cabanis, such a plan meant unwarranted interference with the natural price of labor. Any public assistance program had to be based on encouraging people to work hard, not guaranteeing them wages, and maintaining their self-respect, not making them dependent on assistance. Cabanis understood that certain regions might have an abundance of manpower and only there would he allow an exception to the general rule that public assistance wages to the unemployed be lower than an ordinary day laborer's wage.[49] He apparently believed that the market determined minimum wages justly.

More surprising was Cabanis's agreement with Eden's critique of the Speenhamland family allowances, which offered additional payments for wives and children. This "prodigal" subsidy, he wrote, was "founded on the idea that the poor cannot live without the best white bread, cheese, sugar, and tea."[50] Paradoxically, Cabanis elsewhere consistently stressed the effect of regimen on physical sensitivity, and we have noted his firm support for dietary improvements for prisoners and for the insane. Yet he opposed providing the poor with these nutritional supplements at taxpayers' expense (since he considered fine flour, sugar, and tea as luxuries). Public assistance was intended to foster a return to natural self-reliance and thus should not discourage frugal habits and overburden proprietors.

Public assistance to the unemployed had thus far been an equally unsatisfactory intervention in the natural equilibrium. In 1789 Cabanis had been willing to admit the need for public workshops, but in his essay on public assistance, he thought them a misconceived and misapplied enterprise. We can probably explain his change in attitude by the continual problems of the National Assembly and the Commune of Paris with outdoor public works for men. Established by Necker in the depths of the 1788 crisis and continued by Bailly in 1789, the work projects were suspended and reorganized three times before their definitive dispersal in June 1791 under the watchful eyes of Lafayette's troops. From an ample employment roll of 8,600 men earning a respectable (for unskilled labor) eighteen sous a day at landscaping in 1789, the projects fitfully expanded by the spring of 1791 to a mammoth work force of 32,000, engaged in various road repair and canal construction activities. Despite encouragement from the comité de mendicité, Commune administrators complained about forged enrollment cards, lack of discipline, crime in public parks, illegal sales of cards entitling the bearer to a bonus for leaving Paris, payroll embezzlement by foremen, and, generally, rising expenditures for little useful work. No doubt the economic uncertainty of the time, the evaporation of established authority, and the lack of definite goals produced considerable confusion. The Paris Department official Garnier unequivocally condemned public works in his November 1791 hospitals and public assistance report as a "gross error of beneficence . . . where aid was immodestly asked for and ungratefully accepted," though private industry languished in the same period.[51] The entire experience most likely deterred Cabanis from enthusiasm about workshops and works projects. Even the comité de mendicité, which wished to guarantee everyone a job, retreated from the "dangerous idea that government can relieve the anxiety and activity necessary for the poor to achieve their subsistence."[52]

Cabanis also read Eden's accounts of English workhouses, which were expensive, disorderly, unhealthful, and, by Eden's standards, morally scandalous. Cabanis had previously questioned staff integrity in large, crowded hospitals; he now warned against the dangers of large, overcrowded public workshops. Eden's reports of the high mortality rate and the baneful influence of the "vile and corrupt" on the honest unemployed suggested to Cabanis that workhouse life was like an indefinite prison term, worse even than the degradation of begging. "Most sensible men," Cabanis concluded, "expect no real improvement in the condition of the poor, unless workhouses are completely destroyed or entirely reorganized."[53] The well-intentioned charitable workshop was a social therapy that failed. Cabanis once again warned against distortion of the labor market. Public assistance wages must not tend to raise external wages above their natural level or attract workers to the public rolls. Otherwise, employers might suddenly be confronted with a labor shortage and taxpayers with a swollen assistance budget.

Cabanis at last insisted that aid to the unemployed was in fact a social obligation. The problem was how to preserve the individual incentive to work and at the same time reduce public expense by channeling the entrepreneur's pursuit of profit. To help preserve industrious habits, public assistance must be paid at piecework rates if possible. Ideally, the state would distribute work to be done at home in accordance with the ability of family members. The state also needed to balance approaches for efficient use of funds: buying raw materials from needy artisans would help a flagging industry; manufacturing products that were in demand would minimize useless effort and bring better returns; and employing the poor in familiar trades would improve productive efficiency. Cabanis seemed to know enough elementary economics to realize the impracticality of combining these desiderata but, above all, he wished to avoid the sense of futility of the workhouse. If cottage industry was one approach, another would be entrusting a large works project to a private contractor who would furnish apprentices with food, lodging, and clothing subject to public inspection (as in 1791 in the Hôpital-Général). A state-guaranteed rate of return would insure acceptance of the offer, while surveillance by private interest would keep order more effectively.[54]

PUBLIC ASSISTANCE AND SOCIAL MOBILITY

The social agitation of 1790-1791 and especially of 1792-1795 had hardened Cabanis's attitudes toward public assistance. His ideal of social justice sometimes seemed secondary to his concerns for public order and a favorable economic climate for entrepreneurs. The best hope for promoting natural equality was also to promote natural inequality—to allow the free market to function. But Cabanis was too realistic to advocate a laissez-faire approach to poverty, if for no other reason than the possibility that the poor could become the discontented troops of aristocratic or royalist reaction. In the era of the Consulate, public assistance was becoming primarily communal, while private and clerical foundations were assuming a greater share of all aid to the poor. In this context in 1803, he insisted on a single, centrally administered assistance fund collected from all

144

taxpayers rather than a parish poor rate. Any call for a central fund was a partial return to the principles of secular and national assistance once ineffectually espoused by the National Convention in 1793-1794.[55] A national fund would tap the wealth of prosperous regions to aid less fortunate areas and would restore the goal of effective public assistance to its urgent priority.

As always then, Cabanis balanced the need for state intervention with the need for a natural social and economic equilibrium. The Marxist portrait of the victim or purveyor of false consciousness may be valid to an extent, but not without appropriate modification. Certainly, in his mature works, Cabanis did not adhere to the static "poor are always with us" doctrines that were conventional in the eighteenth century and implicit in the Mirabeau discourses. He prophesied in *Quelques Principes* that a "political constitution based on human nature and the eternal rules of justice must in the long run almost completely eradicate the traces of poverty and distribute without upheaval the means of enjoyment (*moyens de jouissance*) in a more equitable manner. This constitution may very much diminish the number of crimes committed by eliminating both colossal fortunes and extreme poverty."[56] Similarly in a November 1803 review of Volney's physical geography of America, Cabanis remarked that high wage scales in the United States alleviated many causes of dissension prevalent in Europe. He added, "The most serious of these is the enormous quantity of beggars, the rate of wages which is much too low, and as a result, the constant war of the poor and the rich, which must finish by overturning everything, if one does not hasten to favor, everywhere, without violence, a more equitable distribution of the goods of nature and the powers of society."[57] To some extent, Cabanis and his circle were victims of the optical illusion of liberalism— thinking that free trade would help eliminate, rather than aggravate, inequality and not produce any new inequalities. But the awareness of social conflict belies any notion of Cabanis's self-delusion about existing social relations. The most important action, in his view, was an effective national program to

145

relieve the poor. Society itself needed temporary intervention to help it find its natural equilibrium. Long-term social stability was prerequisite to any successful medical and educational reform as well as to the foundation of a science of man. Social stability demanded mitigation of the urgent problems caused by the extremes of wealth and poverty. Hence, the state had to have an enduring constitution and assist the needy, while the educational system stimulated talent and diffused the spirit of enlightenment. In that atmosphere, private and public hygiene could foster human perfectibility.

The Perils of Revolution and the Rational Organization of Medical Experience

Persecution of the Auteuil Circle

rom 1792 to 1795 the heirs of the philosophes could not hope for political and social stability as a context for the establishment of a science of man. Indeed, faced with the defeat of their moderate political program, they had to devote their energies to escaping arrest or surviving in prison. From the dawn of the Republic to the elections of 1798, Cabanis's philosophical writings overshadowed his political or practical concerns. In the heyday of the radical National Convention, Cabanis and his friends remained on the defensive as they lost positions of power and influence.

In the tense period after 10 August 1792, Cabanis was politically active only in Auteuil. Still, we have fragmentary evidence of his fundamental opinions. On 22 August 1792, in a letter addressed to the *Moniteur*, he sought to dissociate himself from the apparently favorable comments by another "Cabanis" residing in Paris about the former royal minister of the civil list, Arnauld de La Porte. La Porte had long ago been implicated in the flight of the King and now was about to be condemned to death for his secret subsidies to counterrevolutionary pamphleteers.[1] Clearly Cabanis wanted no dangerous taint of royalism.

The following March, the National Convention chose Cabanis as one of twelve jurors of the new Extraordinary Criminal Court for political crimes, later known as the Revolutionary Tribunal. In his letter of acceptance, Cabanis com-

147

plained to Gohier, who had just succeeded Garat as the minister of justice, that "groups" in Auteuil were calling La Roche and him "Girondins, Brissotins, Rolandists, or whatever you like." He deplored the "spirit of faction" in the Convention and insisted that he was nonpartisan. The Girondins had been suspicious of the court from the outset, no doubt, and especially after the Convention dissolved a moderate commission designed to oversee court operations. After the treason of General Dumouriez became known early in April 1793, Cabanis temporarily withdrew his resignation, which he had sent on 30 March for reasons of health. We have no record of whether he actually served before his definitive withdrawal on 23 April. This date is worth noting, because the Girondins had arranged to charge Marat before the court with plotting the dissolution of the Convention and encouraging the pillage of warehouses. From 24 April the jury deliberated, and on 26 April, Marat received his acquittal and returned to the Convention in triumph. It was hardly surprising that Cabanis, who was genuinely ill in any case, sought to be free of association with the verdict.[2]

Cabanis's friends among the Convention deputies— Condorcet, M.-J. Chénier, Daunou, Garat, and Siéyès—were aligned with the moderates, to be sure. They were aghast when Robespierre and other Montagnards attacked the Enlightenment heritage. In December 1792, the Jacobin Club ordered destruction of the busts of Helvétius (persecutor of Rousseau) and Mirabeau (now revealed as a correspondent of the Court). In April 1793, Robespierre attacked the philosophes for their servility to the great. In August 1793, the Convention's dissolution of the ancien régime academies expressed a hatred of elitism tainted with aristocracy. In May 1794, when most of Cabanis's friends were already in prison, Robespierre made a notorious speech condemning the arid materialism of the Encyclopedists that left no room for the warm-hearted virtue of the people. After Thermidor, Garat and Daunou, among others, would lead in the portrayal of the Robespierrists as anti-intellectual vandals.[3]

Meanwhile, Cabanis forged closer links with the Condorcet salon. After Condorcet married Sophie de Grouchy, of an old

Norman noble family, in 1786, Cabanis met Sophie's younger and less flamboyant sister, Charlotte (1768-1844). Since 1791, Cabanis had been seeing Charlotte "every day," and the baptismal certificate of their eldest daughter, Geneviève-Aminthe, establishes her birth in Provins on 7 October 1793. There was a formal marriage (with Garat as a witness) only on 14 May 1796, shortly before the birth of a second daughter, in August 1796, who apparently died in infancy. By that time, the Grouchy family was informed of the marriage (they had been hostile to the proposition). The Cabanis's second surviving daughter, Annette-Pamela, was born 25 March 1800 in Auteuil with Destutt de Tracy as godfather.[4]

Cabanis's links with Condorcet became significant when the Convention decreed Condorcet's arrest on 8 July 1793 for his anonymous pamphlet against the new Constitution drafted by the Committee on Public Safety. While the authorities searched Auteuil, Cabanis, who had been reelected to the municipal council on 17 March, hid Condorcet in Mme Helvétius's villa and at Garat's residence. With the assistance of Pinel and the surgeon Alexis Boyer, Cabanis procured a safer refuge for Condorcet near the southern limits of Paris, where he was not disturbed until March 1794. Cabanis even gave Condorcet a forged passport and a legendary vial of poison. It was not until May that the Auteuil circle learned of Condorcet's death, whatever the cause, on 29 March after the failure of an attempted escape.[5] Sophie Condorcet meanwhile occupied herself with a translation of Adam Smith's *Theory of Moral Sentiments* and prefaced it with eight rambling *Letters on Sympathy* (published in 1798) dedicated to Cabanis.[6]

Cabanis's behavior in the Condorcet affair led to increased suspicion by the authorities. A local civil committee member remarked that the village was "tainted by a violent suspicion of aristocracy and that it was necessary to name good sans-culottes" to the council. The resulting illegal municipal elections of 7 November 1793 excluded La Roche and Cabanis from municipal office. Yet Cabanis received the respect of the new assembly, which did not seem particularly bloodthirsty. Finally, in one of the few operations of the *armée révolutionnaire* in the

Paris region, the commandant Charles-Philippe Ronsin himself
and a civil commissioner François-Julien Marcellin, acting on
direct orders of the Committee of Public Safety, arrested La
Roche and Destutt de Tracy, over the protests of the Auteuil
council, as "enemies of the Republic." La Roche was charged
with being a former chaplain to the comte d'Artois, with speaking against Marat in an electoral assembly in 1792, with delay-
ing to remove Mirabeau's bust from the town hall, and with
permitting Condorcet's escape. Destutt de Tracy, no doubt, was
guilty by association with the now disgraced Lafayette.[7] Fortu-
nately, Tracy was saved from execution by Thermidor and
profited from his imprisonment by meditating on the
philosophies of Locke and Condillac.

The Terror certainly struck the Auteuil circle. Cabanis's
former mentor, the poet Roucher, was executed, while Garat,
Ginguené, Daunou, Volney, and M.-J. Chénier all served
prison terms from several months to a year. If Cabanis did not
share their fate, the likely explanation was his provision of free
medical care to the poor of the village. He allegedly refused the
offer of the ambassadorship to the United States so as not to
abandon Mme Helvétius. He helped relieve the tension he felt
during 1793-1794 by translating German works of Meissner
and Goethe (the play *Stella*), eventually published anonymously in 1797. Even before Thermidor, friends of the Auteuil
circle had established what became an important new forum for
their views. In the spring of 1794, literary critics Amaury
Duval, Joachim Le Breton, and François-Stanislas Andrieux,
later joined by Ginguené and the economist J.-B. Say, founded
La Décade philosophique. Here, the Auteuil group could comment on political and cultural affairs, review each other's books,
and perpetuate the spirit of the philosophes.[8]

The Reform of Medicine: Coup d'oeil

MEDICAL SCHOOLS

After Thermidor, the Auteuil circle assumed a leading role in
the reconstruction of cultural and educational institutions. The

political moderates now shared the hope of sufficient political stability to establish enduring professional training schools. And while the stability proved illusory, the institutions often survived political storms. Cabanis once again turned to the issue of organization of the medical profession and the methods of medical practice. Since February 1791, there had been no medical guild in France nor any legally accredited medical diplomas. The corporate monopoly of all Faculties was abolished in August 1792, though at least a few teaching institutions in the provinces continued to function on the margin of the law. Abolition of universities was suspended the day after it was voted, 16 September 1793. The improvised military medical service in 1792-1794 faced appalling shortages of qualified personnel, especially after the battle casualties of 1793. Wartime conditions, including the effectiveness of surgeons in treating fevers as well as wounds, enhanced the prestige of surgeons and forced physicians to study anatomy more carefully. The supreme councils in military medicine no longer questioned the urgent need for large hospitals to accommodate military casualties and to train health officers. Thus, the practical necessities of military medicine supported the civilian impulse to reform already embodied in the Vicq d'Azyr plan.[9]

The Convention Committee on Public Education, including Thouret, approved Fourcroy's plan for a revived Paris School of Health with a single three-year curriculum for physicians and surgeons, emphasis on chemical experiments, dissections, and, most important, clinical and surgical instruction in hospital wards. Regional pressures in the Convention resulted in the creation of three such schools on 4 December 1794 with 25 professors and 300 students in Paris, 16 and 150 in Montpellier, and 14 and 100 in Strasbourg. The Paris professors were an eminent group; included were Pinel, Hallé, Desault, his student Corvisart, Fourcroy himself, and Thouret who became dean.[10]

THE INDEPENDENCE OF THE SCIENCE OF MEDICINE

Before incorporation of the Fourcroy plan in the general public education law of 25 October 1795, Garat, as the commissioner of public education, encouraged Cabanis to complete a more elaborate historical and philosophical study of analysis as it applied to medicine. On 6 July 1795, Garat recommended Cabanis's manuscript "Considérations générales sur les révolutions de l'art de guérir," as "very useful to those studying [medicine]." On 22 September, on behalf of the Committee on Public Education, Fourcroy agreed to review it and on 10 October, he suggested publication of the manuscript as having the "soundest doctrine, and the wisest and most useful opinions for improvement of medical education."[11]

Cabanis delayed publication until 1804 because he intended to improve the manuscript until there were chapters on method for each branch of medicine. In the end, he completed only the historical introduction and an essay on the general principles of analytic method, with sketchy reflections on the branches of medicine and the "accessory sciences." The repetitiousness of some sections, as well as references in the notes, indicate expansion and revision of the draft of 1795.[12] Yet even in 1795 the basic argument must have been apparent. Cabanis pursued two major themes of Enlightenment thought—how to unify the sciences while preserving the uniqueness of each discipline and, secondarily in this work, how to consider the human species part of the unity of nature.

Fourcroy's praise was all the more paradoxical since Cabanis's document differed considerably from the approach of Fourcroy's *La Médecine éclairée par les sciences physiques*. Cabanis consistently argued that medicine must rid itself of unwarranted intrusions from the other sciences. Assuming the validity of medical inquiry (discussed in *Degré de certitude*), the time was still ripe for Hippocratic reform "to place medicine in harmony with the other sciences and to determine precisely their mutual relationships." Hippocrates had furnished indispensable guides to observation in the *Epidemics* and the *Aphorisms*. He knew how to introduce philosophical method into medicine while preserving medicine from unsound theories of natural philosophy. Like Hippocrates, van Helmont, Stahl, and the "famous professors of Montpellier"—Bordeu and

Barthez—had all wished to develop a logic of medicine based on accurate clinical observation. In the modern period, Baconian induction and the empiricist epistemology of Condillac were perfectly congruent with this clinical practice and were necessary to systematize it. Wise physicians refused to succumb to the methods or concepts of "foreign disciplines," whether mathematical, physical, or chemical.[13]

Cabanis did believe that "all truths form a chain with tightly interconnected links." In *Coup d'oeil*, as the "Considerations" were later called, he expressed a variation of d'Alembert's Encyclopedist vision of the "one great truth" synthesizing all of the sciences.[14] With more knowledge, the gaps in the chain of truths would be "filled, the points of contact, or relations among the various points, or of each with the whole continually multiply . . . so that finally all scientific truths will be deduced from a few principles, and they will be as vital to each other as are the members of an organic body." And in the discourses on education attributed to Mirabeau, Cabanis had already drafted the National Academy project. He would envisage the newly-created National Institute as a "living Encyclopedia" in 1796, appropriately representing the "indivisible whole" of arts and sciences. In 1798 he agreed that medical schools should be part of universal higher-education establishments known as lycées.[15] He did not hesitate, in the *Rapports*, to relate the latest physical discoveries on galvanism to physiology nor even to speculate on the phosphorus content of the brain.[16]

Cabanis further developed the relations of laws of the various sciences—each law of simple phenomena was valid for complex phenomena. Thus, crystal growth followed laws of gravitational attraction, vegetable growth had some analogies to crystallization, and "lower species" of animals in some ways acted like "more perfect" vegetables. In physiology, there were merely mechanical laws (muscular motive force), hydraulic laws (fluid circulation), chemical phenomena (digestion, respiration), and laws of crystal growth (bone formation).

Yet the physician had to know these foundations of his discipline without subverting its identity. Cabanis denied, as vigorously as Stahl did, that detailed anatomical knowledge aided medical practice. New instruments or procedures might one day reveal "the intimate fabric of the brain . . . happily this fine anatomy is an object rather of physical curiosity than of medical utility. Though one must not banish it; even though it may some day be used to good advantage, it is perfectly useless today; and we tend to believe that one could always dispense with it." Cabanis did, however, have to acknowledge the remarkable achievements of the Paris School of Medicine in pathological anatomy. The most interesting kind of anatomy, he agreed, was the search for the "cause and seat of disease" in "organic lesions," examined at autopsies and compared with clinical journals. But even here, his concession to an internal approach to pathology was wary. Separating the immediate effects of disease from the effects of maladies long past, from congenital defects, or from alterations caused by death itself would be no easy task. Yet physicians could well hope for the aid of a "living anatomy" that would understand changes in organs due to age or illness.[17]

Similarly, Cabanis wrote that Stahl's opinion on the uselessness of chemistry in medicine was "perhaps almost as much true today." Despite chemical progress, physicians must guard against "specious deductions" from chemistry to physiology and medicine and rely rather on the "genius of observation." Laboratory experiments relating the composition of animate and inanimate bodies would always be less crucial than clinical observation: "not by working with instruments deprived of life can one attain results both certain and applicable [to medicine]. Rather, this new, animate chemistry, whose products are instantly distorted when life ceases, must be practiced by the observation of a sensitive, living nature, at the sickbed, in vast infirmaries." Like Vicq d'Azyr, Cabanis would insist that medicine independently establish its own truths before relating them to chemical discoveries.[18]

He was less sanguine in *Coup d'oeil* than in *Degré de certitude* about past and present effectiveness of medicine. The "madness of theorists" could still kill or maim patients. In fact, the whole history of medicine—its "revolutions," in the traditional sense of cyclical oscillations—had been alternate periods of sound Hippocratic clinical practice and aberrations due to geometric, chemical, and mechanical theoretical systems.[19] Elsewhere Cabanis sketched a fascinating dialectical theory of scientific progress. At first, he wrote, men collected facts for a long period, until "imaginative men" grew impatient and constructed a system outrunning available experience. These efforts, disastrous at the time, advanced scientific knowledge in the long run; for then arose a "conflict of opinions from which the most sublime truths sprang forth." "More precise minds" declaimed against frivolous hypotheses and returned to the "bare study of the facts."[20] Cabanis was thus enough of a historical relativist to respect past scientific speculators even if he always saw the urgency of sound medical theory in helping to save the lives of patients. His view of scientific advance went beyond mere cumulative transmission of past experience and to that extent anticipated the relativism of the Saint-Simonians.[21]

"ANALYSIS" IN MEDICINE: THE LEGACY OF BACON AND CONDILLAC

Perfected scientific method—observation, experiment, and reasoning—was still universal, though analysis did not always proceed the same way or produce the same results. Cabanis pointed out that the well-defined language of magnitude and quantity in mathematics enabled the deduction of a sequence of truths. On the other hand, in medicine, the fleeting, ill-defined phenomena and imprecise signs demanded "talent" and a "happy instinct" as well as "mechanical reasoning methods." But analytical method was precisely the "art of directing talent" so that "average minds may then easily grasp what is now difficult for eminent intellects."[22]

More than ever, Cabanis's *Coup d'oeil* showed how reason should organize the brute, chaotic data of observation. As applied to medicine, analytic method very much resembled the Tables of Resemblance and Tables of Differences in Bacon's *Novum Organum*. Though Cabanis undoubtedly read Bacon,

155

Garat, the philosopher who urged completion of *Coup d'oeil*, had produced in 1795 a succinct summary of Baconian method. In his teacher-training course in "Analysis of the Understanding" (a Lockean title) at the Ecole normale, Garat explained analytic method as a Baconian classification compiling tables of facts where "experiments, phenomena, and other analogous facts are linked by analogies yielding the same results" and other tables where facts "apparently belonging to the same classes and the same analogies lead to contrary results."

> From the emerging clarity of a first well-circumscribed principle, to pass to new experiments which this principle in itself should suggest, to the observation of new facts and new phenomena; to classify and arrange them similarly in dual tables, either by the similarity of appearances and contrast of the results, or the identity of their results, after contrary appearances: to deduce from them principles more extensive than the first, but always limited by the circumference of facts and phenomena embraced; from these new facts, new experiments and new observations, to rise to more all-inclusive principles, and to descend again to the study of facts to arise step by step to increasingly general axioms.[23]

Cabanis repeated in *Coup d'oeil* the analogical procedure of *Degré de certitude*: "The overgeneralized rules drawn from resemblances are corrected by other rules drawn from differences. One descends to individual facts: the distinctions, exceptions arrange themselves; other systems form, embracing greater sectors; and from this collection of successive operations with self-correcting effects or mutually compensating errors, one draws ever more precise and more complete results."[24]

Both Garat and Cabanis used Condillac's definition of analysis as decomposition and recomposition, with the keystone of a "well-made language" denoting the elementary principles. Cabanis considered medical terminology hopelessly confused, despite the abortive effort by Vicq d'Azyr in 1786 to reform anatomical language. Physicians could profit from the revolution in chemical nomenclature introduced in 1787 and 1789 by

Lavoisier, Guyton de Morveau, and Fourcroy. But the chemists based their system on naming elements first, while Cabanis favored naming composite objects, the "true radicals," first because they were immediately accessible to sensation. Otherwise, subsequent observation might show that an element was wrongly named and invalidate the entire system of nomenclature. Sense-objects, by contrast, would always remain evident and could be resolved by derivative signs into their true elements.

In medicine, the composites were collections of symptoms forming a disease, while the elementary, individual symptoms varied in order, duration, and intensity. The clinician encountered the manifestations of disease—a composite such as a cough, pain in the side, expectoration of blood, and acute fever. A precise medical language would name the composite "pleurisy" (probably pulmonary pneumonia to twentieth-century physicians). Though philosophers like Leibniz correctly argued that every case was individual, even a less than ideal provisional classification would be valuable. Clinical observation would then determine whether resemblances to other recorded cases of pleurisy outweighed the differences. Response to therapy might indicate the nature of the disease. For example, for pleurisy the recommended therapy was bleeding, warm drinks to induce sweating followed by sharp drinks and expectorants to purge the stomach and bowels, and mild sudorifics (more sweat-inducers). If the patient did not respond at all to this combination, sequence, and dosage of remedies, he might have another disease or a different species of pleurisy; or, his peculiar temperament might make him unresponsive to a conventional therapy. The medical language needed refinement to differentiate the "truly essential and fundamental phenomena constituting [a disease]" from the nuances of individual cases. In contrast to the naive optimism of *Degré de certitude*, Cabanis admitted that these phenomena might be difficult to discover. In simple matters, it might be easy to observe the dominant, striking sensations, as Condillac suggested, to arrive at principles and deduce the secondary phenomena. But apparent ele-

157

ments of disease did not invariably fall into the same pattern or call for the same treatment. The composite sometimes developed over time, and the observer had to note both persistent and vanishing symptoms. Classification of disease was, then, a demanding task. And after it was completed, physicians would still have to insure proper classification of drugs.[25]

Cabanis then distinguished four kinds of analysis, all useful in medicine at different stages of examination. (1) Analysis of description gave the size, form, and external parts of a structure or substance, situating it amid surrounding bodies or noting its resemblances and differences to related bodies. This static, geographic classification characterized botany and anatomy and, though Cabanis did not say, presumably was useful in knowledge of drugs and in preparing for surgery. (2) Analysis of decomposition and recomposition, characteristic of chemistry, revealed the elements of a substance, or its "intimate constitutive combination of particles." However, in the living realm, such analysis would always be incomplete, since living substances cannot be recomposed. In such cases, conclusions would be only more or less probable. Hence, the limited utility of chemistry in physiology was in part a problem of procedure. Later, Cabanis used the term "decomposition and recomposition of ideas," though he did not immediately relate this category of analysis to the manipulation of signs, or the decomposition of composites in disease, or the recomposition of elements. (3) Historical, dynamic analysis was eminently useful in plant and animal physiology and medical practice since it studied changes in a body to arrive at its properties. Only historical analysis could show whether sequences of events in disease were invariable patterns or whether they were affected by peculiar influences. Classification of symptom patterns would then presumably require use of the historical record of the clinical journal. (4) Finally, analysis of deduction was applicable to ideas more than bodies, and hence more closely followed Condillac's notion of arranging signs in a demonstrative order. With well-chosen signs, as in mathematics, analysis of deduction was certain. Deductions, Cabanis noted, were indispensable to assimilate the observations of decomposition and recomposition and in establishing rational classification and therapy. Cabanis believed he had been true to Condillac's notion of analysis, despite some differences in emphasis, and agreed that in ideal cases deductions would give the most complete analysis. All four forms were interrelated, because deduction applied to description, to decomposition and recomposition of ideas, and to the results of historical analysis. Historical analysis in turn presented description, deduction, and ceaseless decomposition and recomposition.[26]

No combination of analytic methods would remove uncertainty from medicine, nor would medical uncertainty be definable in clear limits. A mathematician could use a very precise approximation for the value of π, and a philosopher might be content with the weight of inductive evidence when reason could not absolutely prove that sunrise would recur; but medical probabilities, similarly inductive, would be lower, given individual or climatic peculiarities that affected a conventionally successful therapy. Despite this uncertainty, once having established the effectiveness of a drug such as quinine as a cure for intermittent fever (malaria), one could confidently prescribe it, given a proper diagnosis, and so much more confidently every time it was effective.[27]

Cabanis never went beyond these principles to elaborate a full treatise on medical method. The implications of *Coup d'oeil* suggested the urgency of collecting tables of symptom patterns, or, if possible, of arrangements of elementary symptoms with columns available for noting modifications of age, sex, temperament, diet, habits, and climate. These tables would in turn be correlated with therapies—the sequence, combination, and dosage of remedies. The resulting science would inevitably be statistical, though Cabanis never admitted it.

Cabanis considered analytic method something of a panacea, as is evident from his hope that even artisans could benefit, as much as physicians, from simplification of their procedures. In this respect, analytic method was a democratic tool, not an occult code for the elite. In one respect, Cabanis's viewpoint seems similar to that of the Convention deputy Joseph Lakanal. He, in recommending the creation of the Ecole normale on 2 October 1794, thought that while free trade would destroy the monstrous inequality of wealth, "analysis applied to all types of ideas will destroy the inequality of enlightenment, even more fatal and humiliating. Analysis is essentially an indispensable instrument in a large democracy; the light it spreads so easily penetrates everywhere; like all fluids, it tends always to seek its own level."[28] Yet, paradoxically, Cabanis could not prevent some social prejudice from creeping into his comment on applying analysis to the ills of more "sensitive" scholars, poets, indeed "all persons not devoted to merely manual labor." For these, the physician would have to be more sophisticated than he was in applying a "few formulas in the countryside and in hospitals."[29] That is, the psychological aspect of physical illness would be more complex among the refined temperaments of the educated. Certainly, Cabanis did not renounce his commitment to providing the best medicine to the poor. But the implication that treating manual workers was easier seems to reek of the myths of the salon.

Cabanis's colleagues and successors in the Paris School of Medicine carried out some of his aspirations. The introduction to Pinel's *Nosographie* (1798) so closely resembled passages of the as yet unpublished *Coup d'oeil* that a reader might suspect Pinel had access to Cabanis's manuscript. Pinel and Cabanis may simply have shared beliefs in the urgency of clinical case studies and in the applicability of Condillac's analysis to a new classification of disease. Pinel, who studied at Montpellier in 1774-1776, cited the same Hippocratic works that Cabanis did as guides to observation. The *Nosographie* paid ample homage to Condillac, and the introduction to his famous *Traité médico-philosophique sur l'aliénation mentale* (1801) even cited the "Ideologists" for refining the classification of mental faculties.

Pinel's nosology hoped to arrive at "constitutive principles" of each group of diseases from which variations would derive.

The observer should be careful to distinguish the basic differences between diseases from the varieties of each species of disease due to age, temperament, climate, prevalence of endemic
illnesses, and occupation. Pinel's classification of mental disturbances was based on analysis of mental faculties (reason, affection, will, and so forth) in the fashion of Condillac and
Destutt de Tracy. Moreover, his approach to therapy was definitely statistical, even if the number of cases was too small for
statistical significance. Given knowledge of the effectiveness of
therapies, Pinel would analyze a number of clinical charts to
show how many times therapies had no effect. Thus he could
deduce differences in species of insanity. Pinel certainly set the
tone for French clinical medicine for at least the first fifteen
years of the nineteenth century.[30]

THE UNITY OF NATURE AND THE SCIENCE OF MAN

It is important to note one further aspect to *Coup d'oeil* beyond
its themes of analytic method and the relationships among the
sciences. Cabanis here first presented his own peculiar image of
the Great Chain of Being. Somewhat like d'Holbach, he developed a theory of the degrees of complexity of beings determining the degrees of complexity of scientific laws. In discussing
disease classification, Cabanis noted the temptation to draw
easy analogies from one set of phenomena to another. At the
simplest level, phenomena "presenting no organization, no
sign of automatic movement, determined by their situation"
were solely subject to the "common law of masses," that is, to
gravitation. Salt crystals and minerals appeared similarly inert
but "combine in a regular order" with "specific laws . . . im-
pressing upon them distinctive and constant characteristics."
Vegetables comprised a third "degree of existence," but the
highest order contained beings with the faculty of sensitivity
and, in most cases, of mobility.

In this tableau, Cabanis chose to stress the conviction he inherited from Montpellier medicine. Sensitivity "separates sen-

sitive beings by a rather distinct line of demarcation from all non-sensitive beings." Indeed, "from the inert mass in the bosom of the earth, to the sensitive being capable of affection and thought, all is doubtless bonded and connected; but Nature herself seems to have drawn lines of separation, and when method fixes them, it consecrates real distinctions, observed among most of the objects so separated, and especially among the most important."[31] Method in the life sciences was different because life was different. Cabanis was not thereby announcing a dualist view of the universe, clearly refuted in the *Rapports* of 1796. But he was also refusing any facile reductionism.

In other sections of *Coup d'oeil*, Cabanis did not hesitate to touch the most controversial aspect of any monism—the relationship between physical and mental in man. To medicine he confided the special mission of integrating human physical history and mental history. "From their methodical combination," wrote Cabanis, "and the indication of their numerous points of contact, results what can be called the *science of man*, or *anthropology*, following the expression of the Germans." Cabanis did not specify his German source—possibly Kant's lectures of 1798 or the Leipzig physician Ernst Platner's *Neue anthropologie* (1771-1772; 2d ed., 1790), both of which sought physiological roots for psychological phenomena while firmly defending the existence of the spiritual soul.[32] Cabanis called "medicine and morals two branches of the same science; together they comprise the science of man." Here Cabanis anticipated Destutt de Tracy's distinction between Physiological Ideology, concerned with sensitivity in the body, and Rational Ideology, concerned with mental and ethical phenomena.

In four pages of *Coup d'oeil*, Cabanis summarized the entire enterprise of the *Rapports*—the dependence of "ideas, feelings, passions, virtues, and vices" on "physical sensitivity." In aiding the moralist and legislator, the physician would show the mental and moral effects of childhood, puberty, old age, sex differences, "primitive dispositions," disease, and habits of regimen. In suggesting rules of diet, physical exercise, and therapy, the physician could help sharpen sensations, elevate ideas, channel passions, and "seize all these invisible reins of human nature." He could identify both the organic lesions producing mental disorders and the imaginative fantasies or changes in habits and climate producing physical illness. A true hygiene could recommend rules on the use of "passions" to preserve or re-establish health and to diminish the incidence of madness and crime. Good sense would become a habit, and moral conduct, a need. For Cabanis, this hygiene was not merely an individual concern but a question for the whole society.

From these brief, but provocative remarks, we can foresee Cabanis's mature version of the science of man. The physician would not be limited to the cure of disease, nor even to the maintenance of health, but would be concerned with the physical perfectibility of the human species. Physical education and changes in physical habits could strengthen certain bodily organs, "create faculties, and even after a fashion new senses, and when these instruments have acted upon several successive generations, all else being equal, men are no longer the same, no longer of the same race."

Thus, one can also see the complementarity of Cabanis's political and philosophical careers. The Mirabeau discourses had stressed not the imprint of temperament nor the modifiability of physical regimen, but rather the power of schooling and civic instruction through plays and festivals. Cabanis would never lose sight of the need for conventional education to develop mind and character. Moral education, too, was "perpetuated with all its successive increments, by a kind of transmission from fathers to children." Cabanis speculated that acquired moral dispositions might be as inheritable as acquired physical dispositions (which Cabanis assumed, like Buffon and Condorcet). If he was optimistic enough to think that "men can after a fashion embrace the infinite," it was because he believed in the mutual reinforcement of man's physical and moral educations.[33] But neither education could be left to nature, any more than could the cultivation of crops. Physical and moral education needed external guidance, as the observation of facts needed the categories of reason.

HYGIENE IN THE CENTRAL SCHOOLS AND THE TRIUMPH OF THE AUTEUIL CIRCLE

During the final months of the National Convention, it appeared for a while that Cabanis was destined to teach hygiene in the curriculum of the newly established secondary central schools. The Auteuil circle, including Garat, Ginguené, and Daunou, had helped draft the new public education law, which originally had a highly innovative curriculum in the moral and political sciences.[34] On 6 April 1795, Cabanis was appointed hygiene professor at an undetermined Paris central school at a salary of 5,000 livres a year through 21 December 1795. Despite the claims in many biographical sketches, he almost certainly never taught hygiene, for, on 22 August 1795, the Committee on Public Education removed hygiene from the central school curriculum with the intention (never realized) of establishing special departmental courses in hygiene and in the art of medicine outside the secondary schools. To be fair, Cabanis asked payment only through 21 November 1795, and no central school professor could be dismissed without a formal act of the department teacher-selection jury and the Directory. Cabanis's salary may be an example of Thermidorian waste, or perhaps of unofficial compensation from friends such as Garat, a member of the Paris jury, for the work of writing *Coup d'oeil*.[35]

We need not revive here the vexed question of the accomplishments of the central schools. Suffice it to say that the Idéologues saw them as important institutions for teaching scientific reasoning, a prerequisite for establishing the human sciences. They also retained hopes of reintegrating the deleted subject of "analysis of sensations and ideas" in the general grammar courses, while the subjects of legislation and history would be vital for teaching the foundations of ethics and politics and the mechanism of social and scientific progress. As a member of the Conseil d'Instruction Publique, an advisory body to the Interior minister, Destutt de Tracy in 1799-1800 had ample opportunity to recommend reforms in the central school curriculum and later composed the first volume of his major work *Projet d'élémens d'idéologie* (1801) as an elementary textbook for the general grammar course.[36]

In 1795 Cabanis could well have expected considerable achievements from the central schools. The Directory was a moderate regime that presumably would encourage learned men and philosophers. In addition, the Paris School of Medicine was launching an ambitious program of clinical instruction. Cabanis himself was about to achieve cultural prominence as a member of the Second Class (Moral and Political Sciences) of the National Institute. He would bring to the Institute the philosophical heritage of the naturalists and Encyclopedists, the medical heritage of Montpellier, the more immediate inspiration of his close friends Condorcet and Volney, and the support of his colleague Destutt de Tracy and the circle of Idéologues.

★ CHAPTER VII ★

Sensitivity: Source of 'Physique' and 'Moral'

The Foundation of the Institute

he Thermidorian Convention consciously sought significant cultural innovation by establishing a Class of Moral and Political Sciences in the unified National Institute of Sciences and Arts. In organizing the Class, the architects of the Institute closely followed the terminology that Condorcet used when he proposed a secondary school curriculum and the formation of a National Society of Sciences and Arts in his education plan of April 1792. The six sections of the Class included the traditional fields of ethics (*morale*) (now conceived as a science), history, and geography, and also the new disciplines of "analysis of sensations and ideas," "social science (a term invented by Garat and Condorcet) and legislation (public law, law of nature and of nations, and political analysis in the style of Montesquieu)," and "political economy."

The future Idéologue circle was prominent among the twelve Directory nominees for the "electing third" of the Second Class—Volney and Garat in the analysis section, Daunou in legislation, and Siéyès in political economy. These twelve nominees to the Second Class joined the nominees to other Classes to co-opt the remaining members, who included the Idéologue Ginguené in analysis and the peripheral Idéologue Roederer in political economy. On 15 December 1795, the electing third filled a vacancy in the analysis section with Cabanis. Thereafter all Institute members elected the nonresident "associates," including the Idéologues Destutt de Tracy and Laromiguière in analysis and the physician Pierre Roussel in

166

ethics. In 1800 the members chose the Idéologue protégé Joseph-Marie Degérando for the analysis section. Thus, seven of the eleven Idéologues in the Second Class were committed to reading memoirs on the "analysis of sensations and ideas."[1]

Destutt de Tracy introduced the term "Ideology" to the Institute on 20 June 1796. By criteria of personal and political kinship, Cabanis, Tracy, Volney, Garat, Ginguené, and Daunou were in the nucleus of the Idéologue circle, while Laromiguière and Degérando had strong links to Auteuil, at least until they took their distance from metaphysical monism after 1802. Siéyès met all the objective criteria for being an Idéologue, yet his personality made him very much a lone wolf. Roederer wrote memoirs on perception and the elements of morality and contributed to *La Décade*, even though in the Consulate he became too close to Bonaparte to sympathize with the Idéologue opposition.

The analysis section was not entirely controlled by the Idéologues, but its essay competition topics clearly demonstrate the debt to Condillac's philosophy: (1) the influence of signs on the formation of ideas (6 October 1796, won by Degérando 27 March 1799), (2) the influence of habit on the faculty of thought (4 October 1799, not awarded in 1801, won 6 July 1802 by Maine de Biran), and (3) decomposition of the faculty of thought (awarded only in 1805 by the new Class of History and Ancient Literature, after the dissolution of the Second Class, also to Maine de Biran).[2]

In the Second Class, Destutt de Tracy began reading the first of his series of memoirs "On the Faculty of Thought" on 21 April 1796, with sequels read on 20 June and 18 October 1796 and 10-15 February 1798 (source of the printed version). Here, too, on 16 February 1796, Cabanis began reading his memoir on the "relationship of the physical organization of man with his intellectual and moral faculties." With supreme confidence in the ideals of Condorcet, he noted that only despots feared the moral and political sciences, while the Republic encouraged savants because they would help establish political stability and tranquillity. In a republic more than in any other regime, public utility, rather than personal passion, had to motivate citizens, and enlightened opinion, rather than the tyrannous force of the guillotine, would insure the practice of virtue.[3]

Moral and Political Assumptions: Condorcet and Volney

Thus, in the interdisciplinary collaboration of the new science of man, Cabanis envisaged the broad concerns of the moral philosopher as well as the solid clinical experience of the physician and the rigorous reasoning of the "analyst" of ideas.[4] While the physiologist studied empirical mind-body relationships and the analyst classified the faculties of the mind and will to understand learning and motivation, the moralist would identify human needs. For Condorcet and the Idéologues, the only empirical first principles of ethics were the facts of physical sensitivity and mental sensation.

But the social goals of the Idéologues required substitution of a natural morality for a religious morality, and a natural politics based on the rights of liberty, equality of opportunity, and property for the ancien régime monarchy governed by the King's pleasure. While the Idéologues perceived their ethics and politics as scientific, they deduced ethical imperatives (natural limits to pleasure-seeking or natural impulses to sympathy and cooperation) as well as political imperatives (the rights of the citizen enshrined in the Declaration of 1789) from the facts of sensitive human nature.

The moral and political philosophy implicit in the works of Cabanis was most directly formulated by Condorcet and Volney. They had both, in a way somewhat different from Locke, united empiricist psychology and natural rights. Condorcet, even before the Revolution, had leaped from the elemental descriptive fact of human sensitivity to enumerate natural rights of personal liberty and security, which implied the injustice of slavery, freedom to enjoy property and to trade without unnecessary interference, equality before a clearly codified law, and political participation in some form for the citizen.[5] These were normative conclusions, allegedly derivable from experi-

ence but actually independent of subsequent empirical discoveries about physical-mental relationships.

With similar reasoning, in August 1793 (at the behest of Interior Minister Garat) Volney published a secular morality
manual for popular instruction, *La Loi naturelle, ou Catéchisme du citoyen français, ou Principes physiques de la morale
déduits de l'organisation de l'homme et de l'univers*. We know
from Cabanis's correspondence with Volney's publisher that
Cabanis himself received the completed authors' copies and
then he transmitted them to Volney. In the 1805 edition of the
Rapports, Cabanis praised Volney's *Catéchisme* as a work "deserving the gratitude of all friends of humanity" for showing
the identity of "rules of conduct for being happy and virtuous."[6] Volney argued that empirically observable natural principles of self-preservation were not always synonymous with
instinctive pleasure-seeking, for true self-preservation required
social cooperation and the restraint of self-interest, while enlightened temperance was necessary to prevent self-destruction.
Cultivating natural faculties of sympathy and practicing virtue,
or the art of being useful to others, were thus in our own self-
interest.[7] Like many contemporary moralists, Volney opposed
self-interest of the individual to the good of the *entire*
society—as if there could never be any subgroups in conflict
with the community at large yet willing to shelter individual
violators of the code of society. Aside from this common defi-
ciency of eighteenth-century morality, Volney had a harsher
view of poverty than Cabanis; he stressed its links to vice and
exhorted the poor to help themselves rather than asserting the
obligation of society to care for the poor. He also made the conventional virtues of his own epoch and culture—sobriety, modesty, prudence, and continence outside of marriage—into absolute ethical standards.[8]

Like Condorcet, Volney attempted to derive the natural
rights of liberty, equality, and property from the "physical attributes, inherent in the organization of man." This line of reasoning was certainly implicit in the doctrines of all the
Idéologues. The origins and sensations of each man were inde-

pendent and self-sufficient, so that liberty was a natural right. All were equal in rights before God and nature because all had the same sense organs. Moreover, as Locke had argued, all had a natural right to own property as a product of their labor, though the amount of property owned would vary in each case.[9] Volney was thus committed to the civil rights won in 1789, rather than to the sans-culotte ideal of 1793, *égalité des jouissances*.

An attempt like Volney's to create a scientific ethic was unprovable with scientifically acceptable evidence and was especially open to controversy in the Revolutionary era. Critics of the Idéologues who were hostile to their moral and political principles would not accept the empirical aspects of their science, whether or not it had more widely acceptable evidence. More radical revolutionaries would never accept the domination of the propertied as a naturally ordained social order, and some conservatives saw threats to religious and political authority in the very attempt to establish a secular morality with an empirical component. Both Left and Right would also contest what they unfairly interpreted as an oversimplified "egoist" view of human motivation.

Early Hostility to "Idéologues": Saint-Martin

There were other barriers to a scientific evaluation of Cabanis's psychophysiology. Since Cabanis nowhere mentioned a spiritual soul, critics' abhorrence of materialism often extended to Condillac's fundamental premise—that sensations are the basis of ideas. Interestingly enough, the first hostile use of the term "idéologue" may even have anticipated the memoirs of Cabanis and Tracy, for Garat's Ecole normale lectures of 1795 in "analysis of the understanding" were vigorously challenged by the philosopher Louis-Claude de Saint-Martin, a disciple of the mystic Martinez de Pasqually and later a translator of Jacob Boehme. In the discussion of 27 February 1795, Saint-Martin denied the validity of the empiricist view of the mind, nor would he allow Garat to take refuge in an agnostic Newtonian phenomenalism, for he asserted that one had to be either a spiritualist or a materialist. Since Garat denied an immortal soul and taught the theory of sensations as the basis of ideas, he was closer to materialism. Saint-Martin continued, "the spiritualists are specially and invariably opposed to the idéologues who believe that we produce our ideas with our sensations, while these ideas are only transmitted to us by sensations."[10] Although the anticipation of the term "Ideology" is uncertain, since the printed Ecole normale debates may have appeared after Destutt de Tracy's invention of the word, Saint-Martin's criticism of Garat anticipates in its essence the charges that Chateaubriand and de Bonald would later level at Cabanis. In short, the human sciences of the Idéologues were inspired by, though not necessarily derivable from, metaphysical monism and definite ethical and political aspirations. Like other would-be founders of the social sciences, the Idéologues suffered from a lack of agreement with their critics on the nonscientific framework for their inquiries.

Physiological and Rational Ideology

Ideology also suffered from the problem of internal coherence, a difficulty apparent to the Idéologues themselves. Recent essays on scientific knowledge have stressed the importance of a scientific "community," with similar training and shared assumptions, in the emergence of a scientific discipline.[11] Yet Cabanis's project was deliberately interdisciplinary. The physiologists were professional physicians who, if not clinicians or experimenters themselves, compiled and criticized clinical observations. The analysts of ideas and the moralists were philosophers in the traditional sense, who excelled in reasoning, even if they were too involved in current events to be confined to their studies. Both groups generally approved the empiricist philosophy of Bacon, Locke, Helvétius, and Condillac but aspired to make it more truly physiological and less metaphysical.

Yet Destutt de Tracy himself in 1796 recognized a distinction between "Physiological Ideology" and "Rational Ideology."

171

The first branch was "very erudite, requiring vast knowledge, but in the present state of our enlightenment" can only hope for "the destruction of many errors, and the establishment of some precious, but still scattered and uncoordinated truths." In modern terms, the physicians were still collecting data that would presumably bring refinements both to theories of learning and motivation and to principles of justice. The second branch, Tracy continued, "demanded less knowledge, having perhaps fewer difficulties, but sufficiently related facts, and aiming at the consequences of these facts, has the advantage of being capable of more direct applications, and already of forming a complete system. To that I limit myself."[12] While Tracy did not reduce his philosophy to a series of verbal equations similar to mathematics, it was more deductive than empirical and could already be applied in education and politics without the nuances of the physiologist.

This de facto division of labor left the physiologists with the greater burden of research and compilation. Moreover, Cabanis was the only physician to be consistently interested in the methods and goals of Ideology. Philippe Pinel, to be sure, devoted several works to analysis in medicine and his renowned treatise on insanity touched on the essence of psychophysiology. Cabanis's disciple Jacques-Louis Moreau de La Sarthe (1771-1826) developed a view of medicine as an integral portion of "anthropology," a term he adopted in 1801, before Cabanis.[13] But the other physicians who joined Cabanis's circle at Auteuil were interested in the science of man primarily in the restricted sense of Barthez—that is, general physiology. The chief surgeon at Saint-Louis Hospital, Balthasar-Anthelme Richerand (1779-1840), published a successful physiology textbook that followed Cabanis's views on sensitivity. Jean-Louis Alibert (1766-1837), also associated with Saint-Louis Hospital, was a dermatologist, although he published an essay on the relationship of medicine to the other sciences, a nosology, and a dualist "physiology of passions" (1825), the latter, long after Ideology was in disgrace.[14] Even the older Montpellier graduate Pierre Roussel (1742-1802), a collaborator on *La*

Décade, was primarily a physiologist known for his important essay on sympathy as well as a work written in 1775 *Système du physique et du moral de la femme*.

The integration of Physiological Ideology and Rational Ideology was problematic because of divergent training and interest. On the side of the Rational Ideologists, Tracy himself made valiant, if not always successful, efforts to assimilate Cabanis's physiology. Tracy, after all, originated the phrase, "Ideology is only a part of zoology."[15] The bright young philosopher from Bergerac, Maine de Biran, was also seriously interested in Cabanis's efforts before he finally took his distance from them.[16] But the others whom Cabanis cited in the *Rapports* —Garat himself, the Consulate official Joseph-Marie Degérando (1772-1842), the philosopher Pierre-Louis Laromiguière (1756-1837), P.-F. Lancelin, and Frédéric-François Jacquemont—concentrated almost entirely on revising Condillac's definition of the mental faculties or relating signs and language to ideas.[17]

Cabanis and Tracy hoped that they would demonstrate complementary approaches to human perfectibility. Like dualist physicians before him, Cabanis hoped to affect "ideas and passions" by showing that sound physical habits modify the state of the brain, the nervous system, and the internal organs. In modern terms, he was interested in individual hygiene and, assuming the inheritability of improvements, the biological evolution of the species. Tracy, like Garat, was interested in instilling sound mental habits. By perfecting language and improving pedagogy, he hoped to develop faculties of mental attention, memory, and judgment. This was the domain of cultural evolution, par excellence. Tracy and Cabanis could never perfectly integrate theories of biological and cultural evolution. But while Cabanis produced only the *Rapports* as a major work of Ideology, one cannot blame Tracy for a narrow focus. In fourteen years he completed five volumes of the *Eléments d'idéologie*— on the mental faculties, or Ideology proper (1801), grammar (1803), logic (1805), and a double volume on the will, including political economy and moral philosophy (1815). Having already

173

constructed an "encyclopedic" tree of the sciences in an article of 1797, by 1805 Tracy was using Ideology in the broad sense as encompassing all the sciences. The study of the human mind was thus the master science which included all others. The schema of 1805 included legislation (explored in Tracy's *Commentary* on Montesquieu's *Spirit of the Laws* [English ed. 1811, French ed., 1817]) and the first principles of physics, geometry, and calculus.[18] After discussion of Cabanis's *Rapports*, we shall consider how well Tracy's work related to it.

Rapports du physique et du moral de l'homme

The arrangement of the *Rapports* indirectly recalls Condillac's advice on method. Like a rhapsody in analysis, the *Rapports* decomposed the simple, generative principle of physical sensitivity from physical and mental experience, considered it in all its fixed and modifiable aspects, and recomposed it with a view to achieving a socially desirable "acquired" temperament. The work retained its unity despite the six years between the reading of the introductory memoir and the publication of the full text.

The second and third memoirs dealt with the uniform in human nature, a "physiological history of sensations," and were read on 7 and 12 Thermidor IV (25 and 30 July 1796) and published with the first volume of memoirs of the Class of Moral and Political Sciences in Thermidor VI (July-August 1798). The fourth through the ninth memoirs treated the inherent and environmental variations of sensitivity. Three of these, on age (7 and 12 Fructidor IV [24 and 29 August 1796]), sex (22 Fructidor IV [8 September 1796]), and temperament (22 Ventôse V [12 March 1797]), were included in the second Institute volume, published in Fructidor VII (August-September 1799). After Cabanis joined the faculty of the Paris School of Medicine and became more politically active, his academic pace considerably slowed. In fact the conclusion of the sixth memoir almost intentionally marked a pause, given its clear statement of ultimate objectives. Subsequent memoirs did not appear until Thermidor x (July-August 1802), though the Institute records indicate that Cabanis read the seventh memoir, on the effects of disease, on 7 Frimaire and 7 Nivôse ix (28 November and 28 December 1800).[19] The eighth and ninth memoirs, on regimen and climate, completed Cabanis's discussion of the influences on sensitivity.

The metaphysical tenth memoir placed sensitivity in the context of all universal forces in a long essay on "animal life, the first determinations of sensitivity, instinct, sympathy, sleep, and delirium." The last two memoirs, on "influence of the *moral* on the *physique*" and on acquired temperaments, were so brief as to suggest that Cabanis's ill health had prevented him from thorough exploration of the subject. Finally, the 1802 preface placed the work in the context of Enlightenment empiricism and Ideology, while the new edition removed republican rhetoric from the introductory memoir. Besides this obeisance to the political atmosphere of the Consulate, there was hardly any change in tone from the first to the second half of the text.

Some readers of the *Rapports* question whether Cabanis contributed anything truly original or significant to his subject. Philosophes and naturalists had, after all, long since attempted to view man as a natural being. Cabanis's measured eloquence could not match the vigorous sallies of the style of the baron d'Holbach. La Mettrie had already dared make man into an unusual kind of mechanism. As a theorist of the moral and political sciences, Cabanis was not a well-travelled student of climates and governments like Volney, nor did he aspire to the mathematical ingenuity of Condorcet. Studying physical-mental correlations had also been a medical pastime since Hippocrates. Cabanis was not so erudite in medical literature as Antoine Le Camus, though he excelled in keeping pace with recent clinical observations and recent laboratory experiments. He was not himself an innovative physiologist or an eminent physician with an extensive Parisian or Court practice like Bordeu or Barthez. Moreover, Diderot had already synthesized philosophical monism and medical vitalism. In 1796 and 1798 editions of La Mettrie and Diderot could appear in Paris without fear of censorship.

Yet precisely because he stood at the intersection of philosophical and medical traditions, Cabanis's *Rapports* provided a highly subtle metaphysics and a nuanced view of the unity of nature and of knowledge. Not only did he interweave disparate intellectual strands; he proclaimed his handiwork from the heights of official culture. At the Institute, Cabanis did not need the temperament of an *esprit fort*, launching anonymous pamphlets to shock the *bien pensant*. Unlike Diderot, he did not need to consign his work to posterity.

Moreover, the *Rapports* was not merely the work of an epigone but a fascinating link between the Enlightenment ideals of science and universalism and the indecipherable, concrete self of the Romantics. It represents the coexistence of the states of mind (anticipated by Diderot), recently called by Gusdorf the "esprit éclairé" and the "âme sensible."[20] More than the Enlightenment philosophes, Cabanis was calling for a new discipline, the application of a view to man that would establish the legitimacy of an autonomous science of human behavior.

Cabanis began his *Rapports* with a plea for the unity of the sciences and their methods and a hope of describing the "constant and universal nature of man," but he never was willing to pay the price of d'Holbach's reductionism. Human sensitivity was not merely animal sensitivity; its varied circumstances would alter the intelligence, passions, and needs of a *homo economicus* or *politicus*. Ideology would study not only the invariable relationships of men in society but the rich range of their highly idiosyncratic physical dispositions. Thus, the human sciences could not achieve the precision of the physical sciences, even if they had the same "degree of certainty" in Condorcet's sense.

Cabanis was not merely duplicating the treatises of private hygiene that had appeared earlier in the eighteenth century. He made clear his conviction that public morality, the educator, and the legislator also required the advice of the physician. The obedience of the *physique* in man to the "powerful and varied action of a host of external agents" was the basis of a science. For "observation and experience can teach us to predict, calculate, and direct this action, and man would thus become in his own hands, a docile instrument, whose mainsprings and movements, that is, all his faculties and operations, would tend directly to encourage their own development, a more complete satisfaction of needs, an improved state of happiness."[21] Teaching sound physical habits to men was a social mission as well as an individual one and it would be best fulfilled at first by constituting the theory of relationships between physical and mental habits.

While Cabanis aimed at a natural morality and politics, free of the religious scaffolding of "accidental opinions," he did not advocate mere acquiescence in the existing temperament of individuals. The art that he proposed was intended to "modify, correct, and improve" the instruments of nature, to "develop faculties, change or correct their use, create, after a fashion, new *organs*."[22] The medical therapist would use physical habits to restore equilibrium, sharpen sensitivity, or to develop a more sociable temperament. Nature's work was always modifiable to some degree.

PHYSICAL SENSITIVITY:
UNKNOWABLE, VERSATILE PRINCIPLE OF LIFE

In the preface and introductory memoir of the *Rapports*, Cabanis accepted the major assumptions of empiricism as already proven. Locke, Bonnet, Condillac, and Helvétius had already shown that "physical sensitivity is the source of all ideas and habits in the mental and moral existence (*existence morale*) of man." But while these philosophers gave the "analysis of intellectual faculties and affections of the soul," they did not develop the physiological principle that physical sensitivity was also the "ultimate term one arrives at in the study of vital phenomena." Here Cabanis presented the common physiological argument that impressions preceded all movements, whether in the brain or elsewhere in the body. The nervous system was thus necessary for all phenomena of life and mind. Cabanis repeated, without citation, a major contention of d'Holbach: "The *physique* and the *moral* are thus confounded at their source, or rather the *moral* is only the *physique* from certain particular viewpoints."[23]

On the one hand, Cabanis made sensitivity the *sine qua non* of life: "nous sentons, nous sommes." Yet this eighteenth-century *Cogito* proposed no Cartesian "essence" of life and thought. Sensitivity was merely the most important *phenomenon* of life. As in the works of Bordeu, Fouquet, and Barthez, sensitivity was a physiological unknown, or "general experimental cause." Following the Newtonian paradigm of explanation of forces, Cabanis noted that hypotheses about the essence of sensitivity would be as vain as hypotheses about attraction.[24]

Yet Cabanis was not merely concerned with verbal descriptions of life. He was ready to explore laboratory experiments that attempted to unravel the "manner of action" of the nervous system. Unlike Lacaze and de Sèze, Cabanis was not abusive toward such physiological inquiries. His sixth memoir recorded at length, with corrections in each edition, the controversy between Luigi Galvani and Alessandro Volta concerning nerve and muscle electricity. Cabanis hoped that their work would "lift some of the veils covering the mystery of sensitivity" and would "furnish views directly applicable to medicine, hygiene, and the physical education of man." In 1791 Galvani had claimed the discovery of "animal electricity" in muscle contraction when the tin leaf around a sectioned nerve touched a muscle attached to a copper plate. In 1792 and 1794 Volta denied the presence of a special "galvanic fluid" and claimed that the difference in electrical potential between the metals produced ordinary "electric fluid." Volta appeared justified, since no meter then available could have shown a rest potential in the nerve. While Cabanis accepted Volta's views, he left in the text the hypothesis that "electricity modified by vital action is the invisible agent which, ceaselessly flowing through the nervous system, carries impressions from the sensitive extremities to the different nervous centers, and from there reflects the impulse determining motion in the motive parts." Cabanis never matter-of-factly reduced the nerve fluid to electricity in the fashion of d'Holbach. Even Bonnet, hardly a materialist, had been receptive to theories of electric fluid in the nerves. And Cabanis emphatically added that "this fluid does not behave in living bodies and their remains after death as in our laboratory or shop instruments, nor as in clouds and mists." Life altered the character of electricity.[25]

Such qualifications did not forestall critics from labeling Cabanis a "materialist." The *Rapports* Preface disingenuously claimed to engage only in physiological inquiries and remain indifferent to metaphysics. But Cabanis never disguised his hostility to religious dogma or his refusal to admit the spiritual soul. In fact, Cabanis saw no difference in kind between living and nonliving matter. If chemists could one day determine the composition of atmospheric air and water, asked Cabanis, why could they not "recognize with the same precision" the "elementary principles forming organized bodies?" Even highly complex matter was not exempt from the necessity inherent in its properties.[26]

THE LEVELS OF UNIVERSAL AFFINITY

While all these assertions testified to a monism, or a belief in only one kind of substance in the universe, they did not suggest reductionism in which the properties of life were merely those of inert matter. Use of the label "materialist" suggests a mechanistic, clockwork universe and ignores the rich legacy that Cabanis had absorbed from vitalist medicine as well as his subsequent evolution in the *Letter* to Fauriel. The metaphysics of the *Rapports*, though monist, offered a refinement of the levels of complexity of a single substance and of scientific laws already sketched in *Coup d'oeil*. In the tenth memoir, Cabanis presented all physical forces as manifestations of a single universal force at various levels of affinity. Yet in a sense, Cabanis stood Newtonianism on its head. Buffon, for example, had sought to encompass all physical forces under variants of the laws of Newtonian attraction. Cabanis suggested the opposite possibility—that complex living sensitivity might be present in primitive form in ordinary matter. More akin to de Sèze, Barthez, and Maupertuis, Cabanis admitted that such questions were beyond scientific solution but reasoned that if one wished to find a "single common determinate cause" for all physical phenomena, it is probable that one would be guided by the most complex rather than by the simplest. He wondered, "Is it by sensitivity that one will explain the other attractions, or by gravitation, that one will explain sensitivity and the intermediary tendencies between those two terms?"[27] Cabanis answered this question only in the uninhibited speculations of the *Letter to F[auriel] on First Causes* (1806 or 1807), when he decisively chose the primacy of sensitivity.

Even in ordinary matter, subject to gravitation alone, Cabanis saw an inherent tendency ("by the automatic development of the properties of matter") to a harmonious, orderly motion governed by a single motive principle. The celestial bodies, he suggested, "may have long existed in other mutual relationships," but "this great whole may be itself susceptible of further improvement in unforeseen ways." Even at the simplest level of matter, Cabanis saw dynamic cosmic progress. While he rejected Final Causes, or direct reference to a deity, he clearly implied that this development of harmonious motion was an improvement. Though he did not cite a source for this idea, the earliest version of Laplace's hypothesis of planetary formation from the rotating solar atmosphere was readily available in 1796 in the popularized *Exposition du système du monde*.[28]

All other active forces, chemical affinity, the "instinct of plants," and animal sensitivity similarly displayed "a direct tendency of bodies toward each other, acting only according to more or less complex laws, because of the conditions of the isolated elements, and the circumstances of their encounter, resulting in all the new properties manifested in the different combinations." Cabanis was probably aware of the importance of "affinity" in the New Chemistry. In 1786 Guyton de Mor-veau had defined "chemical affinity" as the "force with which bodies of different nature tend to unite." Fourcroy in 1782 had noted that in the formation of chemical compounds, "two or more bodies that unite by affinity of composition form a new being which has new and distinct properties from those belong-ing to each body before the combination." Yet Guyton de Mor-veau, his predecessor Macquer, and the Swedish chemist Tobern Bergmann all hoped eventually to derive chemical affinities from complex laws of Newtonian attraction.[29] Cabanis was also familiar with the origins of the usage of the term "affinity" in Hippocrates and Stahlian chemistry to mean like seeking like. In Diderot's Encyclopedia, the Montpellier physician-chemist Venel had vigorously rejected the reduction of chemical properties to Newtonian mathematics and physics and had interpreted affinities as indecipherable sympathies.[30]

Cabanis synthesized this ancient, qualitative affinity of like seeking like with the chemists' notion of the emergence of new properties in compounds distinct from the properties of ele-ments. In a review of Berthollet's *Essai de statique chimique* of 1803, Cabanis was clearly skeptical of the argument that affin-ity was an obsolete term reducible to laws of mass action or other laws of general physics. To Cabanis, Berthollet's quan-titative "combining tendencies" were qualitative affinities by another name.[31] When Cabanis cited Bergmann's "elective at-tractions," he noted that chemical attraction was "not a blind force, indifferent to the tendencies taken; it begins to manifest a kind of will; it makes choices."[32] For Cabanis, chemical affinity remained irreducible to Newtonian attraction.

Having established this gradation of forces, Cabanis extended the notion of special affinities to embryo formation and growth. Like Maupertuis and Buffon, he believed embryo development to be an epigenesis, or a successive formation of the major or-gans. The affinities involved were those of like seeking like. Was there, he wondered, a nucleus (*noyau*) in the embryo to-ward which "analogous principles travel with choice, around which they are arranged and disposed in an order determined by

181

their nature and mutual relationships?" The force of sensitivity was here "determined by organization" and derivative from the "general laws which govern matter." Sensitivity emerged in "certain circumstances in which the elementary principles, in virtue of their respective affinities, mutually penetrate, become organized, and by this new combination acquire qualities they previously lacked." Nature was one, and sensitivity arose from physicochemical reactions. Yet sensitivity was also a different degree of being than the merely physicochemical. Enlightened physicians, Cabanis insisted, knew that the "animal economy is only submitted to the laws of other bodies from several viewpoints of little importance."[33]

This spectacle of a single universal force did not lead Cabanis to "diminish astonishment and admiration" for the order of the whole. He claimed that he intended no more impiety than did Newton in the synthesis of the laws of celestial and terrestrial motion. Indeed, insofar as the word "force" came to Newtonians with psychic overtones, Cabanis was a legitimate heir to the Newtonian legacy.[34] We must recall that, though the unity of nature was a metaphysical hypothesis, Cabanis marshalled empirical evidence to support the interrelationships among the levels of complexity in nature—chemical decomposition of plants and animals, observation of spontaneously generated animalcules from decomposing organic matter or even from inanimate matter, variation in living species, the organic sympathies, both "primitive" and "accidental," in human sensitivity, and the physical sympathy of the members of the same or related species.

TRANSFORMATION IN NATURE:
SPONTANEOUS GENERATION, LAMARCK, LACÉPÈDE

To demonstrate that plants consumed oxygen in respiration and purified the air by removing carbonic acid gas (carbon dioxide) in sunlight, Cabanis recalled the experiments of the Dutch chemist and physician to the Habsburgs, Jan Ingenhousz (1730-1799), and of the Genevan botanist and an associate of the history section of the Second Class, Jean Senebier (1742-1809).[35] Other chemists, such as Fourcroy, had decomposed the "mucilage" of vegetables into nitrogen, oxygen, carbon, and hydrogen. Plants were not only composed of chemical elements but they tended to "animalization"—that is, to become organized as animals—because of the activity of an unknowable "vivifying faculty." This obscure claim merely meant that, given the action of specific conditions, such as humidity, any known insensitive vegetable substance would "almost instantly give birth to particular animalcules," sensitive and living animal matter. Cabanis concluded that there was clearly an "uninterrupted chain" linking vegetable and animal substances. Otherwise, to explain such spontaneous generation, one would have to assert the unlikely hypothesis that life was diffused everywhere, but only disguised by the external circumstances of inanimate bodies.[36]

Several experiments seem to have convinced Cabanis that life could be spontaneously generated, both from organic and inanimate matter. In abbé Rozier's *Journal de physique* (July 1784) and in the *Nouvelles expériences* (1789), Ingenhousz described the formation of colonial, filamentous algae. According to Ingenhousz, the "green matter" that Joseph Priestley observed when sunlight acted on the walls of sealed, inverted, water-filled bell jars was a cluster of animalcules, or "true insects." In both stages of development, the creatures yielded "dephlogisticated air" (oxygen), in effect transmuting water into air. Like Needham, Ingenhousz asserted that there was a "plastic force inherent in nature."[37] For him, there were no troublesome pantheist implications, however—only an awe at the generation of salubrious, air-purifying organisms from putrefying matter.

Cabanis himself in the preface to the *Rapports* regretted that he could not yet present the results of an incomplete series of "experiments on animal and vegetable degenerations and transformations."[38] In the tenth memoir, he indicated his belief that animal parasites were degenerations of the substance of the host. More important, he observed the transformation of the "oleo-mucous substance" in decomposing pulverized almonds into myriads of microscopic animalcules that survived as long as they had a food supply. Medical experience further persuaded him that some intestinal worms were a product of animalization of "mucous matter . . . fortuitous generations directly caused by the weakness of the [digestive] functions, or indirectly by the irregular mixture of humors." Once again, rather than assume that there were particles susceptible of organization everywhere, Cabanis thought it more plausible to believe that appropriate physical and chemical conditions created a higher order of affinities with new properties. The phrase "fortuitous generation" suggested Maupertuis and the phrase "aberrations" of nature suggested Lucretius as much as either suggested the current hypotheses of Lamarck.[39]

The experiments of an Imperial War Commissioner in Limoges, Jean-Baptiste Fray (or Frey), opened even broader vistas to Cabanis. In 1804 Fray sent Cabanis a long manuscript, "Essai sur l'origine des substances organisées et inorganisées," which proposed a true abiogenesis, a production of vegetables and animals from the action of light and heat on a sealed mixture of gases or purified distilled water. Cabanis advised Fray to publish only the experiments without the speculative commentary, and in fact, this extract did appear in Berlin in 1807. In the 1805 edition of the *Rapports* Cabanis hoped that the Institute would review a work that "appears to give us such great hopes." In fact, Cabanis did not live to see the Institute review, which occurred only upon Fray's solicitation after he had published his entire book in Paris in 1817. In October of that year, the chemist Gay-Lussac and his colleague Bosc tersely reported that Fray's jar "containing nitrogen and hydrogen in distilled water" was "inadequately sealed." While Fray solicited another review as late as June 1819, the *Procès-verbaux* of the Academy of Sciences do not record any further action.[40]

If the 1807 publication accurately reflected the 1804 manuscript, one can understand its appeal to Cabanis. Fray, like Cabanis, believed in a single universal force encompassing attraction, chemical affinity, and organization. Even though he called this force an "instructive and intelligent principle" endowed by God to conserve matter, he offered only a more theistic version of Cabanis's metaphysics of 1806-1807 as expressed in the *Letter* to Fauriel. In addition, Fray maintained that the laws of organic matter were sufficient to explain intelligence, and his physiology of the nervous system bore marked resemblances to Cabanis's views.[41]

One can also understand Cabanis's caution in encouraging Fray's hypothesis of "organic globules" or "monads" existing everywhere, which spontaneously generated both small creatures and, possibly, highly developed animals in uninhabited areas, with the composition of the air and water determining the species.[42] Cabanis was not beyond admitting the possibility of spontaneous generation of large animals, at least at one time in the remote past. But in the *Rapports* he had explicitly rejected the "organic molecules" of Buffon or any such hypothesis of potentially living particles. One cannot imagine Cabanis recommending to the Institute a hypothesis that would effectively restore belief in two kinds of matter.

Having alleged experimental proof of the transformation from the chemical to the living or from plant to animal, Cabanis also discussed the dynamism within living species. His limited transformist theory owed much to the medical literature on climate, to Buffon's discussion of variation in the *Histoire naturelle*, and, probably, to Maupertuis's essays. While the *Rapports* were being written, two of Cabanis's colleagues in the Institute were considering variations in species or analogies between fossils and living species.

The botanist and invertebrate zoologist Jean-Baptiste de Lamarck had long been convinced of a hierarchy of simple and complex living forms in the plan of nature and had also speculated on the geological and chemical changes affecting life.[43] Yet his relation with Cabanis remains problematic. Both were allegedly members of the Société des observateurs de l'homme in 1800 though neither seems to have participated actively in this group.[44] Cabanis did not share Lamarck's relentless opposition to the New Chemistry, an attitude that helped isolate Lamarck from the French scientific community.[45] Yet the chronology of Lamarck's works makes some influence on Cabanis possible. Lamarck's first transformist views, acknowledging change of one species into another, appeared in the opening discourse of his zoology course at the Museum of Natural History on 11 May 1800, published in 1801 as a preface to the *Système des animaux sans vertèbres*. A more refined theory, including the spontaneous generation of life, appeared in *Recherches sur l'organisation des corps vivans*, published in Thermidor x (July-August 1802) in the same month as the *Rapports*. The influence of Lamarck's May 1800 discourse on Cabanis's ninth and tenth memoirs, which Cabanis claimed to be writing in late 1800, remains a possibility.[46]

The 1800 discourse reiterated a scheme introduced in the *Flore françoise* of 1779—that is, the graduated complexity of the "large families" of living creatures. Lamarck suggested that the response of a species to changes in climate or milieu could alter its organization. The feet of birds, for example, developed claws for perching, became webbed for swimming, or became elongated for wading. Nature produced these changes with time and circumstance:

> The faculties become extended and strengthened by usage, diversified by new, long-preserved habits, and imperceptibly the conformation, consistency, in a word, the nature and state of the parts as well as of the organs, participate in the consequences of all these influences, which were conserved and propagated by generation.[47]

Lamarck already suggested here the mechanism of use and disuse and repeated the commonly accepted tenet of the inheritance of acquired characteristics. He hinted at a more thoroughgoing transformism in noting that the order of complexity in living creatures "makes one suspect the path (*marche*) of nature in the formation of all living beings."[48]

Lamarck never shared Buffon's belief in direct change induced by the environment. In the elaboration of the 1800 discourse in 1802 and in the *Philosophie zoologique* of 1809,

Lamarck stressed the reaction of an organism to needs created by the environment. He indicated that the most important hierarchy of the significant families was due to an "inner natural tendency to complexity" in any climate or environment. According to one recent study, Lamarck could not accept the natural extinction of species or the likelihood of geological catastrophes or great migrations. Hence, there was only one satisfactory explanation for the differences between living marine mollusks and fossils—the transformation of species and the spontaneous generation that would assure the survival of small organisms.[49] In Lamarck's eccentric chemistry, the subtle fluids of electricity, sunlight, and heat would act on the containable fluids of the organism, which in turn would become sufficiently agitated to induce changes in organs and systems.

Cabanis and Lamarck thus both believed in the graduated complexity in nature, in a dynamic Chain of Being in which species were changeable (though species was not the significant unit for Lamarck), in spontaneous generation, and in a significant role for the environment in transformism. Cabanis believed that needs created faculties but he was closer to Buffon's view of environmental change than to Lamarck's theory of inner tendencies to complexity, and of course Cabanis was not interested in the mechanism of fluid chemistry. Cabanis and Lamarck thus had parallel, but not identical, outlooks.

A more likely stimulus to Cabanis came from the naturalist and physicist B.-G.-E. de la Ville-sur-Illon, comte de Lacépède (1756-1825), whom Cabanis met at Roucher's salon before the Revolution and again as a colleague in the Institute and in the Senate. Like Lamarck, Lacépède edged toward transformism in the "Discours sur la durée des espèces," published with the second volume of his *Histoire naturelle des poissons* in 1800. Lacépède accepted Cuvier's explanation of geological catastrophes as causes for the disappearance of fossil species. He also cautiously refused to admit that any species had truly disappeared, given the vast areas of earth and sea that were still unknown. But he spoke of the possibility of degradation of a species by a long series of "insensible nuances and successive alterations" changing its external features or internal organs. The potentially radical idea was that "such a great number of modifications in its forms and qualities" might mean that a species had "metamorphosed into a new species." Such metamorphosis occurred artificially in hybridization but could also occur naturally because of changes in climate and milieu, "chance circumstances" that "maintain, fortify, or increase" particular traits.[50]

Cabanis anticipated both Lamarck and Lacépède when in 1796 he related the growth of *human* needs, habits, and faculties: "each *need* relates to the development of some *faculty*; each faculty by its very development, satisfies some need; and faculties grow by exercise, as needs increase with the ease of satisfying them." We might find such phrases in Diderot's *Le Rêve de d'Alembert* or even in Condillac's discussion of human faculties, but Cabanis cited no work of physiology or psychology, but rather Siéyès's draft Declaration of the Rights of Man, which had distinguished the needs and faculties of man in society.[51] By 1802 Cabanis was arguing that climate, diet, and habits created new needs that changed the faculties of all living species. This reasoning seemed more attuned to the work of Lacépède than to Lamarck. Cabanis cited Cuvier's memoirs on species extinction due to geological catastrophes and also mentioned Lacépède's explanation of the "relative imperfections of an organization only weakly guaranteeing their [species] duration." Again, reminiscent of Maupertuis, Cabanis speculated that "certain fortuitous changes" in living species might be "fixed in the races, and perpetuated to the last generations." In a simple statement of adaptation and selection theory, Cabanis argued that species that have escaped extinction "have had successively to bend and conform to sequences of circumstances, from which apparently were born, in each particular circumstance, other entirely new species, better adjusted to the new order of things."[52]

Cabanis apparently considered change within each genus and family, as from *Eohippus* to the modern horse. He never suggested a broad evolution, as from amphibians to mammals, or speculated like Diderot on a single animal prototype for all surviving species. Like Diderot and d'Holbach, Cabanis left open the possibility that the "first production" of large animals was spontaneous, though he genuinely believed that there was still generation of microscopic animalcules. A note of 1805 reiterated that these generations were not supernatural nor in defiance of the "properties of matter, or the laws which control all beings."[53] Cabanis's belief in the generation of large animals sounded as much like the "equivocal generations" of Lucretius from mother earth as the spontaneous generation of Lamarck. He was still far from a modern theory of evolution.

Yet Cabanis had broken the static categories of the old Chain of Being. Modifiability of species related directly to modifiability of the human individual. Like Buffon, Cabanis spoke of an internal mold to describe the individual strength of affinities in the body (metabolic forces, in this case) and of the natural healing force.[54] In complex animals, the original affinities at embryo formation determined the strength of centers of sensitivity or the relative dispositions of organs and systems. In the human species, physicians called this characteristic organic state "temperament." Thus, the major theme of the *Rapports* was the levels of affinity in human physiology, subconscious and conscious sensitivity.

PHYSICAL AND MORAL SYMPATHY

The hierarchy of forces was complete, however, only at the level of interaction among individuals. Like the Condorcets, Cabanis asserted that the force of instinctive, subconscious physical sensitivity was at the origin of moral sympathy. He claimed to have evidence that the aura of light rays from the eyes of animals, the odors of each species, and the warmth of animal heat were powerful physical excitants to sympathy. In the human species, voice modulation in speech and musical tones had similar organic effects even before their significance as linguistic or cultural symbols. Moreover, the most powerful existing animal sympathies, sexual love and the maternal instinct, had an obvious organic basis.[55]

Like Shaftesbury, the Scottish moralists Francis Hutcheson and Adam Smith (whose *Moral Sentiments* appeared in Mme Condorcet's translation in 1798), and Rousseau, Cabanis believed in natural moral sympathy.[56] Sympathetic affection was partially instinctive and organic and apparently "independent of reflection." Of course, a "series of unperceived judgments" and the conventions of culture conditioned identification with others' joys and sufferings and transformed it so that it "scarcely resembles pure instinct."[57] Still, moralists needed to recognize the physical basis of the common observation that people enjoyed their "purest and sweetest" pleasures when they were compassionate and helpful to others.

Cabanis could have found belief in the equivalence of virtue and happiness in many eighteenth-century moralists, even in the works of the baron d'Holbach, but basing ethics on the most refined natural affinity—physical sensitivity—introduced a more optimistic tone into a monist metaphysic. Here was no neutral, coldly mechanical, clockwork universe. Rather the impulse to social virtue was built into the natural order of physical forces. To be sure, Cabanis had previously stressed, in his essays on hospitals and public assistance, the imperious and superbly efficient motive of self-interest. But the coexistence of Rousseauist sympathy with utilitarian self-interest eased the task of the moralist. Virtue and reason did not always have to struggle against an intractably selfish human nature. Cultivating sympathy, as well as enlightening self-interest, would promote social harmony.

Cabanis also believed that natural sympathy facilitated the educator's task. In seeking to please others, one tended naturally to imitate both their external actions and their mental operations. This imitative faculty was precisely the means of learning, in adults as well as in children. Physical sensitivity helped insure intellectual development as well as moral development. It is little wonder that Cabanis wrote that the "principle of perfectibility of the human race is found in its very organization."[58] In both philosophical and political works, Cabanis ascribed an ethical good to a natural order. Yet for neither individual nor social health could the natural order spontaneously prevail. The physician, the moralist, and the legislator had to aid healing, teach ethics, and educate for good citizenship.

EXTERNAL SENSATIONS AND INTERNAL IMPRESSIONS

Against this background of cosmic unity and beneficence, the *Rapports* demolished the barriers between body and soul. Cabanis did not accept Condillac's hypothetical statue-man, awakening one sense at a time, which avoided the concrete reality of sensation and the nervous system. Perception and comparison of external sensations could not be understood by isolating each sense, as Condillac had done in his *Traité des sensations*. The external senses supported each other and related by sympathy to the internal organs. Taste and smell, for example, were essential companions. Nor could sounds affecting the ear fail to influence the stomach and diaphragm, just as sight affected abdominal impressions, and smell inspired reactions in the intestines or the genital system. Since Condillac avoided physiology, he refused to deal with subconscious impressions or instinct except as unperceived judgments.[59] He found the whole notion of obscure sensation troubling because of his distaste for innate ideas. How could one *feel* without consciousness, especially if *movement* followed the feeling? Condillac insisted that all movements and mental determinations resulted from true sensations and judgments. If the judgments were unperceived, they had become too rapid and habitual to be noted.[60] The establishment of nonconscious determinants of behavior—mechanisms of emotions and drives—would be a fertile field for psychological inquiry in the nineteenth and twentieth centuries.

Cabanis's most significant contribution to the empiricist model was his emphasis on subconscious impressions from the

191

internal organs or from within the nervous system. His discussion illustrated his belief in the unity of nature as well as in the uniqueness of life. On the one hand, automatic determinations from internal impressions circumscribed human freedom and assimilated the human species to the animal world. But on the other hand, sensitivity was an active faculty that raised all animal life above the merely mechanical. Sensitivity as a positive, organic response was a notion of Stahl and Bordeu more than of mechanical philosophers. The discussion of involuntary motions owed more to Whytt than to d'Holbach.

Cabanis followed a long tradition on the subject of internal impressions. Medieval scholastic literature had used the term "internal sense" for memory and emotion. Descartes had listed corporeal hunger, thirst, and "natural needs" as "sens intérieurs." In the mid-eighteenth century, Le Camus added to the "sensations intérieures" (the above-mentioned appetites) a special category of "reflected" sensations for dreams and hallucinations. Both Descartes and Le Camus wrote of the involuntary motions later labeled reflex phenomena.[61] Bordeu and de Sèze had seen a kind of sensitivity, a "taste" or "choice," in strictly organic secretions. Finally, philosophers routinely adopted the physicians' usage. Turgot's Encyclopedia article "Existence" (1756) referred to a sixth sense, or "tact intérieur," including internal pains in the intestines or joints, nausea, faintness, hunger, thirst, and the emotions. D'Alembert, three years later, thought that the "sens interne," active in strong emotions, was especially centered in the stomach region.[62]

Even before the *Rapports*, Cabanis discussed the issue of the minimum conditions for conscious sensation. In a review of the opinions of two German physicians and one French colleague on the persistence of consciousness in the brain after execution by the guillotine, Cabanis rejected the idea of pain in the alleged movements of decapitated heads. No stranger to the grisly subject of guillotine efficiency, as a member of the Paris Hospitals Committee in 1791, Cabanis had to endorse the tests of the blade on cadavers. In his review, he observed that whether one believed in irritability or not, residual convulsive movements could not produce pain. The experience of nerve ligatures and of paralytic patients who had limb mobility without sensation showed that movement, though not pain, could exist without the integrity of the nervous system. Haller himself agreed that post-mortem muscular movement was not conscious. Whytt had shown that nervous sympathies and consciousness demanded a fully functional brain and spinal cord. Cabanis concluded that a severed head no longer had a conscious *moi* and could be declared instantaneously dead.[63]

In 1796 in the *Rapports*, Cabanis saw Haller's distinction between sensitivity and irritability as merely verbal. Haller himself conceded that nerves normally activated voluntary muscles. Moreover, as Moravia has recalled, Haller's *Elementa* admitted a trace of nervous activity in some involuntary motions, though he held "irritable force" responsible for most involuntary motion. The vitalists agreed with Haller that the soul had no consciousness of nerve-muscle relations in involuntary motions but they insisted that *all* motions required nervous sensitivity. Cabanis supported the simpler hypothesis of one principle of sensitivity, following the "Stahlians, semi-animists, new solidists of Edinburgh [Cullen], and the most learned physicians of Montpellier." In post-mortem muscular movement, he maintained, there was only a trace of sensitivity or an isolated impression in the nerves.[64] Cabanis thought, no doubt, that the single principle of sensitivity would make a distinct soul seem superfluous.

Cabanis revised his views in a note of 1802. He now distinguished a "faculty of contraction apparently inherent in the muscle fiber" in post-mortem movement from "co-ordinated organic movements," "nerve sympathies," and "instinctive determinations," which took place throughout life and were subconscious "sensitivity without sensation."[65] This latter level of sensitivity was the realm of internal impressions. In short, if irritability existed, it was unimportant in the ordinary course of life. Moravia has given an excellent detailed analysis of Cabanis's critique of Haller. Cabanis remained convinced that all living motive forces, even involuntary motions, depended

193

upon nervous sensitivity and the integrity of the nervous system.[66] Though Cabanis was close to the reflex concept in relating such movements to the spinal cord and inferior nervous centers, he never cited the physiological contributions of Johann August Unzer or Georg Prochaska.[67]

Cabanis distinguished two kinds of internal impressions—one from the nerve-endings in internal organs, relating to organic functions and development, and the other from within the nervous system itself. Both varieties were more powerful than external sensations, the first because of the continual functioning of internal organs, and the second, the most indelible of all, because of proximity to the center of sensitivity in the brain.[68]

The first category comprised a wide range of autonomic phenomena, drives, reflexes, and animal instincts. Cabanis's discussion ranged from the obscure impressions of circulation, secretion, peristalsis, and muscle tone to the instinctive self-conservation of animals or other unlearned behavior, such as bird nest construction. In addition, Cabanis attributed the intoxicating effects of alcohol and narcotics to the internal impressions in the stomach and the intestines rather than, as a modern neurologist might say, to direct effects on the central nervous system.[69]

Because many internal impressions were ordinarily subconscious, they were most easily discovered in pathological malfunctions, as in abdominal disturbances or lesions, which forced themselves upon the patient's awareness. But the symptoms of pathology offered clues to normal physiology. Disturbances in the female reproductive system, for example, could become obvious when internal impressions produced the delirium of "hysteria." Like many colleagues, including his friend Roussel, Cabanis firmly believed that hysteria was a frenzy of the uterus.[70]

While Cabanis could easily prove that internal impressions had mental and behavioral consequences, he could not define the origins of the impressions precisely or present a true anatomy of the peripheral nervous system. Still, he classified centers of internal impressions in accordance with ideas of

Whytt and Barthez on organic sympathies and of Bordeu on federative organic physiology. He even cited van Helmont's notion that the seats of the *archei* were partial selves responsible for operations unperceived by the common self. While the brain received all conscious impressions, three principal subcenters of sensitivity first concentrated internal impressions. In excited or pathological states, these impressions might reach the brain, but otherwise they remained subconscious, sometimes to be "reflected" immediately toward motive fibers. Hence arose the involuntary vital motions.

Bordeu had designated the precordial (heart) and epigastric (stomach and diaphragm) regions (the latter was Lacaze's "phrenic center") as centers of partial sensitivity. Cabanis adopted the term "phrenic region" for the diaphragm and stomach and distinguished two other subcenters, the hypochondriac region (liver, spleen, upper abdominal plexuses, upper small intestine), and the genital and urinary systems, and lower abdominal intestines. This third center was partly glandular and controlled most phenomena of sexuality, sex differences, and individual feminine disposition to hysteria. Of course, Cabanis had no idea of cerebral coordination of the endocrine system, but he did suggest a direct nerve liaison between excited internal organs and a corresponding characteristic region of the brain. Derived from Bordeu and Cullen, this schema added to the geography of the nervous system a rudimentary theory of cerebral localization.[71] The centers of sensitivity furnished the key to individual variations discussed in subsequent sections of the *Rapports*; for there could be many kinds of relationships of strength and weakness among the subcenters and the brain. The primitive affinities at embryo formation would fix some relationships, while external agents could modify others.

The development of subcenters was also related to the complexity of the nervous system. In simpler animal species with simpler needs of conservation and nutrition, there might be fewer subcenters and fewer corresponding spheres of influence in the nervous system. On the other hand, in the human species, the predominance of the brain with respect to the sub-centers continually reasserted itself. In simpler species, despite the smaller number of subcenters, internal impressions and instinct dominated external impressions and intelligence. The very term "instinct," a Latin derivation of a Greek term for "internal stimulus," fittingly described the predominance of internal impressions in unlearned animal behavior. Pursuit of animals by an untrained hunting dog and the sucking of infant mammals (including human infants) were both examples of instincts related somehow to cerebral organization. The communication and intelligence of more complex animals made them closer to the human species than they were to simpler animal species completely under the sway of instinct.[72]

Even the human species, however, could not escape the primitive residue of instinct. At birth the human infant already had a nutritive appetite and had experienced the internal impressions of pressure and resistance enough to constitute a true *moi*. Cabanis agreed with Locke in rejecting innate ideas but he could not accept the phrase *tabula rasa* for the human mind at birth; by then internal impressions had produced inclinations and needs in the fetus, at least a rudimentary will, and the sentiment of frustration. While sucking was a true instinct, the nutritive appetite, both in the sense of the pangs of hunger and the pleasure of eating, stimulated the digestive system after birth and affected the organs of taste and smell. The human species also shared the animal instinct of self-conservation in dangerous situations (what moderns later called the fight-or-flight reflex), partially determined by the impressions of the circulatory and nervous systems. Nutrition and self-conservation were also intimately related. Finally, the imperceptible tonic contractions and active extensions of the muscular system formed an instinct that was dependent on the nervous and circulatory systems (thus on self-conservation, which brought extraordinary energy to the muscles) and on the state of the diaphragm and digestive systems (which also provided strength to the muscles). The instincts thus called into play an interaction of the centers of sensitivity.[73]

Cabanis often noted the effect of organic disease on ideas and passions as well as the characteristic internal impressions produced by age, sex, and temperament. For example, disturbances of the hypochondriac center in nervous diseases led to stubbornness in ideas and inclinations, the development of sad and fearful passions, a disposition to concentrated attention and meditation, and various errors of the imagination.[74] Yet these were empirical correlations rather than a systematic, Baconian-style table of presence, absence, or intensity of internal impressions in each circumstance. Quite possibly, Cabanis's modesty induced Tracy's pessimism about Physiological Ideology; for Cabanis admitted that the problem of a general analysis or classification and decomposition of internal impressions was "evidently insoluble at least in the current state of our knowledge."[75] Physicians knew too little of changes in the sensitivity of internal organs and their relationship with the brain to assign each organ (or even each center) its characteristic category of impressions. Cabanis was content to assert that the subconscious conditioned the mental and moral, just as a modern psychologist might assert the physiological origin of emotions without a detailed correlation with cerebral structures and biochemical hormone action.

Such a portrait could only stress the kinship of animals and men. Yet the laws of all animal life were more complex than the laws of ordinary matter. To the Montpellier physicians and to Cabanis, sensitivity was an active functional response, warning the animal of pain and providing him with pleasure. Cabanis followed Whytt, Cullen, and Bordeu in stressing the stimulus threshold—the "certain determinate intensity (*vivacité*)," depending on individual temperament, below which no nerve impulse will occur.[76] Descartes and Haller had already admitted this physiological fact, but the vitalists and Cabanis interpreted it as showing how sensitivity transcended mechanics. The brain had to react for sensation, as much as for voluntary motion. Even if the sensory influx reached the brain, there was no true perception without attention. Sensitivity was no passive registration of incoming impulses, but rather a disposition, partially fixed, partly alterable, of the receiving network. Distracted attention could explain why a wounded soldier felt no pain while he remained in the thick of the fray or why Mesmer's vaporous patients could suddenly claim to be cured. While internal impressions could trigger reactions by subcenters, the brain itself had to react to generate a true feeling or a distinct idea.[77]

The vitalist physiology could act in service of a metaphysical monism. Sensation itself was an active function, just as thought was an activity, and it could not be isolated from its physiological correlates—the brain, the entire nervous system, and the internal organs. Condillac's dictum that thought was only a transformed sensation could now appear in a new light. No active force was needed to intervene and transform sensation into thought. Sensation was preeminently physiological, and no soul was needed to unify the self.

Cabanis's most striking examples of active sensitivity came from the second variety of internal impressions depending upon the "cerebral or nervous pulp" itself. Nerve and brain functions supposed a continual spontaneous activity and energy that produced the normal phenomena of dreams and the pathological phenomena of delirium and hallucinations. Even sleep itself was not passive, but required a flow of nervous power and of blood to the brain, while sleepwalking illustrated lively brain activity.[78] In sleep, internal impressions and memories had no competition in the brain from immediate external sensation. Internal impressions thus produced the confused associations of dreams. A particular nervous disposition might lead to chronic nightmares, while a lively imagination or organic needs might elicit dreams arousing the genital system. Activity in the inferior centers once more corresponded to activity in the brain.[79]

On the basis of anatomical observations by Morgagni, among others, Cabanis also saw abundant evidence of relation between cerebral activity and the physical state of the brain. Excessive cerebral rigidity might lead to mania, while softness could produce imbecility, and irregular consistency or pathological lesions could produce oscillations between inertia and fits of frenzy. Pinel himself had admitted some cranial malformations

198

in imbeciles. Cabanis claimed that some autopsies of the insane revealed abnormalities in the sexual organs (possibly a reference to syphylitics), which illustrated the importance of all centers of sensitivity to sanity.[80]

In addition, Pinel's recent inquiries into madness had shown that "bad habits" were a more prevalent cause than organic lesions. In such cases, according to Cabanis, the internal impressions of hallucinations had often virtually neutralized external reality. A manic temperament was an example of internal impressions run wild. Madness, properly speaking, was the "invincible predominance of a certain order of ideas, and their incoherence with external objects." Madmen literally lived in a state of wakefulness resembling a dream.[81] Even madness often illustrated cerebral activity that only exaggerated the normal. In no metaphorical sense, Cabanis called the inspiration of genius an "incomplete delirium." The gifted and imaginative were subject to domination by lively impressions from within the nervous system. Even the most purely spiritual mystic state related to the dispositions of the organs of the body.[82]

DESTUTT DE TRACY ON FREEDOM OF THE WILL

Critics might still be discontented with Cabanis's portrayal of sensitivity as an active faculty. With little or no difference in degree between human and animal sensitivity, and with sensitivity involved in involuntary motion or uncontrollable hallucination, what room was there for the notion of free will? A subconscious reflex act or an addled mind hardly seemed to provide a paradigm for human freedom. Cabanis never discussed the moral problem of freedom. His Idéologue colleague Destutt de Tracy grappled with this issue in one section of the "Mémoire sur la faculté de penser" of 1796. There he noted that sensation and perception of desire were actions but that they were sometimes "performed necessarily under compulsion." "Clearly," Tracy argued, "we are passive when we perceive sensation without desiring it, and active when we experience it after having sought it by a special act of our will." The will was always determined by desires, and desires were always motivated. Freedom existed in Locke's sense when one had the "power of satisfying our desires" without constraint. Tracy also distinguished our primary desires determined by our organization from complex desires reflecting the varied experience of each individual. Like Condillac, Tracy reasoned that we might change our complex desires by new sources of impressions, new knowledge, and new physical and mental habits. He concluded, "One cannot therefore say that our most complex desires are the mechanical results of our organization. . . . The will influences their formation, in this sense it is free."[83] One was morally responsible for acquiring knowledge about the consequences of actions.

In the *Projet d'élémens d'idéologie* of 1801, Tracy discarded the notion of the will as a separate faculty and presented it as a variety of sensations, sensing desires. The will was absolutely passive in the sense that, as a result of organization, it had to desire the pleasurable and to judge the pleasurable as such. The "organs producing [desires]" created physiological necessity, while previous operations of mind and will created psychological necessity. For all that, one could still apply attention to or recall some sensations rather than others, and one could learn to "rectify" the judgments determining our will. Thus, one still deserved praise or blame for failing to make the will "benevolent and enlightened."[84]

Tracy never specified *how* the will gained the power of control that he recommended. But clearly, both Cabanis and Tracy wished to formulate a moral art and, like Volney, they were no advocates of surrender to instinctual pleasures. They expected natural checks on unbridled hedonism, and Cabanis, for his part, mentioned with Stoic fervor the utility of inevitable physical pain, which "elevates and tempers courage, in which we can always find refuge, if we know where to look, from the misfortunes of human destiny."[85] If Cabanis was thus not a vulgar hedonist, he was not resigned to inevitable fate under all circumstances, either. His entire work was geared toward human perfectibility. In his empiricist and monist concept of human nature, there was a place for self-discipline, for conscience, and for freedom.

Tracy's subsequent publications seemed to stress the determination rather than freedom of actions. In the *Traité de la volonté* of 1815, he treated desires, and indeed "all intellectual phenomena," as if they were "only a series of facts or appearances, corresponding to, and, as it were, parallel to, the series of mechanical, chemical, and physiological acts which actually occur."[86] In this respect, organization produced the same necessary consequences in the human species as in animals, whatever the apparent consciousness of freedom of the will. If man had a soul, so did animals, since there was only a difference of degree. While Tracy defiantly supported this "truth" whatever its consequences for morality, he once again claimed that it did not threaten the foundations of morality. For the necessity of human desires still did not mean that men were prisoners of their bodies. They were still capable of "actions tending toward humanity, praiseworthy and virtuous," in which their organic tendencies toward self-interest were submitted to "justice and reason."[87] Morality in this view simply did not depend on activity or free will.

Tracy's critical correspondent Maine de Biran demanded precise distinctions between active and passive faculties of the understanding and will. Even if physiological sensitivity were not merely mechanical, Biran could not call it active. The experience of effort, based on muscular movement, was, for Biran, the foundation of the free, active, responsible self. To Biran and other dualist critics, organic life in itself could never generate the activity of the will or of the ego.[88]

THE STOMACH-BRAIN ANALOGY: THE CIRCLE OF LIFE

Thus, the hostile reaction to Cabanis's notion of sensitivity would not be appeased by his links to the vitalists, for the activity of a mere organ was not the same, in the view of these critics, as the activity of the mind. Cabanis gained posthumous notoriety for his provocative parallel of the functioning of the brain and stomach. For his part, Cabanis wished to show the analogy between the highly specialized, active brain and the less complex, but also active stomach. The brain, he reasoned, is a "particular organ, specially destined to produce thought, just as the stomach and intestines digest, the liver filters bile, the parotid, maxillary, and sublingual glands produce salivary juices." No one knew the mechanism of thought, but then neither did they know how the stomach digested nutritive substances. The offending paragraph followed:

> We see food, with its own characteristic qualities fall into this organ [the stomach] and leave it with new qualities, and we conclude that the stomach, in fact, altered the food. We also see isolated and incoherent impressions arrive at the brain by means of the nerves; the organ begins acting, acts upon them, and soon transmits them metamorphosed into ideas, externally revealed by the language of physiognomy and gesture, or the signs of speech and writing. We conclude, with the same certainty, that the brain after a fashion (*en quelque sorte*) digests impressions; that it organically performs the secretion of thought (*fait organiquement la sécrétion de la pensée*).[89]

The dramatist Laya, in his review of the *Rapports* in the *Magasin encyclopédique*, found the phrase "secretion of thought" a beautiful image, but nineteenth-century dualists could hardly contain their revulsion at this apparent degradation of human intelligence. The physician L. Cérise, editor of the 1843 edition of the *Rapports*, found even the terms "organe moral" and "centre pensant" to be barbarous violations of grammar.[90] A German historian of medicine and bibliographer thought the metaphor sufficiently informative about Cabanis to consign him to oblivion.[91]

We may legitimately ask whether Cabanis equated thought with a corporeal fluid secreted by the brain. The anatomist Malpighi, the Iatrophysical physicians Baglivi and Boerhaave, as well as Buffon and Diderot, all accepted the idea that the brain secreted nerve fluid. More recently, William Cullen, in works translated by Cabanis's teacher Bosquillon, questioned the dominant view by noting that the nerve fluid persisted in decapitated animals, and that no one was certain of the nature of the fluid. He himself speculated, however, that there was indeed a "subtile, very moveable fluid, included or inherent in every part of the medullary substance of the brain and nerves" that seemed to him to be "of the nature of Newton's aether."[92]

Certainly Cabanis's speculations on nerve transmission did relate them to the "subtle fluid" of electricity, though he never identified them with the Newtonian tradition that assimilated the various subtle fluids of eighteenth-century physics to the aether mentioned in Newton's *Opticks* and letters. Even so, these subtle fluids were different from ordinary, ponderable matter and were therefore not similar to the secretions of an ordinary gland. In addition, Cabanis insisted that nerve electricity had special animal properties irreducible to ordinary electric fluid. Finally, on the page immediately following the stomach-brain analogy, Cabanis warned that philosophers knew only the phenomena of sensitivity, not its nature or essence. Therefore it was a "general fact of living nature," unlikely to be subsumed under some "more general fact of nature," which itself in any case would not have a determinate essence.[93] Thus, Cabanis attached himself not to the Newtonian "aether philosophers," but to the Newtonian paradigm of the inexplicable force, known only by its effects.

Destutt de Tracy, in the "Extrait raisonné servant de table analytique" that he compiled for the 1805 edition of the *Rapports*, summarized the stomach-brain analogy by calling the brain the "digesteur spécial, ou l'organe sécréteur de la pensée."[94] In 1842 Frédéric Dubois d'Amiens, secretary of the Academy of Medicine, in his critical examination of the *Rapports*, omitted the phrase *en quelque sorte* from his exposition of the passage, "le cerveau digère les impressions." A year later, the physician Cérise made the identical omission in his introductory essay to the *Rapports*.[95] Such petty inaccuracies by friends and foes alike might have been coincidental, but gross misunderstandings have arisen from similar "insignificant" errors.[96]

Critics of the reduction of the *moral* to the *physique* could more justifiably attack the eleventh memoir, a disappointingly brief essay on the influence of the mental on the physical. The effect of intellect and emotions, or "affections of the soul," on nervous, circulatory, digestive, and other systems was a conventional subject in a physiological treatise. Physicians such as Gaub forestalled materialist interpretations by stressing the independence of the mind in some mental-physical correlations. Even Cabanis's own disciple, the hygienist Jacques-Louis Moreau de La Sarthe, envisaged in 1801 an "anthropologie morale" (counterpart to an "anthropologie physique") that would assess the effect of passions, affections, and emotions upon the body.[97] And Cabanis himself in the posthumously published lectures on Hippocrates, prepared for the School of Medicine in 1797, emphasized the need for the physician to accelerate cures by properly consoling patients and learning the "good use of passions in treating several diseases."[98]

Yet in the eleventh memoir, Cabanis was determined to assert the vanity of two explanatory principles in psychophysiology. After a brief discussion on how emotional anguish hindered digestion and how anger and courage increased muscular strength, he abandoned the subject of passions detached from organic roots and went on to define the influence of the *moral* on the *physique* only as "the influence of the cerebral system, as organ of thought and will, by sympathetic action exciting, suspending, and disturbing the function of other organs."[99] The brain governed the entire body as the reservoir and distributor of sensitivity, and the nervous system gave the brain extensive communication with other organs and greater energy than other organs could command. But the brain was only a sector in the unbroken circle of life. It shared the dispositions of the internal organs, most especially of the stomach (hardly a surprising conclusion, in view of Cabanis's model of the action of intoxicants directly on the stomach rather than the brain).[100] In the 1844 edition of the *Rapports*, the editor, the physician Louis Peisse, could not help but comment that Cabanis's focus on brain disturbance minimized the distinction between a blow on the head, or other temporary indisposition, and a true mental illness.[101]

When Cabanis discussed "affections of the soul," he referred to "changes already determined by physical habits"—as if the physical was always the primary locus of change. In the tenth memoir, he had criticized Pinel's terminology, "traitement moral" for the insane, because of the vagueness of the term *moral* and the temptation it allowed to attribute the influence of ideas and passions to a principle other than physical sensitivity.[102] In Cabanis's science of man, after all, the physician would base his therapy, for mental and moral problems as well as for disease, not on a psychological theory of personality structure, but on the knowledge of the correspondence of organic dispositions and sympathies with disturbances and passions.

Cabanis's metaphysical framework of the single force, diversely manifested, demonstrated his debt to the naturalists and philosophes committed to the idea of unity of nature and a tightly linked Great Chain of Being. Cabanis's most original contribution to psychophysiology, his discussion of internal impressions, was an attempt to use clinical or empirical evidence to support the notion of degrees of the force of animal sensitivity. At the same time, sensitivity was an active faculty, as it had been for the dualist vitalist physicians. But Cabanis's reputation was sealed by his adamant refusal to admit a special category for the mind or soul—no matter if he celebrated the order and beauty of nature and the power of the human intellect in contemplating the manifestations of the single universal force. Critics saw in his *Rapports* a shameful degradation of man to the physical and organic as materialistic and morally scandalous as the work of d'Holbach. If materialism were not enough of an offense in itself, Cabanis was also, to conservatives and Catholics, guilty by political association with the circle of the Idéologues of advocating the dangerous ideas of liberal individualism and secular education.

Yet Cabanis in the *Rapports* did more than establish the universal functioning of sensitivity as the source of assumptions about human needs, motivations, and sympathies. The moralist and legislator needed to accept sensitivity as the first principle of ethics or politics. But they could not act wisely to help individual development or social harmony without departing from the perspective of a uniform human type; and the central section of the *Rapports* considered men and women in all their diversity.

CHAPTER VIII

The Perfectibility of Temperament

*Fixed and Variable Temperament: The Vision
of Condorcet and Volney*

he uniform operations of sensitivity opened uncharted fields of the unconscious and established the invariable first principles of morality. Yet the variations of sensitivity were the key to improvement of the human species; this was the future research area of the clinical and abnormal psychologist. Cabanis's discussion of these variations in the *Rapports* was a modernized version of the traditional Hippocratic concern for the organic and environmental influences on disease. Lacking evidence of pathogenic microbes, physicians had investigated all possible combinations of atmospheric as well as corporeal constitution. Medical therapists as different as Le Camus and Barthez had agreed that the prevention and cure of disease depended on strengthening, opposing, or modifying the natural effects of age, sex, temperament, climate, and regimen. These variables reappeared in all of Cabanis's medical discussions of case histories. He expected physicians and public health officials to adapt their hygienic rules to individual or local circumstances. While Cabanis gave no systematic instructions for curing the affections of mind or will, his remarks implied that the influence of sensitivity as charted in the *Rapports* would be data for the science of man just as they were data for medicine itself. Accumulated clinical observations would provide moralists and legislators with a basis for generalizations and a guide to peculiarities.

The theoretical basis for the applied science of man was the modifiability of temperament, in the broad sense of the resultant of variables affecting physical sensitivity. The ancients had classified temperament according to dominant humors, the Iatrophysical school according to solid-fluid balance or tension of solids, the Montpellier school, according to the state of sensitivity or of a vital principle. To Cabanis, the "state of the nervous system and of the cellular tissue" was crucial for all organic dispositions. Just as Barthez stressed radical sensitive and motive forces, Cabanis stressed the primitive internal mold peculiar to each individual, or the underlying pattern of affinities and sympathies that fixed the relationship of the various nerve centers.[1] Both internal development and external agents changed this primitive state. The inevitable aging process altered sensitivity throughout the life cycle, while the irrevocable imprint of sex forever fixed a certain sensitive-muscular balance. Illness temporarily changed temperament and sometimes, especially when physicians intervened, even left permanent effects. Finally, physicians, moralists, and legislators could best hope to modify exposure to climate and regimen. While Cabanis recognized the right of all the indigent sick to medical treatment, however, he did not go so far as to designate travel to change climate or to improve diet as a natural right. Indeed, we have seen his opposition to the use of public funds for nutritional supplements for the employed poor. But the applied science of man affected problems of public health as well as private hygiene. Cabanis recognized, but did not resolve, the problem of unequal access for the poor to the means of therapy.[2]

In addition to the ancient framework of the temperament theory and its recent modifications, a powerful stimulus to Cabanis's empirical correlation of physical and mental variables came from his friends Condorcet and Volney. While no one can prove Cabanis's access to Condorcet's manuscripts, he did help edit Condorcet's works from 1800 to 1804 and he needed to refer only to the published works to find ambitious efforts to determine the variations of sensitivity.

In the reception speech at the Académie française in 1782,

Condorcet had stressed that only the certainty of results in the moral sciences was less than the certainty of results in the physical sciences, while the degree of certainty with which one could estimate probabilities was the same in each case.[3] The same year at the Académie des sciences, Condorcet hoped that all sovereigns would encourage research on diverse populations in order to explore the "relationship among the physical constitution of man, his mental attributes, the social order, and the nature of the climate." Mathematicians would tabulate the results of a long series of inquiries to increase their "degree of certainty."[4] In 1793 in the *Journal d'instruction sociale*, Condorcet proposed that savants throughout the world attempt systematic correlation of the influence of climate, soil, diet, habits, occupations, and social institutions on fertility, marriage rate, life expectancy, height, physical strength, mental attributes, character, and behavior. New classification methods (a kind of proto-Dewey decimal system) would facilitate determination of mutual relationships of variables.[5]

In the posthumously published *Fragment sur l'Atlantide*, Condorcet suggested that governments create statistical bureaus to collect such information by an exhaustive census or by sampling techniques, where skilled surveyors were required. The result would be that medicine and hygiene would provide the "greatest means of perfecting the human species" by demonstrating the influence of temperament, child-rearing, schooling, exercise, regimen, habits, occupation, illness, and climate on intellectual faculties, quality of mind, and passions. Since physical weakness and mental debility might be related, one might recommend physical exercise or other changes in regimen to affect intelligence and character. Such therapeutic measures would acquire a definite role, to be supplemented by pedagogy and other philosophical methods of reasoning.[6]

Condorcet's famous *Esquisse d'un tableau historique des progrès de l'esprit humain*, written in 1793 and published posthumously in 1795, celebrated a medical and hygienic utopia in its last section, the "Tenth Epoch."

May not our parents who transmit to us the strengths and weaknesses of their constitution, our distinctive facial features, as well as our own susceptibility to certain physical ailments, also pass on to us that part of our physical organization determining intelligence, intellectual vigor, spiritual energy, or moral sensitivity? Is it not probable that education, in perfecting these qualities, will simultaneously influence, modify, and improve the organization itself? Analogy, analysis of the development of the human faculties, and even certain established facts all apparently lend substance to such conjectures which would further push back the bounds of our hopes.[7]

Thus, education itself would produce organic improvements through the inheritance of acquired characteristics, though Condorcet added in the *Atlantide* that all traits might not be transmissible.[8] Since the human sciences would improve moral faculties as well as physical and mental abilities, Condorcet thought that human moral energy would ultimately be channeled toward the public good, so that "any action violating another's right will be physically impossible, as cold-blooded barbarism is to most men today."[9] Condorcet's buoyant vision was maintained by his wife and by Daunou when they took the initiative to have the *Esquisse* circulated in 1795 with generous subsidies from the Convention.

The impact of Condorcet's doctrine of perfectibility on Cabanis was clearly visible when in a 1799 letter to *La Décade*, Cabanis invoked the image of a society where "advantages attached by each man to the habits of virtue will be so well demonstrated; that one will mock the wicked as fools, whenever one will judge it unnecessary to tie them up as madmen."[10] The image was less of totalitarian social control than of the virtual disappearance of immoral action. Yet Cabanis, for all his interest in the accumulation of medical case histories, never openly acknowledged that perfectibility would be achieved by statistical methods. Indeed he ignored Condorcet's work on the probability calculus applied to decision-making.

Cabanis was also probably aware of Volney's plea in his history lectures at the Ecole normale in 1795 for empirical studies of the "relationships between dispositions of the body and states of mind." Indeed, Volney almost epitomized the medical tradition of correlating mind and body. After noting the effects of food, drink, and digestion on feeling and thinking, he continued:

> The well-regulated or poorly-regulated functioning of the corporeal mechanism is the powerful governor of the functioning of the thinking organ; consequently, what is called a defect of mind or character is often only an effect of temperament or function which would sometimes require for its correction only proper regimen. Such a work, if well-composed and well-edited, would show the cause of a good number of vices and virtues in physical habits, and would thus furnish us precious rules of conduct, applicable according to temperament, and would lead us to a spirit of indulgence, so that we would ordinarily see, in those men called quarrelsome or malevolent, only men who are sick or poorly constituted, and who must be sent to the mineral baths.[11]

Volney here outlined the project of the *Rapports* in charting the variations of sensitivity. But he also echoed the tolerant outlook of La Mettrie's *Homme machine* and anticipated Cabanis's defense in 1799 of the philosophes who advocated perfectibility: "Convinced that the wicked only reason poorly, and that those who reason poorly are only unfortunately organized or poorly reared people, their [the philosophes'] indulgence is unfailing."[12] Thus, the catalogue of individual diversity would foster compassion for ineradicable handicaps as well as teaching techniques of perfectibility.

Age and Sex

Cabanis's memoir on age was a study in developmental psychophysiology in which he discussed the state of the nervous system and the facility of organic function in childhood,

211

adolescence, maturity, and old age. The introduction offered a theory of chemical changes in animal substances of different ages. Cabanis probably derived his views from the experiments of Fourcroy and Berthollet in decomposition of animal substances. They had found more nitrogen in more animalized substances, such as the "fibrin" of muscular tissue in older animals. Cabanis noted that the dilute fluids and imperfect solids of young animals yielded gases similar to those of the chemical decomposition of plant "mucilage." By contrast, the "gelatin" of animal cellular tissue and fibrin, a compound of "nervous pulp and cellular tissue," represented a higher degree of animalization manifest in older animals.[13]

Thus, physical and chemical changes affected the nervous system, which, in turn, influenced mental and moral phenomena. In childhood, vivid sensations, intense internal impressions, and irritable muscles corresponded to impetuous actions and convulsive passions. Well-toned muscle solids and well-regulated sensations brought the increased physical strength and mental confidence of youth and maturity. Educators had to realize that the especially impressionable memory of children under seven made those years the time of formation of the "most important habits . . . the most general feelings and ideas of human nature."[14]

This medical perspective reinforced the emerging eighteenth-century image of childhood and adolescence as distinct states. Cabanis cited Rousseau's *Emile* favorably several times (*Emile* itself cited the pediatrics of physicians such as Desessartz) and agreed that children needed instruction adjusted to their stage of development.[15] Since Cabanis himself was more concerned with public education than with private tutoring as in *Emile*, he had stressed in the Mirabeau discourses and again in 1799 the importance of appropriate elementary textbooks for primary education.[16]

Finally, Cabanis accounted for the mental and moral problems of old age. Weakness of the nervous system brought lethargic sensitivity, painful internal impressions, lassitude in all functions, difficulty in remembering recent events, and, in its wake, timidity and prudence, even occasionally the "second childhood" of senility.[17] The aged could not always attain the happiness inspired by physical well-being but they at least had the consolation of pleasant memories. Society had to recognize its responsibilities to the indigent aged no less than to indigent children. Cabanis had previously cited Siéyès in asserting the indebtedness of society to the elderly for services rendered.[18]

Cabanis's memoir on the sexes was congruent with the increased medical literature on the reproductive system and on the concept of femininity in the eighteenth century. More uninhibited discussion of sexuality reflected the decline of religious taboos on the body or instinctual drives but it hardly altered the stereotyped social role recommended for women.[19] Cabanis thought sex differences were based on "unknown circumstances by which the embryo itself is formed, lives, and develops." These affinities at conception determined the "particular disposition in the primitive formation of the nervous system" as well as muscle and bone structure. He identified a clear physiological focus in the genital subcenter of sensitivity for the sex drives emerging at puberty. The strong influence of the sex drive was due to links of the reproductive system to the brain via the spinal cord and to specific genital-abdominal sympathies. Moreover, all glands had a mutual sympathy affecting available "energy" in the brain. Gonadal secretions obviously affected other body characteristics as well, such as voice, body hair, and facial expressions.[20]

Even from the naturalists' viewpoint, Cabanis insisted that for each animal species, the "character of its needs, pleasures, occupations, sociability, perfectibility . . . particularly spring from the circumstances or conditions of reproduction" and from the dispositions of reproductive organs. In the human species, such organic dispositions influenced general brain activity and, specifically, feelings of "benevolence, tender and gentle sociability." Testifying to the Enlightenment rehabilitation of the passions, Cabanis asserted that moderate activity of the "organs of generation" was "the fertile principle of the greatest thoughts, the most elevated feelings."[21]

213

Despite this completely organic psychology, Cabanis's description of psychosexual phenomena, including the anticipation of notions of sublimation and repression, has a peculiarly modern tone. He saw adolescence as the age of "all romantic ideas and illusions" in mental and moral life, a time when

> all loving affections are so easily transformed into a religion, a cult! One worships invisible powers as if adoring a mistress, perhaps solely because one does adore, or needs to adore, a mistress; everything stimulates such extremely sensitive fibers, and the insatiable, tormenting need to feel cannot always be sufficiently satisfied with real objects.

For Cabanis, then, rehabilitating the body was a way of preventing misguided flights of imagination into the world of spirits. Cabanis's medical observations of convulsive hysterical fits in women also led him to link such disorders with total repression of the sex drive. While Cabanis was thoroughly conventional in his view of marriage and the family, he thus recognized sexuality as a primary force ignored at great risk. Even the natural changes of menopause in the female reproductive system brought on waves of passionate, uneasy, unappeasable feeling.[22] The implicit conclusion, then, was the need for moralists and physicians to assuage the insecurities of menopause and to help preoccupy the lively imaginations of adolescents, so vulnerable to religious enthusiasm.

Cabanis's anticlerical views were even more obvious when he denigrated the monklike virtue of abstinence. The only explicitly moral remark in his entire discussion of sexuality was his condemnation of castration of young men (for the choir by Christians and for the harem by Moslems) as "cruel and disastrous to society." Such individuals not only lost sex drive, but became weak, cowardly, and corrupt.[23] Thus, a healthy reproductive system was crucial to emotional stability and even to a balanced intellectual life.

The greatest practical application of the influence of sex on sensitivity was doubtless due to the radical distinction between the male and female organism. On this issue, Cabanis was an implacable advocate of nature uncorrupted by culture. Like Diderot and Rousseau, he developed his ideas about woman's place from prevailing medical theories on female organic characteristics. Especially important was *Système physique et moral de la femme* (1775; 2d ed. 1783), the work of the physician and Montpellier graduate Pierre Roussel (1742-1802). Inasmuch as Roussel frequented the salon of Mme Helvétius, occasionally wrote for *La Décade philosophique*, and was an associate of the ethics (*morale*) section of the Second Class of the Institute, he may also be considered an Idéologue. Both Roussel and Cabanis stressed the peculiarly strong sensitivity of the female reproductive system, the weak muscular fibers, and an anatomy requiring increased effort in walking. The weaker cerebral pulp of women produced more rapid, lively sensitivity, which easily exhausted the radical forces of the nervous and muscular systems.[24]

The muscular weakness and sedentary inclinations of women were allegedly advantages in heightening sensitivity for the ordained functions of conception, childbirth, and lactation. In fact, the emotional counterpart of such sensitivity was the strong maternal instinct and responsiveness to children. But physiological imperatives also led women to desire a strong protector and to learn to charm male aggressivness into tender solicitude. By contrast, male muscular strength fostered a desire for exercise, bold displays of courage, even domination. Thus arose the inexorable "law of nature": "Man must be strong, defiant, enterprising; woman must be weak, timid, dissimulating." Like Auguste Comte later, Cabanis suggested the female intellect was unsuited for "long and profound meditations" but was particularly apt where great sensitivity was required— "that part of moral philosophy directly concerning observation of the human heart and of society." Cabanis lyrically described the role of women in their "proper" sphere. In his essay on hospitals, he declared that a woman's "delicate hand is made for caring for our ills, and her light and tender imagination, for consoling us in our suffering."[25] The destiny of women did not imply inferiority to men but rather activity in traditionally female occupations.

Cabanis rejected scholarly and political roles for women despite his encounters with remarkably gifted women in the salons of Paris and Auteuil. After all, he wrote encouraging letters to Mme de Staël and did not spurn the "Letters on Sympathy" offered by Mme Condorcet.[26] Still, he insisted that women lost their beauty and charm when, through "unfortunate destiny or the disastrous admiration of undiscerning friends," they acquired literary or political aspirations. He warned that careers for women would undermine the family, the basis of civil society. As if deliberately contradicting Condorcet's defense of the intellectual equality of women, Cabanis argued that their meager accomplishments in philosophy and the sciences were a matter of temperament, not poor education.[27] "Les femmes savantes," he acidly commented, knew nothing thoroughly, and their necessarily brief attention span insured confusion and superficiality. Of course, Cabanis was here perfectly in tune with even the most egalitarian thinkers of the radical Revolution, who similarly excluded women from their claims.[28] Perhaps Cabanis regretted Mme Roland's meddling at the time of Girondin ascendancy. The most likely explanation of his attitude, apart from sincere medical conviction, was the character of the two women he most admired—Mme Helvétius and his wife Charlotte de Grouchy. Contemporary testimony described both as intelligent, refined, charming hostesses who exercised their "domestic empire" without intruding upon serious intellectual discussion.[29]

Cabanis only once deigned to poetically discuss the passion of love, apart from this "arid and cold exposition" of sexuality. He rejected both the "cold gallantry" of chivalry and the "frenzied torrent" of feeling provoked by artificial social barriers. For him, love was best the "consolation, not the arbiter of life." He even hoped that the new "social art," in a society of equality and "public reason," would promote happiness without the artificial "enthusiasms" of other eras. Thus, Cabanis was not for

216

enshrining the great influence of the genital center of sensitivity through an idealization of instinctual drive. His disdain for the Dionysian certainly marked him as a man of the Enlightenment, despite his emphasis on the need to know the uniqueness of each individual self. Doubtless, aspects of the Enlightenment and of Romanticism could coexist in the same author. But the neoclassical ideal of sober happiness and passionless love seemed to be Cabanis's reaction to overzealous proponents of the emergent Romantic ethos. Cabanis's colleague Destutt de Tracy would undertake a more elaborate anatomization of love, and Stendhal would respond with a decidedly Romantic work that idealized both courtly love and the frustrations that heightened passion.[30]

"Primitive" Temperament and Illness

The third inherent influence on mind and character in Cabanis's work was "primitive" temperament. Despite his rejection of a humoral theory, Cabanis retained the four ancient categories (sanguine, bilious, phlegmatic, melancholic) which correlated body build and coloring with rapidity of movement, reaction to illness, and character traits.[31] He recognized the contributions of Boerhaave and Stahl in highlighting solid tension, fluid density, solid-fluid balance, energy in muscles and blood vessels, and relative volume of internal organs. But Cabanis insisted that the determinant phenomenon was the "manner of action of the nervous system, and its effort upon the organs." Citing observations of the Swiss physician J.-G. Zimmermann (1728-1795), the opinions of Bordeu, and the notes of his own mentor Dubreuil, he concluded that the "difference of temperaments especially depends upon the difference of centers of sensitivity, of relationships of strength, weakness, or sympathetic communications among various organs." Each of the classical temperaments displayed a distinctive internal mold that, from birth, directed the activity of the heart, liver, and genital system.[32]

Nevertheless, like Barthez, Cabanis wished to use external

criteria to help identify these internal differences. Great chest capacity, for example, would normally indicate the more active respiration of the sanguine individual, though in some cases it might indicate the engorgement characteristic of phlegmatics. The large chest of the sanguine facilitated respiration and improved circulation, animal heat, and general well-being so long as fibers were flexible enough and the cellular tissue moderately moist. This temperament also had suitably rapid, vivid impressions and suffered no constriction in any center of sensitivity. On the other hand, the phlegmatic had difficult circulation, softer fibers, little energy in the liver and genital organs; hence, dull sensations, slow movements, and a serene, inactive character.[33]

The distinctions of Lacaze and Barthez, as well as Haller's observation of muscular types, prompted Cabanis to add two varieties to the four of the ancients. In the sensitive temperament, typical of learned men, artists, and sedentary artisans, the cerebral and nervous system, rather than the muscles, was dominant. Women generally also had a sensitive temperament, but their weaker fibers permitted only "superficial and fleeting" determinations. Conversely, the muscular temperament, typical of outdoor laborers and, in the extreme case, of the athlete, had muscular dominance, strong and active inclinations, and weaker sensitivity to impressions. Vigorous exercise in fact had the moral consequence of lessening the natural capacity to sympathize with fellow human beings.[34]

Cabanis admitted that any temperament classification designated only ideal types, in reality "mixed and nuanced" in every individual in "infinitely multiplied" combinations. Still, the therapist needed a blueprint to know the extremes of individual strengths and weaknesses. The physiological science of man, after all, sought to modify organic sympathies, to balance the effects of age, sex, and primitive temperament with the accidental factors of climate, regimen, and therapy in illness.[35]

Just as Cabanis was receptive to a chemical theory of aging, he favored more physical and chemical knowledge about the nervous system. Besides discussing galvanism, he was convinced that phosphorus content affected nerve functioning. Cabanis took his evidence partly from medicine and partly from natural history. Medical students and physicians observed an especially strong luminescence emitted from the decomposing cerebral tissue of cadavers. We now can attribute this phenomenon to luminescent bacteria. But in the eighteenth century, naturalists, including the author of "Phosphore" in Diderot's *Encyclopédie*, linked the energy of some sea animals to phosphorescence. Lavoisier had demonstrated in 1789 that putrefying organisms yielded a self-inflammable gas, phosphoreted hydrogen. Cabanis, among others, erroneously concluded that phosphorescence itself was a slow combustion, or oxidation, of phosphorus in decomposing flesh. Hence the post-mortem luminescence of the brain in higher animals might be an index of nervous energy. Cabanis asserted that he observed a special brightness in decomposing cerebral tissue of maniacs and a less intense luminescence in the case of leucophlegmatics.[36] In addition, excised nerves showed persistent electrical discharges at the same time observers could see phosphorescence. In 1802 Cabanis inserted a note of praise for the chemist Berthollet, the pharmacist Nicolas Deyeux, and the physician Dupuytren, who had all attempted the chemical decomposition of animal matter and organic systems.[37] Cabanis hoped that one day the variations of age, sex, and original temperament, including the traditional observations of solid and fluid states, would correlate with phosphorus and nitrogen content as well as with oxygen assimilation (in modern terms, metabolism).

Cabanis thus anticipated the significance of chemical and metabolic variations for individual differences. But here, too, he was not ready to abdicate to the physical sciences. He still maintained the primacy of "physiological and medical circumstances." He was also confident that the most important conclusions about nervous activity would come from "contemplation of the living man" rather than the "examination of humors and dead organs, where the scalpel and chemical analysis find only unfaithful imprints of life."[38]

The fourth inevitable phenomenon affecting sensitivity,

ideas, and passions was disease, the special target of the physician. Here Cabanis carefully explained that behavioral changes might be due to disturbances of the nervous system, of internal organs, or of various solids and fluids. Once more he linked languor or hysteria to disorders of the genital subcenter of sensitivity. Brain inflammation might bring on a frenzy, while inflammation of the uterus and ovaries might produce nymphomania. Diseases of the hypochondriac subcenter might lead to obstinacy, sad or fearful passions, or overactive imagination. As in the medical writings, Cabanis stressed that therapy for a disease cannot be uniformly applied but must be adjusted to the age, sex, temperament, and habits of the patient, as well as to the climate.

In his twelfth memoir, Cabanis briefly discussed cases in which the crises of an acute fever or a chronic affliction would leave persistent changes in deep-seated organic dispositions. In most illnesses, the concentration of sensitive forces favored melancholia, a turning inward of the patient upon himself. At least for the duration of the disease, there was a general shift in normal temperament, as from sanguine to bilious, bilious to melancholic, melancholic to manic.[39] Some nervous "vapors" might produce extraordinarily strong feelings and acute intellectual faculties. Certain acute fevers had even occasionally ended a state of congenital imbecility. While Cabanis tantalizingly argued that therapy could imitate nature in improving the constitutions of patients with congenital defects, he left details for a special work on the "physical improvement of man," a treatise Cabanis projected but did not live to complete.[40]

Volney and Cabanis on Climate

The practical applications of the science of man seemed most evident in discussing the modifiable factors of climate and regimen. From the era of Hippocrates, there had been abundant medical literature on salutary and harmful climates and physical habits. Cabanis found Hippocrates' *Airs, Waters, Places* a medical middle term between the philosophical extremes of

Montesquieu, who attributed too much to climate, and Helvétius, who thought culture far more significant. He profited
from a series of investigations in physical and cultural anthropology by his friend Volney.

Each of the two parts of Volney's *Voyage en Egypte et Syrie*
(1787) contained an inventory of the physical state of the
region—topography, soil, winds, and natural history (mineral,
vegetable, and animal)—and the "political state"—native races,
occupations, commerce and economic life, political administration, religion, social customs, and other aspects of culture.[41] In
1795 Volney prepared a manual for diplomats for the Foreign
Affairs Commission during the rule of the Thermidorian Convention, *Questions de statistique à l'usage des voyageurs*. Here
appeared the same subdivision of physical and political states,
with much more refined categories for demographic, health,
political, and economic variables.[42] Previously, in the *Voyage*,
Volney announced the goal: to "seize the relationships and
causes, reveal the overt or covert, remote, or immediate
motive" producing the character and customs of a people.[43]
Like Condillac, he recommended decomposing the complex, observed reality into classifiable facets and recomposing the totality.

In both the *Voyage* of 1787 and the *Tableau du sol et du
climat des Etats-Unis* (published in 1803 and reviewed by
Cabanis the same year), Volney stressed the importance of climate for well-being, though he also argued that the adaptability
of men made them less vulnerable to physiological disturbance
because of climate than other species. He particularly rejected
the idea that climate predestined a people to freedom or slavery
and instead emphasized the importance of religion and government. In Egypt, Islam and despotic rule hindered economic development, while in the United States, a free government was
favorable to prosperity. Moreover, in North America in similar
climates the Anglo-Americans were far different from the
French-Canadians.[44]

In the Ecole normale history lectures of 1795, Volney developed an even more dynamic theory of physical-political rela-

tionships. He suggested a plan to study the effect of migrations on a history of the same people as well as a study of the coexistence of climatic and cultural variables. Knowledge of the effects of changes in "habits, exercise, regimen, and food" would also be a "necessary element in the science of governing, or organizing a social body, and constituting it to relate to the movement of nature." As Condorcet believed, one could thereby determine the "moral and political constitution of a nation" from a "tableau of well-authenticated (*bien positifs*) and well-verified facts."[45]

Like Cabanis, Volney thought of the legislator as a therapist adjusting the law to the natural temperament of a people and to the temporary phenomena of a crisis. Volney retained a cyclical theory of history rather than a view of inevitable progress. Yet he continually suggested that history, the "physiological science of government," would provide innumerable case studies to legislators for the formulation of a theory of "preservation and perfection of peoples."[46]

Cabanis's memoirs on climate and regimen reflected some of Volney's concerns. Like Volney, Cabanis defined climate broadly as the "totality of physical circumstances attached to each locality." To deny climatic influence would thus be to minimize not only latitude, air temperature, winds, and other weather phenomena, but also soil and topography, with all their consequences for endemic disease, available natural resources, feasible occupations, and practicable regimen. The very influence of climate on regimen would make it important enough. Indeed, if the climatic environment did not influence sense-impressions, the senses would not be functional. If impressions everywhere had a "common character . . . inseparable from human nature or essential to its development," men could not adapt to the variety of their environments and would be so impervious as to be hardly educable at all.[47]

With this argument, Cabanis sought to reduce any view that environmental influences did not affect sensitivity to the absurd. Yet an adherent of Helvétius would still have argued that the adaptation to cultural, social, and political experience was far more crucial than to climate. Cabanis adopted the cautious view of Hippocrates himself, who attributed the docility of the Asian temperament more to political despotism than to barren terrain or the dry winds of the desert.[48] Cabanis himself remarked that the Greek and Turkish inhabitants of modern Greece did not have the physical or mental characteristics of the ancient Greeks described by Hippocrates, despite similarity of climate. He admitted in the *Letter* to Fauriel that laws, institutions, and administration were powerful in habit formation.[49]

Like Condorcet and Volney, Cabanis argued that the invariable first principles of human nature were independent of climate. One could thus neglect climate when "co-ordinating those external and general laws, justified in all times and places, by their natural occurrence in human organization and the constant disposition of sensitivity." Implicitly, this view safeguarded the universality of the natural rights of man and citizen and the universal principles of self-interest and sympathy that founded political economy and ethics. Volney had argued that men adapt to every climate, so that religion and politics were far more important factors in their social behavior. But Cabanis praised Hippocrates for knowing that climate "counted for much." He insisted that climate "may still furnish some guidance for the choice of certain institutions which cannot be the same, or produce the same effects, in all countries."[50] Men under similar governments, with similar education and experience, would still react differently because of climate.

Cabanis's ninth memoir proceeded to provide empirical evidence to illustrate the effects of climate. From the observations of Buffon and other naturalists, Cabanis recalled the variety in animal species in each climatic zone, according to temperature, soil, available food, and manner of life. Some phenomena allegedly demonstrated the crucial effect of climate: dogs acquired immunity to rabies or lost the propensity to bark when transported to areas where such immunity and habits were present in indigenous canines. Agronomists and animal breeders could also testify both to degenerations and improvements in horses or sheep transported to different climates.[51] Cabanis thought this evidence bolstered his theory, since, of all impressions, climate acted in most constant fashion and was the most likely to modify organic dispositions. In both animals and men, organic dispositions, relating to needs of hunger, sleep, and excretion, became habitual, and constantly acting impressions would induce new habits.

Like Lamarck, Cabanis also assumed there was sufficient evidence to prove inheritance of acquired characteristics. He cited observations by the naturalist Charles-George Leroy of untrained offspring of trained female hunting dogs who would often point in the presence of game. The habits induced by climate would also be inheritable:

> Particular faculties, developed to a greater extent, may be propagated from generation to generation; and if the determinate causes of the primary habit continue to act, during several successive generations, a new acquired nature is formed, which can only be changed if these same causes cease acting for a long period, and especially if different causes impress upon the animal economy another series of determinations.[52]

Climatic action could modify traits accessory to primitive organization, and, however much its action at any moment, these traits would become fixed in the inheritance transmitted to offspring.

Given this mechanism for climatic effects on animals, one could enumerate influences of climate on refined human sensitivity—skin color, bone structure, muscular development, solid-fluid balance. Buffon's plausible climatic theory of racial diversity was even based on the convergence of races "by a chain of intermediaries, whose nuances or imperceptible gradations always meet at the point of contact." Travellers' reports suggested that the Portuguese who settled in the Cape Verde Islands off the west African coast in the late fifteenth century gradually acquired the coloring and racial features of native blacks. Cabanis accepted these reports at face value as testimony of the climatic differentiation of the human species. Furthermore, regional peculiarities existed even within each nation, and there were observable differences between mountain and valley people.[53]

Cabanis proposed a study of the correlation of climate with temperament, disease, habits, and occupations. More medical observations and travellers' reports, including Volney's description of Egypt, furnished material for an extended account of the effects of air temperature, pressure, humidity, and gas composition in the nervous system. At the beginning of a discussion of four of the traditional six non-naturals in his eighth memoir, Cabanis lauded the ancients for relating temperamental change to temperature and the seasons. Warm climates, for example, extended nerve endings and favored a sensitive temperament, though they also might induce spasms in the nervous system. Hot, dry air might excessively stimulate the subcenters of sensitivity. The age of puberty arrived earlier in these regions, while the climate fostered a restless search for stimuli of increasing intensity. The mental consequence was a lively, passionate, poetic imagination, but the moral consequences were increased alcohol and drug consumption and unabashed sensuality that led to the degrading subjection of women to imperious male masters.[54] Cold climates, by contrast, discouraged reflectiveness and increased the appetite for food, the tonic energy of the muscles, the inclination to exercise and, generally, to vigorous and industrious behavior. Cabanis even thought a temporary excess of oxygen in air would heighten vital activity, though, if prolonged, it would exhaust the nervous system.[55]

While temperature thus affected sensitive-motor balance, Cabanis also tried to correlate climate and the four classical temperaments: gentle seasonal change favored the sanguine, heat and drought, the bilious; cold and fog or wind-swept tropics, the melancholic; and swampy regions, the phlegmatic. The wise therapist adjusted drugs and dosage to climate and prevailing temperament. A disease cured by a strong stimulant to the nerves in the north might require a muscular tonic in the south.[56]

Cabanis was easily able to show the impact of climate on food available and on the range of occupations limited by the terrain. Again apparently inspired by Volney's parallels of physical and political geography, Cabanis related topography and life style. Mountain people would always tend to be herdsmen or dairy farmers, residents of the plains could choose to farm grain, fruit, or vegetables, while hunters, and in some areas, savages, would occupy the forests. Just as Volney emphasized that fertile land could induce indolence, Cabanis developed the idea that residents of fertile areas would be light-hearted and pleasure-seeking, while rugged or barren terrain would inspire sober industry and orderliness. Vaguely anticipating a "challenge and response" thesis à la Toynbee, Cabanis attributed the ingenious farming, craftsmanship, and sailing of the Dutch to the challenge of their soggy soil and their location suitable for trade.[57]

Indeed the saga of the Low Countries introduced the idea that "climate itself can in several respects and to a certain point be modified by the hand of man." "Active and learned industry" had conserved the soil, directed the course of rivers, and constructed canals to create artificial sources of wealth and happiness. Indeed the progress of civilization everywhere modified climate—swamps and unhealthful forests could be cleared to become fertile prairies, and arid hillsides could become productive vineyards. Cabanis wrote in an era that followed a period of land clearing and reclamation even in so "developed" a country as France.[58] Yet he was not overoptimistic about the resources of "art" in a refractory climate. Human effort could not change latitude, topography, or distance from the sea and only with difficulty could it change river direction, water supply, or access to water transport. Climate would continue to act when human labor flagged.[59]

Thus, while climate was a modifiable variable even without travel, Cabanis did not share Condorcet's vision of man as the equal of nature. The ineradicable imprint of climate seemed a formidable challenge to the power of science and technology. Legislators would have to be vigilant to take advantage of the benefits that nature provided and adjust institutions to the temperament induced by climate. Cabanis was obviously aware of the fragility of any human ecosystem. But he was no Cassandra about the depredations of human industry. On the contrary, he mentioned only the benefits to the condition of the soil, water, and air from human action upon the environment.

Cabanis was also aware that dependence on climate could be modified not just by land reclamation or canal-building but by international commerce, which made various regimens potentially accessible to all climates. Yet he assumed that the most widespread influence of certain crops, such as opium, would still be local in their effect on the habits of cultivators. He was also pessimistic about the suitability of perishable foreign food products for commerce; in any case, they would be available at prices suitable only for the very rich. Cabanis here approached the subject of social variability of dependence on climate. A "very enlightened friend" reminded him that "the effect of climate is not the same for the rich as for the poor." Cabanis concurred that among the different classes of artisans and laborers, "its influence is even more or less powerful according to the various gradations of social status (*degrès de l'état social*)." Local products would always be more consistently accessible to the "poor, and unhappily everywhere the most numerous class."[60] While Cabanis was as much a prophet of perfectibility as Condorcet and was a spokesman for the benefits of commerce, a true economy of abundance still seemed to him a utopian vision. His caution was remarkable in view of the increasing distribution of sugar, cocoa, tea, and other colonial commodities among various classes. He made no predictions about improved agricultural production, food storage, or means of transportation, nor did he discuss in greater depth the other obvious problems of using climate for hygiene—the inability of the poor easily to travel to attain the benefits of a therapeutically desirable climate. But access to climate in the broad sense was still a concern of legislators, insofar as they could influence it, and not just a privilege of individuals.

Regimen and Occupation

Regimen was the most unquestionably controllable of all influences on sensitivity. The treatise of private hygiene on the non-naturals—including exposure to air, habits of diet, exercise, sleep, and occupations—was a conventional medical genre.[61] At the Paris School of Medicine, Cabanis's colleague Jean-Noël Hallé repeated his plea for a comprehensive discipline combining private hygiene with the public health studies that were usually assigned to "legal (forensic) medicine." Cabanis was thus on traditional ground in his memoir on regimen, which he defined broadly as the "totality of physical habits, whether necessitated by circumstances, formed arbitrarily by art, or by the taste and habit of individuals." While natural variation provided empirical evidence of climatic influence in animals, artificial breeding illustrated the effects of regimen. Delicate human sensitivity and retentive human memory were even more amenable to habit formation than the sensitivity of animals. A wise regimen of physical habits would insure sound mental and moral health. Cabanis saw a need to develop principles valid for similar individual temperaments and circumstances so that ultimately the species itself would be "indefinitely perfectible; after a fashion, capable of everything."[62]

Of the six non-naturals, Cabanis did not discuss "evacuations and retentions" or "affections of the soul" but he did cover the familiar subjects of air, food and drink, rest and motion, and sleep and wakefulness. He made clear his expectation that changed physical habits would modify "internal impressions and habitual dispositions of organs" and thus, by sympathy, the centers of sensitivity, which stimulated ideas and passions. After the discussion of the factor of air, mentioned previously, Cabanis stressed the need for a true dietetics, as the ancients had wished, but consonant with modern findings. He asserted that animal nutrients strengthening and activating the muscles would be salutary in cold climates, while a vegetarian diet was inadequate everywhere, even in the tropics. With some malice, Cabanis noted that monastic experience illustrated the harm of vegetarianism and fasting. "Emaciating the monk" was a regimen fit for assuring abject obedience, but it aggravated melancholic dispositions, stirred unhealthful "ecstasies," and violated "all the laws and feelings of human nature." Cabanis thus implied that some alleged religious experiences were merely the result of malnutrition. Further, he maintained that overconsumption of fish could induce nerve, skin, or glandular disorders, while the poor, forced to live on chestnuts and buckwheat, would have slow muscular response and dull sensitivity.[63] A "philosophical hygiene" would avoid such threats to health and well-being.

Cabanis also warned against the abuse of alcohol and narcotics. Any intoxicant might, in extreme cases, as with some notorious criminals, lead to a combination of "ferocity and stupidity." Distilled spirits, consumed in greater quantities in cold climates in an effort to strengthen sensitivity, actually weakened the sensitive system and produced a prolonged feverish state within the body. Similarly, prolonged use of narcotics exhausted sensitivity, debilitated the brain, and heightened susceptibility to paralysis or apoplexy. The particular drug and dosage produced behavioral effects ranging from total apathy to the "wildest frenzies." Strangely enough, Cabanis believed hashish far more dangerous than opium. On the other hand, the "intellectual beverage," coffee, recommended for scholars, artists, and men of letters, gently stimulated both sensitive and motive forces and counteracted the influence of both narcotics and alcohol. Food, beverages, and drugs all affected the stomach and thus, through sympathy, produced marked effects on the brain.[64]

Sound regimen would also adjust exercise and sleep to individual temperaments. An extreme muscular or athletic temperament demanded vigorous exercise, though at the price of weakening sensitivity and fostering inclinations to violent, precipitate action. Exercise was a temporary tonic for scholars and artists but, if prolonged or strenuous, would bring about lively, rapid, external sensations that distracted one from the internal impressions suitable for involved reasoning or meditation. Moderate exercise and a longer period of sleep would give men of sensitive temperament a new reservoir of excitability to renew their exhausted nervous systems.[65]

Though Cabanis admitted that "affections of the soul" were

229

"indeed capable of producing changes in the state of organs," he avoided the topic, ostensibly because he wanted to focus on the effect of physical habits, and probably so as not to lend credibility to the concept of an independent noncorporeal force. His final subtopic was the mental and moral effect of various "manual and mechanical" occupations. Cabanis once again endorsed the benefits of work in general, which would bring an income guaranteeing an interest in social stability. Developing the idea of a "medicine of labor" proposed by the Italian physician Bernardino Ramazzini in 1700, Cabanis arrived at the elements of an occupational sociology.[66] Yet we must recall that he never explicitly related work-induced temperament to social class. The peasant in the next hut, after all, might have a temperament with all the bilious impetuosity of an ex-noble general of the armies of the Republic.

He did see, however, a marked alignment of outdoor unskilled heavy manual laborers (lumberjacks, porters, longshoremen, ironworkers) with the muscular temperament. Their exertions gave these men a courageous, ingenious, adaptable character. Unfortunately, such exercise also resulted in coarse sensibilities and "less social" dispositions. All the same, as Adam Smith had already argued, the outdoor labor of the farmer exposed him to diverse external stimuli and required a versatility for changing seasonal tasks. Thus, farmers acquired a considerable number of ideas from their surroundings.[67] In fact, Cabanis had a decidedly uncomplimentary view of societies without the stabilizing influence of agriculture. He thought a people of hunters inevitably became pitiless, warlike, and crafty—almost numb to the sympathetic emotions of humanity and, among primitives, prone to cannibalism. Even shepherds, who appeared in so many literary Arcadias, were, with few exceptions, xenophobic "hordes of brigands" who were ignorant of "territorial property," which was the basis of "civil laws."[68] Thus, Cabanis reinforced the eighteenth-century myth of the sensible, peace-loving farmer, tied to property in land, while definitively rejecting Rousseauist primitivism.

Cabanis thought that sedentary indoor artisans (shoemakers,

tailors, embroiderers), by contrast, benefited from shelter in bad weather and acquired a sensitive temperament. Fewer striking external impressions resulted in the dominance of internal impressions, an enhanced reflectiveness, and refinement of the social instinct. We might wonder if Cabanis would have repeated the conventional belief that outdoor workers were more inclined to precipitate action if he had studied the Paris police dossiers on Revolutionary crowds. Modern historians have shown a disproportionate number of locksmiths, cabinet-makers, and other indoor artisans among the sans-culottes active in the *journées* of 1789-1795.[69]

Cabanis did see negative aspects to indoor work, such as enervation of the muscles and, in large shops, the division of labor that assigned repetitive, specialized tasks. And the poorly ventilated air of closed workshops, never as wholesome as the outdoor atmosphere, could dull the nervous system. Aware of chemists' calculations of oxygen needs in hospitals, Cabanis warned that overcrowding, apart from its moral perils, corrupted the air. And noxious vapors might arise from the by-products of an industrial process. While Cabanis was otherwise an active proponent of industrial freedom, he reminded employers that to prevent "moral disorders," they had better pay as much attention to proper ventilation, lighting, and clean facilities as they routinely did to harsh discipline and repression of abuses.[70] Cabanis was always suspicious of closed work-shops, and one cannot imagine him an enthusiast for the factory system, yet he never meant his warnings of the potential threats to health to denigrate the economic and social benefits of commerce and industry. On the other hand, his reflections opened up vistas of industrial psychology that were rarely explored until the twentieth century.

As in the economic theories of Adam Smith (and, a year later, in the first treatise of J.-B. Say), Cabanis supported the true productivity of "enterprises of industry and commerce" as well as of agriculture. He even associated the diffusion of the spirit of enlightenment and the Revolutionary ideals of liberty and equality with the growth of commerce and industry. In ancient times, commerce and industry had been the glory of the most enlightened Greek city-state, Athens. Similarly, in the period of expansion of commerce and industry from 1500 to 1800, there had occurred, first, the religious reformation, which broke the monopoly of a single church on European culture, and then, the increasing independence of the "industrious" from the "rich," which prefigured the reign of "social equality." While not outlining a theory of history, Cabanis, like Condorcet, saw the emergence of ideas as related to economic and social change. All the more beneficent, then, were the changes helping to ensure the triumph of progressive ideas.

In the end, the "relationships" that Cabanis observed between physical sensitivity and the six factors of age, sex, temperament, illness, climate, and regimen could lead to precise journals charting the state of the nervous system and "organic dispositions" of individuals. Sufficient observation would presumably lead to rules, as in general clinical medicine, for adjusting medical therapy, altering regimen, or changing exposure to climate.

The "Well-Tempered" Individual

While Cabanis's concluding memoir offered few suggestions on producing an acquired temperament, the conclusion of the sixth memoir unhesitatingly outlined the future objectives of the physiologically based science of man. As an heir to a philosophical tradition valuing scientific perfectibility, Cabanis offered the goal of mental and physical equilibrium—the socially desirable, balanced temperament. As an heir to a medical tradition conscious of human diversity, he refused to extinguish sympathy for the deviant extremes of wayward temperaments. More cautious even than a neo-Cartesian physician such as Le Camus, Cabanis believed that the primitive imprint of temperament could be strengthened or weakened but that only in rare cases could it be transformed. The most effective alterations of physical sensitivity would ensue when climate and regimen concurred, but when their concurrence ceased, the natural temperament would usually return. Indeed, the only infallible alterations of temperament came from the intermarriage of individuals of different stock. For that reason, Cabanis thought all endogamous peoples had better preserved, more distinctive natural temperaments.[71]

As a standard and as a limit, Cabanis envisaged a "well-tempered" individual whose sensitive and motive forces would be perfectly balanced and in whom stable equilibrium of centers of sensitivity and of bodily functions would guarantee physical and mental well-being. Though such a "normal" individual was the objective of therapy, the ideal in fact could not exist. Each individual would inevitably have idiosyncrasies, and the inherent dynamism of temperament would assure that new needs would continually arise with new faculties and the fresh exigencies of the impinging environment. Hence, physical and psychic equilibrium would always suffer at least temporary imbalances.

Nevertheless, Cabanis was an inveterate optimist on the relationship between environment and inheritability. He believed that a philosophical hygiene would be aware that each individual at birth was the bearer of inherited acquired characteristics of his ancestors. Thus, the ultimate aspiration of altering temperaments was nothing less than the perfection of "general human nature," the "physical education" of the entire human species, which might "approach ever more closely a perfect type." Indeed, asked Cabanis, how could men neglect human physical education when they devoted so much time to plant and animal breeding? Was it "more essential to have peaches agreeably fragrant and tulips agreeably speckled than wise and good citizens?"[72]

Cabanis's science of man would have an ethical component as well. While physical and mental health was its prime concern, the social value of the entire enterprise was at least partly its promotion of moral action and political awareness. The new regime of the Revolution had already brought about equality of rights. The science of man would work toward eliminating the artificial inequality of capacities. As in his social and political writings, Cabanis stressed the vanity of efforts to "reduce all individuals of the [human] species to a rigorously uniform common type." If differences in strength and talent persisted in horses bred in the same stable, surely there would persist among citizens of the same country differences in character, vital energy, and habits of mind and will. But the science of man gave the key to affecting mental and moral habits through organic dispositions and temperament. Natural inequalities would remain, so that all men could not be made suitable for all positions in society, but proper guidance could make all men equally fit for social life. As in Condorcet's "social mathematics," Cabanis's long-term political objective was fitness for citizenship—not equality of enlightenment and skills, but equal capacity to play a political role. Thus, the educational methods Cabanis advocated elsewhere could complement and reinforce the efforts of physicians.

Cabanis could not directly apply the theories of the *Rapports* in his administrative and political career because the practical problems he faced often preceded his formulation of a theory. We have seen, however, how his deeply rooted feelings of moral sensitivity and sympathy were one justification of his advocacy of social assistance and how a political philosophy of natural rights could be related to the nature of a sensitive being. We will explore in a subsequent chapter how the notion of perfectibility was fundamental to Cabanis's ideas on education.

There were structural similarities in Cabanis's theoretical and practical views—the intervention of the therapist to modify temperament toward a more desirable norm or toward a more natural equilibrium paralleled the intervention of the legislator to assure the elimination of artificial inequalities in society. The observed natural diversity of sensitivity in his theory could also be used to argue that the natural inequalities of property must also be maintained.[73] But Cabanis himself expressed determination to *eliminate* those diversities that, because of ignorance or temperamental imbalance, prevented meaningful participation in the political process. We will later discuss his theory of government, which indicated both the range and the limitations of his concept of "fitness for social life."

The *Rapports* provided a storehouse of information for individuals concerned with private hygiene, for moralists interested in the physiological origins of motivation or mental illness, and for officials or legislators responsible for public health and social policy. Cabanis did not provide a systematic summary of all the practical implications of his theories, however. He intended that physicians or educators dealing with children, adolescents, or the aged continually bear in mind the peculiarities of stages of development. His warnings against artificial frustration of the natural sex drive were certainly contrary to the prevailing ethic, but on the other hand, his discussion of the role of women was eminently conventional and potentially retrogressive. Individuals could follow the precepts set forth in the *Rapports* allowing them to adjust regimen to temperament, occupations, and climate. In addition, public health officials could assess the dangers of alcohol and drugs, and legislators might attempt to calculate realistically the possibility of human modification of climate or to mitigate the socially unequal access to choices of climate and regimen. But most of these implications were left to the interpretation of the reader. The *Rapports* was intended as a work of science, and the only explicit recommendations were matters of clinical or psychosomatic medicine for a professional audience.

Reactions to the Rapports

Unfortunately for Cabanis, the reaction to the *Rapports* was usually as much a matter of doctrine as of science. The Idéologue circle certainly was favorable to the Institute memoirs as well as to the complete edition published in 1802. And in the spring of 1800, the grammarian and writer François Thurot saluted the Institute memoirs in *La Décade philosophique* as a "positive science of morals." He wistfully hoped that there could be increased ability to predict "revolutions in the moral order" as there already was predictability for the physical world of nature.[74] A subsequent initialed review of the *Rapports* in *La Décade* exceeded Cabanis's claims by hailing the ability of mankind to "neutralize primitive dispositions" and "denature the most decided temperaments."[75] In 1805 the Idéologue physician and biographer of Cabanis, Jacques-Louis Moreau de La Sarthe, announced his confidence that studies like the *Rapports* would hasten the progress of medicine, legal medicine, and "physiological philosophy."[76] Physiologists such as Cabanis's disciple Richerand and the Montpellier vitalist Charles-Louis Dumas both drew on the *Rapports* for their textbooks.[77] And in 1808 the former Idéologue protégé Maine de Biran indicated that ten years earlier, he had been fascinated by the *Rapports*, although he was revolted by the stomach-brain analogy and already thought that Cabanis used a "metaphor" as if it were a "thesis of physics."[78]

Certainly the *Rapports* had its detractors even during the Directory. In a pamphlet of 1797, the distinguished literary critic La Harpe attacked atheistic, materialistic works that reduced "spiritual faculties to physical sensitivity."[79] And in the education debates in the Council of Five Hundred in 1799, the moderate Grenoble lawyer Pison-du-Galland warned against a godless educational system and caricatured materialism as a philosophy "confounding soul and body, which would make of us a machine, ruled like the animal by the impulse of fleeting appetites; which makes our will a passive instrument of chance, a blind collision of the elements."[80]

In the early years of the Consulate, the Catholic revival spurred heated critiques from the political Romantics. Chateaubriand's *Genius of Christianity* (1802) railed against hypocritical moralists who, in denying the spirituality of the human soul, undermined the foundation of virtue: "Our recent *idéologues*, in separating the history of the human mind from the history of things Divine," would neglect the theological purpose of all metaphysics. Every correlation of body and soul only proved to Chateaubriand the triumph of the spiritual "celestial flame" against physical constraints.[81]

Similarly, in 1818 the ultraconservative political theorist Louis de Bonald laboriously defended the view that man is an "intelligence served by organs" against Cabanis's view that man is a corporeal being whose organs produce intelligence. In suicide or war, de Bonald argued, the soul could order destruction of the organism. Cabanis's materialism "ruins morals without being useful for physics, and can only profit atheism." Without the immortal soul, "reason would cease its activity, even the passions all their illusions; there would be no more honorable enterprises, noble projects, high hopes, consolations for misfortune, restraint in prosperity, and all society, struck dead, would immediately cease, like a river whose waters were frozen by cold."[82]

To philosophical critics as well as political opponents, the "materialism" of the Idéologues appeared their most detestable conviction. The battle over materialism was also, of course, the battle over free will, moral responsibility, and effective social controls. Critics in their haste to attack sometimes created the illusion that the Idéologues were a more coherent movement than they actually were.

Cabanis and Destutt de Tracy

Certainly the two Idéologue leaders, Cabanis and Destutt de Tracy, had common goals. They both followed the basic teaching of Condillac that held that all mental processes derived from sensation, and they accepted the validity of Condillac's rules of analytic method, which led to decomposition and recomposition of mental faculties by Tracy and the development of analysis in medicine by Cabanis. Both parted company with Condillac and with religious orthodoxy in refusing to postulate an immaterial soul. And both wished to update Condillac by supporting his notion of sensation upon a physiological basis. Cabanis and Tracy also shared ethical and political positions unacceptable to Catholic conservatives—such as the deduction of individual natural rights from sensitive human nature. Conservatives could certainly not accept their common concern to found a secular, natural morality and to teach it, along with other branches of Ideology, in the public schools.

Cabanis and Tracy paid high tribute to each other and consid-

ered that they were engaged in a common enterprise. In 1802 a
letter of Maine de Biran affirmed that "the two friends seem to
have only one opinion in everything, they live only for their
household and their dear *ideology*, whose progress interests
them above all."[83] In 1801 Tracy himself announced his desire
to dedicate his *Projet d'élémens d'idéologie* to a "true friend to
whom I am particularly indebted for what may be good in my
writing."[84] In 1805 he admitted that, fearing unfavorable criticism, he had not yet disclosed the friend's identity. In the
Logique he dedicated the first three volumes of the *Elémens
d'idéologie* to Cabanis and thanked him for "fruitful" conversa-
tion and early access to unpublished sections of the *Rapports*.
He added, "The success which I most prize, is that my work
may be inscribed a consequence of yours, and that you yourself
may see in it only a corollary of the principles you have expounded."[85]

While Tracy constantly invoked the primacy of physiology
and continually attempted to use physiological evidence, he
sometimes departed from Cabanis's interpretations. The differences may have seemed negligible to adversaries but they certainly altered the message of the *Rapports*. Tracy gradually assimilated the physiology of internal impressions. In his memoir
of 1796, he recognized that some "pains or pleasures" in the
"interior of our body" were also "true sensations." Moreover,
he claimed, involuntary, unlearned movements, such as an infant's sucking, were in the category of "un je ne sais quoi
properly called, without attempting to explain it, *instinctive determination*."[86] In the *Idéologie* of 1801, Tracy seemed more
confident and explicit in his physiology. He equated the simple
feelings of "primary desires" with "internal sensations," such
as "colic, hunger, thirst, stomach ache, headache, dizziness, the
pleasures caused by all natural secretions, the pains of their disturbances or suppression." In short, organic function and dys-
function produced internal sensations. Later, he argued that
one did not perceive some movements because of habit; this was
somewhat at variance with Cabanis's view that some involuntary movements were controlled by subcenters outside the

brain. More pointedly, Tracy asserted that there was no difference in the simple sensation of the joyous state caused by good news or a glass of wine or of the pain caused by a stomachache or sad circumstances. Here, Tracy seemed to slide beyond what Cabanis intended, for he concluded that the pleasant or painful state of any passion, such as love or hatred, was also a true internal sensation.[87] His usage seemed to hark back to Descartes's catalogue of internal senses. Cabanis had argued that organic dispositions affect ideas and passions (fitness to meditate, for example) but he did not merely equate an internal impression with a passion, which was a resultant of impressions, memories, and judgments. Passions may have had instinctive origins but, for Cabanis, they were not merely instincts nor merely simple sensations.

In 1801 Tracy more boldly stated that "vital force" (as in the muscles) "can be represented only as the result of attractions and chemical combinations that, for a time, give birth to an order of particular facts, and soon, by unknown circumstances, return under the control of the more general laws of unorganized matter."[88] There was an analogy to Cabanis's theory of orders of affinity in this view, but none of Cabanis's subtle warnings on the irreducibility of life to inert matter. Tracy, after all, was not so deeply indebted to Montpellier medicine.

Cabanis and Tracy no doubt influenced each other on the problem of an individual's discovery of the external world. In 1796 Tracy had maintained that the faculty of motility in the subject and the resistance of external objects gave knowledge beyond mere perceptions. Cabanis meanwhile reduced sensitivity in the fetus to impressions almost entirely internal in nature, though he believed that there were rudimentary "inclinations and determinations" even in the fetus. By 1801 Tracy had adjusted his views to make knowledge depend on sensations of voluntary movement, which preceded sensations of resistance. Cabanis, for his part, agreed in 1802 that effort and resistance were fundamental to knowledge, though the weight of the fetus's own members would be sufficient to produce this sense of effort, hence a rudimentary will, an incipient *moi*. Thus,

Tracy made the idea of will somewhat more corporeal, while Cabanis adjusted his terminology to take into account Tracy's emphasis on resistance.[89]

Yet Tracy also supported physiological interpretations different from those of Cabanis. When he praised the physiologist-philosopher Pinel for admiring Ideology, he called the art of curing the demented equivalent to "manipulating the passions and directing the opinions of ordinary men; it consists in forming their habits." Tracy stressed the psychotherapeutic aspects of Pinel's "moral treatment," which later fascinated other Idéologue physicians, such as Alibert and Moreau de La Sarthe. Cabanis certainly advocated change in regimen and occupational therapy for the insane, but he was most confident in the use of physical agents to affect physical dispositions. Tracy's brief reference to Pinel's work endorsed a physiological approach about which Cabanis had considerable reserve.[90]

In the *Logique*, Tracy's aim of perfecting rational instruments revealed some concern with the obstacles created by the body. Errors in human judgment, argued Tracy, came from the distortion of pure ideas by accessory impressions at different times, leading to lapses of memory and flawed comparisons. But these accessory impressions came precisely from the "predominance of action of certain organs," from the variations of sensitivity caused by age, sex, temperament, and illness. Tracy saw the only antidote to such influences in separating accessory impressions from the pure idea, or the reason or good sense that all men share. Unfortunately, men were often unaware of the distorting impressions and therefore subject to illusion. Men were commonly victims of their passions, and in extreme cases of true delirium and madness, the distortions inhibited sound reasoning.[91]

Of course, Cabanis would have agreed that analytic method must be the same in all climates and for all regimens. A logic had to stress the uniform in human reason, not the diverse. But Tracy introduced the variable influences on sensitivity as if they were so many threats to a sound mind, so many unwelcome distractions. To Cabanis, individual diversities were the given, the

invaluable guideposts for the effort of the physiologist and philosopher to sharpen the reasoning ability of an individual and to
moderate his passions. Age, sex, temperament, and illness were
not foggy lenses obscuring clear ideas; they furnished themselves an accurate index of peculiarity from which the physician
could deduce a personalized corrective prescription. The physiological, so basic to Cabanis, seemed an intrusion rather than a
foundation for the *Logique* of Tracy.

Finally, in the introduction to his unfinished ethical treatise
published in 1815, Tracy tried anew to base ethics on physiology but in the process, he abandoned Cabanis's project of affecting internal impressions. After borrowing the descriptions of
the behavior of bees from the naturalist Constant-Duméril,
Tracy resorted to the terminology of the anatomist and physiologist Xavier Bichat (1771-1802) to distinguish human organic
life (respiration, circulation, digestion, secretion, excretion)
from human animal life (sensation, movement, speech, and
reproduction—though Bichat placed reproduction separately).[92]
Admitting the analogy to the ancient distinction of animal and
rational souls, Tracy ascribed the well-known phenomena of
moral conflict to the diverse passions fostered by each kind of
life. "Organic life," or the "life of conservation," for the most
part involuntary and controlled by the spinal cord and the
ganglionic system, produced the instinctive inclinations and the
disposition toward self-interest, which often conflicted with the
interests of others. "Animal life," or the "life of relation," for
the most part voluntary and controlled by the brain, fostered
the inclination to sympathize with fellow human beings. While
Tracy did not decry self-interest as such, he expected the
moralist to accentuate the "benevolent passions" while mitigat-
ing the harmful consequences of conflicting interests.[93]

Tracy was certainly following a long Enlightenment tradition
in distinguishing self-love and benevolence, though he was
more pessimistic than most eighteenth-century moralists in opposing the two inclinations. Cabanis certainly never underesti-
mated the power of self-interest, though he thought it would
easily be "enlightened" to serve others. More important, when

Cabanis spoke of cultivating moral sympathy, he optimistically noted its basis in instinctive animal affinity. Thus, moralists could use regimen and climate to favor a change in temperament most conducive to moral sympathy. In Tracy's schema, which was also used in Richerand's physiology in 1802, instinctive and rational life would be in constant conflict. By placing the best hope of virtuous conduct in acting upon the life of relation, Tracy swept away Cabanis's hopes for moral perfectibility through physiology—affecting the brain through the dispositions of internal organs. For Cabanis, the organism was unified. Some instincts were self-conserving, but others were social, and both could affect the conscious life of relation. Cultivation of the social instincts was intended to be an important task of the science of man.

Perfect coherence among the Idéologues would have been as difficult as a consensus today in a learned symposium on the human condition among a panel including a physiological psychologist, a physical anthropologist, an educational psychologist, a psychotherapist, and a philosopher of the mind. But the diversities in expression and emphasis between Cabanis and Tracy were nonetheless real because they were both labeled materialists by adversaries. The Rational Ideology of Tracy had an even less physiological allure in the studies of Degérando, Laromiguière and Maine de Biran. The latter philosopher began by taking Cabanis quite seriously and ended as a convert to Catholic dualism. The Physiological Ideologists, for their part, were physicians who attempted with varying success to generate some interest in the broader connotations of a science of man. When external and official hostility to Ideology proved more formidable than internal incoherence, the effort to combine Rational and Physiological Ideologies would be stillborn.

Despite the difficulties of the Idéologue circle, a remarkable literature on psychophysiology and its implications for human perfectibility arose between 1796 and 1802. Cabanis's *Rapports* was one of the most important treatises in a collection of works that stressed the power of habit. The works of the medical Idéologues Pinel and the lesser-known Alibert, Richerand, and

Moreau de La Sarthe, the early works of the philosopher Maine de Biran, and the outstanding anatomical and physiological works of the surgeon Bichat all brought attention to the problem of using analysis in medicine to attempt to found a science of man and to understand the range and limitations of human capacities.

CHAPTER IX

Approaches to Psychophysiology

The Medical Idéologues: Pinel

hile the medical literature on tempera-
ment had always encouraged *physique-
moral* comparisons, the goals of the
Idéologue leaders stimulated parallel efforts by their colleagues. Cabanis himself
never created a "school," but his *Rapports* helped provoke
a cluster of studies on the power of habit and perfectibility.
The same philosophical and medical issues that fascinated
Cabanis—the place of man in nature, the usefulness of analytic
method in the human sciences, and the irreducibility of life—
helped shape the framework of these investigations.

The younger physicians in the Idéologue circle of Auteuil had
a less rigidly unitary view of the organism than Cabanis. They
were more cautious than he about the use of physical regimen
and climate as a means of regulating not only the physical temperament but also the elevation and energy of ideas. Philippe
Pinel's pioneering clinical work with the mentally ill suggested
to physicians, as well as to Tracy, the power of habit through
psychological conditioning as well as through physical agents.
And the sophisticated physiology of Xavier Bichat, who was not
really an Idéologue, suggested a division between most internal
organs and the central nervous system that challenged
Cabanis's hope to improve temperament.

While the younger Idéologues accepted the validity of Condillacian empiricism and analytic method in medicine, they also
stressed the vitalist aspect of Cabanis's Montpellier heritage and

refused to discard the fundamental division in the Chain of Being between body and soul. Divergent metaphysical assumptions prevented the cooperation necessary to establish a science of man. The human perfectibility envisaged by the younger Idéologues did not necessarily extend to political liberalism in the fashion of Cabanis and Tracy.

Certainly the most impressive methodological model for the younger generation was the most distinguished physician in the Auteuil circle, Philippe Pinel (1745-1826). Introduced by Cabanis and Roussel to Mme Helvétius, Pinel always remained devoted to analytic classification of disease. We have previously noted his similarity to Cabanis in citation of Hippocratic works, in his emphasis on case histories to determine essential symptoms, and in his remarkably parallel approach to the history of medicine. When Pinel applied the principles of his *Nosographie* of 1798 to ''species'' of mental illness, he followed Tracy's subdivisions of the faculty of thought. Convinced that there was no one principle of the mind, Pinel believed, contrary to Condillac, that medical evidence justified a separation between the will and the understanding.[1]

Pinel chose to publish his first memoir on classification of mental illness in the periodical of a dynamic group of younger physicians and Paris medical students, the collection of the Société médicale d'émulation. Established 23 June 1796 by Bichat and the surgeons Jacques-Louis Moreau de La Sarthe and Jean Burdin, and enjoying the blessings of the Institute and the Interior Ministry, the Société was a means of diffusing medical knowledge no less prestigious than the Société de santé founded three months earlier by senior physicians in Paris. The sixty resident members included at least six medical Idéologues (Pinel, Alibert, Cabanis [who was inactive], Roussel, Moreau, and, in an VI [1797-1798], Richerand).[2] Alibert was the first secretary-general, Pinel was president in an VII (1798-1799), and Richerand was also an officer. Moravia has already stressed the commitment of this group to empiricism, although we cannot assume that the non-Idéologue majority gave priority to the aims of Cabanis. Elder physicians such as the School of Medicine dean Thouret, Cabanis's teacher Bosquillon, Fourcroy, and Barthez (as correspondent) later joined the group.

Pinel developed his views on mental illness in a memoir for the Société médicale d'émulation in 1800 and extended them later that year in his *Traité médico-philosophique sur l'aliénation mentale*. He announced his indebtedness to all "modern psychologists," including Locke, Harris, Condillac, Adam Smith (in Mme Condorcet's translation), and Dugald Stewart. He warned, however, that Locke and Condillac had not been physiological enough—that madness was not merely a matter of erroneous association of ideas. The "idéologistes" had begun to analyze the understanding, but there was still a need for a careful tableau of the "moral affections," in the fashion of the English physician Alexander Crichton. Only then would there be a full correlation of passions and physiology. He also warned against "metaphysical discussions and the digressions of idéologisme," which might hinder a strict "science of facts."[3] While Pinel thus accepted the point of departure of Tracy, he did not wish any nonmedical assumption to disturb his classification.

The species of mental illness included, first, "melancholia, or delirium without fury"—the domination of all of a patient's faculties by a particular fixed idea. Such a condition could lead to ardent enthusiasms or precipitate violent action but it could also produce a suicidal depression. Except for a specific obsession, the melancholic had other faculties of the understanding intact. The second category, "maniac fury without delirium," also left intact perception, judgment, imagination, and memory but produced profound disturbances of "affective faculties" and deep-seated impulses to violence. In lucid moments, however, the patient was quite coherent and rational. "Manias" could be periodic or continuous, and regular intermittent manias seemed the most difficult to cure. The third species, "mania with delirium," often periodic, almost always stemmed from an overexcited nervous system. It produced exaltation of passions and enthusiasm and sometimes the assumption of another identity but, if one allowed for the patient's erroneous premises and judgments, it did not disturb the coherent reasoning of the patient. The fourth species, "dementia," paralyzed the thinking faculties, disturbed the relationship of ideas to external objects, and produced superficial and disparate emotions, often with incoherent babbling, crying, and agitation. Finally, the often congenital "idiotism" resulted in a stupor of all affective and intellectual capacities, with poor external sensitivity and little speech. Like Cabanis, Pinel admitted that cranial malformation could cause "idiotism," but a profound psychological shock could have similar results.[4]

In fact, the provoking factor had no direct relation to the species or severity of mental illness. Pinel cited Cabanis in arguing that insanity was sometimes only an extreme manifestation of aspects of a normal sanguine temperament. After many dissections, though, Pinel concluded that organic lesions were neither necessary nor sufficient for mental illness. Nor could the relation in some cases of mental illness to cranial capacity lead to the dangerous assumption of the incurability of most cases.[5] The nosology of mental illness implied treatment adjusted to each species. And just as hospital reformers had emphasized the segregation of patients according to disease, Pinel recommended that asylum directors separate the species of mental disease. In particular, convalescents must not observe those who suffered fits, and idiots and epileptics required isolation.[6]

Pinel certainly indicated that there was no possible justification for the indiscriminate Hôtel-Dieu routines of baths, bleeding, and purging, since patients without organic lesions would be unlikely to benefit from such uniformly applied physical remedies. In fact, Pinel advocated three broad categories of therapy. First, he recommended a "medical treatment," with purgatives, such as decoctions of chicory with magnesium sulfate, to prevent fits and to assist some melancholics, and antispasmodics, such as camphor, opium, or cold baths, to relieve prolonged or violent fits, especially in mania without delirium. Second, Pinel, like Cabanis, advocated a "physical regimen" to break an unhealthful pattern of habits. Proper diet, comfortable room temperatures, and occupational therapy would strengthen the natural healing process in the body and help counteract the dominance of melancholic fixed ideas. Work would occupy the calm moments of periodic maniacs and would be a substitute for someone whose "state of fortune seemed to prohibit a change of climate."[7] Pinel, too, thought that mania might be linked to "errors and illusions of ignorant credibility," such as fears of hellfire or belief in miracles, oracles, or possession by demons. A consistent occupation might put an end to the excesses of contemplative devotion.[8] Third, except in cases of idiotism or periodic manias, however, Pinel characteristically insisted on the use of "moral philosophy" to reason with the patient and to change his environment. The precedent set by the English Quaker brothers Tuke at their "retreat" for the mentally ill at York, as well as the work of Crichton, no doubt helped influence Pinel's choice of methods. Pinel stated his preference for the moral maxims of Plato, Plutarch, Seneca, Tacitus, and Cicero over all the artful pharmaceutical formulas of tonics and antispasmodics. He ruefully added that this approach worked best for "cultivated minds." But he still had such confidence in the resources of nature that he would use drugs "only when the insufficiency of moral remedies is proven to me." Even where drugs were needed, the moral treatment might enhance their effects. Its essence was "counteracting the human passions by others of equal or superior force." The use of guile and flattery, and even an apparatus inspiring fear, by an ingenious supervisor would benefit a mentally disturbed patient. A "wise and energetic repression" might be necessary where gentleness would not suffice, but never harsh or inhumane treatment.[9]

Pinel was willing to experiment with the use of drugs on rarely curable melancholia, dementia, and idiotism. But Cabanis placed more hope in the use of physical agents to redirect the dispositions of a center of sensitivity and even, if possible, to cure organic lesions. In Cabanis's view, physical agents followed more reliably known laws than any moral treatment. Hence, Pinel's place seems secure as a forerunner of psychotherapy, while Cabanis's legacy is entirely to psychosomatic medicine.

Alibert: The Power of Habit

Pinel's "moral therapeutics," based on a theory of the passions and the conditioning of habit, clearly impressed the younger generation of Idéologues, including the surgeon of the Hôpital Saint-Louis, Jean-Louis Alibert (1766-1837). From a judicial family of Rouergue, Alibert came to the Ecole normale in 1795, met Cabanis, Roussel, and Bichat as a student at the School of Medicine (1795-1799), and later became a noted dermatologist. In the first volume of the memoirs of the Société médicale d'émulation, Alibert argued that medicine could profit much by cooperating with metaphysics and with a "history of sensations, ideas, and passions." He repeatedly praised Condillac's empiricism, though he avoided a radical reduction of mental faculties to transformed sensation. Indeed, he affirmed that "man is endowed with an intellectual principle" that "reflects and combines." At the same time, he recognized that useful mental habits were not merely an educational matter. Like Cabanis, he rejected Helvétius's cultural theory of the mind, affirming that temperament kindled both passions and genius; consequently, medical knowledge, to Alibert, would refute the "system of that philosopher who recently did not hesitate to relate all [mental differences] to the different occupations, choice of methods, or chance circumstance."[10] Alibert ventured the thought that the greatest creations of the human mind "relate to an as yet undiscovered radical energy of the sensitive system."

Alibert wrote a long essay explicitly on the power of habit as the "major phenomenon and primary instrument of the human economy." Going beyond Cabanis's claims, Alibert thought habits of diet and exercise could "triumph even over temperaments" and "mold, after a fashion, the *physique* upon the *moral*." Like Volney, he thought adaptation to circumstances limited climatic effects on temperament. But he acknowledged that habit formation in childhood was undeniably important and that a consistently moderate regimen could temper the effects of strong passions. Thus, Alibert was certainly a partisan of physical remedies. He warned physicians that habit could mask disease by imparting new symptoms and that habit in chronic ailments could nullify the effects of repeatedly prescribed medication. The wise physician would consider habit in his diagnosis and therapy. In fact, Alibert speculated that the distraction from certain habitual dispositions was probably responsible for certain spectacular cures, such as the exploits of Mesmer.[11]

Alibert's discussion of habit bore the imprint of the Montpellier medical theory on sympathies. He hoped that physicians would one day unveil the mystery of organic sympathies independent of the nerve network. He cited favorably the "Note on Sympathy," published the previous year by his colleague Pierre Roussel, who believed that "sympathies may be for animate beings what attractive and chemical affinities are for inanimate matter, the link uniting organs destined to form a society."[12] For Alibert, too, organic dispositions and the imitative propensities they encouraged were a hidden source of self-improvement and sociability. Alibert thus endorsed a version of Cabanis's theory of orders of affinity. He did not hesitate to proclaim as a medical aspiration to "perfect men for governments," just as statesmen must "perfect governments for men."[13]

Alibert was a less radical philosopher than Cabanis, however; he had never been a metaphysical monist. His *Physiologie des passions* (1825) explicitly warned against knowing man by his "organic envelope" and placed the "foundations of ethics in the soul."[14] Alibert always echoed something of the sentimental deism of his friend Bernardin de Saint-Pierre. Many nonmaterialists were discontented under the Restoration. By contrast, Alibert had become sufficiently eminent to serve as *médecin ordinaire* to Louis XVIII and Charles X, and, as a loyal servant of the elder Bourbons, he lost his position at Court after the Revolution of 1830. Thus, his Condillacian empiricism and belief in perfectibility did not inevitably lead him to liberalism or republicanism.

Richerand: Conservative Empiricist

Similarly, Balthasar-Anthelme Richerand (1779-1840) was both a follower of Cabanis and later a political ultraconservative. He came from a family of such modest fortune that he could not afford the fees for the doctorate, and in 1804 the Interior Minister Chaptal granted him a special fee exemption. Richerand studied at the Paris School of Medicine from 1796-1798 and thereafter offered private lectures in physiology. His successful physiology text (1801) and the patronage of Cabanis and Fourcroy launched his remarkable career. In 1802 he became assistant chief surgeon at Saint-Louis and, at age twenty-eight (1807), the government appointed him professor of external pathology at the Paris Faculty, despite the candidacy of the distinguished clinician Dupuytren.[15]

Richerand's physiology shared many of the tenets of Alibert on the power of habit. He too was concerned about decreased sensitivity to drugs and the general physiological principle that habit eventually weakens both painful and pleasurable sensations. On the modifiability of man, Richerand took a curious middle-of-the-road position: "Social education," he agreed, could alter character, though most often character was the effect of organization. Like Tracy later, he saw a struggle of instinctive against rational determinations but Richerand added the struggle against the "received ideas of convention, duty, religion." Passions, he thought, were not mere organic appetites, but intellectual elaborations of basic desires. He accepted Cabanis's temperament classification and agreed on the possibility of acquired temperaments. He also agreed that age, sex, illness, climate, and sensitive-muscular balance differentiated sensitivity, and even that physical causes were predominant in insanity.

Richerand was thus ready to accept the basic Idéologue tenets. He matter-of-factly acknowledged that "all phenomena of the understanding stem from physical sensitivity," and that the "physical retains the mental in a strict and necessary dependence." He accepted the possible influence of internal impressions on reason, and he was unafraid to cite Cabanis's analogy of the action of the brain on impressions to the action of the stomach on food.[16] In 1802 he referred the reader for further discussion of mental faculties to Tracy's *Projet d'élémens d'idéologie*. All of these statements remained in the tenth edition of his physiology text (1833), long after Ideology had ceased to be a vital philosophical movement. Yet even in 1802, Richerand had staunchly maintained the irreducibility of life and had called sensitivity a "faculty of the soul."[17] Empiricism and belief in strict physical-mental correlation were no indications of monism or materialism.

Like Alibert, Richerand flourished under the Restoration. Ennobled in 1815, he received the title of a baron and the post of consulting surgeon to Charles X in 1829. Apparently shaken by the Revolution of 1830, in 1833 he advised his readers that he was preparing a political essay, which finally appeared anonymously in censored form four years later as *De La Population dans ses rapports avec la nature des gouvernemens*. Though primarily concerned with the harmful effects of overpopulation and urbanization, Richerand penned a bitter diatribe against the "sophists" of the eighteenth century, including Rousseau and Montesquieu, and their doctrines of popular sovereignty. Despite his own rise from obscurity, Richerand lost no opportunity to condemn the power of the multitude, the influence of industrialists and bankers, the dangers of a free periodical press, and the parliamentary dominance of lawyers. Even the newly reestablished Academy of Moral and Political Sciences (1832) seemed to him an invitation to sedition. Thus, while still acknowledging Cabanis as his mentor in his physiology text, Richerand lapsed into a reactionary ultraroyalism, remote from the liberal politics of Cabanis, Tracy, Daunou, and Siéyès.[18] Idéologue aims sought to reconcile natural rights and free exercise of faculties with perfecting human nature through medicine, hygiene, and education, but the goal of increasing fitness for political participation had lost all appeal for Richerand in the tense social conditions of the 1830s.

Moreau de La Sarthe: The Use of the Passions

A more consistent application of Pinel's approach to the power of habit came from the hygienist, assistant librarian of the Paris School of Medicine, and biographer of Cabanis, Jacques-Louis Moreau de La Sarthe (1771-1826). A surgeon in a military hospital in Nantes in 1789, Moreau had to give up his practice because of a hand injury incurred in a surgical accident. Thereafter, he was absorbed by the theoretical and literary aspects of medicine. He attended Pinel's private lectures in comparative anatomy in 1792 at the Société d'histoire naturelle. Moreau's hygiene lessons at the Lycée républicain in 1799 confirmed his alignment with Physiological Ideology, and he wrote prolifically for *La Décade philosophique* from 1800 to its disappearance in 1807.

The ill-fated patron of the sciences Pilâtre de Rozier, victim of a balloon explosion, had established the Lycée in 1781. In 1785 the royal family gave official patronage to this center for public lectures in chemistry, anatomy, physics, and history. Surviving the Revolutionary turmoil, the Lycée had expanded its offerings by 1800 and boasted a distinguished faculty, including Cuvier in natural history, Roederer in political economy, and the young Idéologue Degérando in moral philosophy.[19] Moreau's course outline revealed a lively interest in the art of perfecting human nature by wise regimen and of assuring the ultimate improvement of the species.[20]

Early in 1801, more than a year before Cabanis inserted the term "anthropologie" in the Preface to the *Rapports*, Moreau designated two broad subdivisions of the science of man. First, "anthropologie physique" would encompass natural history of man and human anatomy; physiology, or the science of human organization; hygiene, or physiology applied to the preservation of human life; and medicine, or physiology applied to healing the sick. These categories were certainly compatible with

Cabanis's objectives in the *Rapports* and with Tracy's notion of Physiological Ideology. Secondly, an "anthropologie morale" was not remote from Tracy's schema of sciences related to Ideology, despite differences in subdivisions: "experimental division," or biography, history, and travellers' reports; ideology, or analysis of intellectual faculties; speculative ethics, or analysis of sentiments (Tracy would have unified the second and third categories); and applied ethics, leading to "public economy" and "legislation" (in modern terms, economics and political science).[21]

Interestingly enough, when Moreau established this schema in a review of Pinel's treatise on insanity, he placed Pinel's contribution in the "partie morale" of anthropology. Moreau was fascinated with the analysis of sentiments and he clearly sensed a divergence between the physiological focus of Cabanis and Pinel's delicate balance of passions. Like Pinel, Moreau explicitly emphasized the influence of the *moral* on the *physique*, the "history of feelings," which he classified as profound "passions," fleeting "emotions," and "affections." Moreau hoped for some objective index to feelings. He found a plausible guide in the attempt of the Swiss physician Lavater to relate character and temperament to facial features and expression, the art of physiognomy. From 1805 to 1809, Moreau annotated a ten-volume edition of Lavater, adding a historical introduction on physiognomy since the Renaissance and a description of the recent study of Gall on cranial configurations. In 1803 Moreau also undertook a *Histoire naturelle de la femme*, with systematic classification of feminine passions and a catalogue of the effects of anger, fright, and similarly intense feelings on respiration, circulation, and digestion.

Moreau expected "mental remedies" to be useful in both physical and psychological ailments. "Courage," he claimed, "protects from contagious disease; the fanaticism of martyrs makes them nearly insensitive to the cruelest torments; and confidence in any medication whatsoever appears to be the only specific for hydrophobia."[22] Moreau thus wished to expand Cabanis's therapeutic approach to use of the *moral* to

perfect the *physique*. In his sketch of Cabanis under the heading
"Moral" in the medical section of the *Encyclopédie
méthodique*, Moreau was quite appreciative of Cabanis's
work.[23] He disdained some earlier efforts to alleviate mental
disturbance, however. For example, he called Le Camus's
hygiene "ridiculous" and thought it rightfully mocked in Voltaire's *Dictionnaire philosophique*: "Ah! M. Camus! Vous
n'avez pas fait avec esprit la médecine de l'esprit."[24] On the
other hand, he approvingly cited the case histories of Pinel's
moral treatment. Like Alibert, Moreau foresaw political consequences to the new art: hygiene would present government
with a "physiological theory of ethics and happiness."[25] And
like Cabanis, he prophesied that improved therapies would
achieve a long-term physical education of the species.

Bichat: The Immutability of Organic Life

The most original contemporary physiologist, Xavier Bichat
(not properly a member of the Auteuil circle despite Picavet's
label), a surgeon and pupil of Desault at the Paris Hôtel-Dieu,
adopted an outlook that directly limited the range of *moral-
physique* interactions.[26] Not only did he deny the feasibility of
Cabanis's program to use physical agents to educate the mind;
he also cast doubts on Moreau's plans to use the passions to influence physiology.[27]

Bichat's recognized skill as a pathological anatomist and
pioneer in the interpretation of autopsies lent significance to his
remarks on habit. Tracy did not hesitate to adapt Bichat's
physiology to ethics. And the social theorist Saint-Simon established three categories of specialization of skills—motor, rational, and emotive—which corresponded to Bichat's division
of animal functions.[28] Later Auguste Comte, who adopted
Bichat's rigorous separation of the life sciences from physics
and chemistry, assigned him a place of honor in the Positivist
Calendar.[29]

The well-known definition of life as the "totality of functions
resisting death" firmly aligned Bichat with the legacy of Stahl

and the Montpellier vitalists. Like the clinicians suspicious of the accessory sciences, Bichat insisted that physiology be independent of mathematical methods (to the point of contesting the value of the Lavoisier-Laplace measurements of animal heat).[30] But even so redoubtable an opponent of obscurantist vitalism as Claude Bernard acknowledged that Bichat's label "vital properties" was genuinely descriptive and physiological rather than a refusal to explain or a mystical invocation.[31]

Yet Bichat broke with the Montpellier clinicians on the traditional Hippocratic notion of unity in the organism. He divided the Hippocratic circle of life into two functionally distinct semicircles at the diameter of consciousness and voluntary control. True, the two basic vital properties, sensitivity and contractility, were manifest in both sectors, in the "organic life" of the ganglionic nervous system and internal viscera, and in the "animal life" of the cerebral nervous system and the brain. But organic life was fully active from birth, while animal life alone was educable by habit.[32]

In discussing sensitivity and contractility, Bichat cited Cabanis only once—on the imperfect organic life of the human fetus.[33] Bichat was, in fact, somewhat insouciant toward his learned physiological predecessors; he never mentioned Haller, although he did acknowledge Aristotle and Buffon. Cabanis complained in 1802 that Bichat borrowed ideas from the Institute memoirs without citing them.[34] But Bichat's reluctance to cite Cabanis might have been more deliberate than inadvertent, for Bichat used Cabanis's premise of *physique-moral* relationships to reach markedly different conclusions.

Like Cabanis, Bichat noted the effect of the physical conditions of internal organs upon the passions and he briefly mentioned the influence of sex, climate, and the seasons on animal life. His theory of aging could have had educational applications. Bichat would have directed children to music and drawing because of the predominance of nervous sensitivity in their temperaments; and he would have taught the "sciences of nomenclature" and the arts to adolescents imbued with a lively imagination and retentive memory, while he would have postponed teaching the exact sciences until students reached an age when their judgment was mature. Bichat thought all men occupied a place on a continuum of constant available energy divided among animal functions, so that strength of one organ or system presupposed weakness of the others. Varying Cabanis's contrast of sensitive and muscular temperaments, Bichat distinguished the predominantly sensitive from the active or rational, and hence inspired Saint-Simon's triadic division of sensitive poets and priests, active administrators and workers, and rational scholars and scientists.[35]

Bichat added his prestigious voice to the views of Pinel and Moreau on the effect of passions upon physical functions. Anger, joy, and fear all caused changes in circulation, secretion, respiration, and digestion. Bichat also agreed with Cabanis that affections of the internal organs would cause sympathetic reactions in a part of the brain. Consequently, involuntary muscle spasms and facial expressions may show how the passions appropriate the sphere of animal life. To Bichat, character was precisely the relative ease with which the active, willing brain regained control over fits of passion.[36]

In contrast to Cabanis, Bichat never suggested improvement of the human species through manipulation of the physiological influences on mental life or through direction of the inevitable physiological effects of passion. For Bichat, the superiority of human reason and judgment that was cultivated in the mind, indeed all the grandeur and perfectibility of man, was a development of animal life. Even so, not all phenomena of animal life were salutary. Habit did indeed perfect the judgment, but also progressively weakened the feelings of pleasure and pain. "Inconstancy" and the insatiable desire for novel sensations were thus unfortunate consequences of our "natural organization."[37]

While repetition of external stimuli affected the higher faculties, habit did not control organic life. Bichat admitted that habits might modify tastes and desires and he obscurely mentioned unnamed medical works "considering the influence [of habit] from different viewpoints than I have." But he believed it

257

fortunate for human survival that organic life needed no education. Those functions such as hunger and excretion which acquired periodicity and a semblance of habit occurred at mucous membranes endowed with a *tact interne* analogous to the sensitivity of animal life.[38] On the other hand, the predominance of an organic system constituting temperament and the equilibrium of reason and passion constituting character were fixed with the "primitive structure of the parts." Bichat continued, "Because, as we have seen, both the physical temperament and moral character belong to organic life, they are not at all susceptible to change by the education which modifies so prodigiously the actions of animal life." Education might therefore moderate character, but it would never completely alter it. A physician would be pursuing a chimerical aim if he attempted to change character by controlling organic life: "he might as well try to change the force of contraction of the heart or the arterial pulse."[39]

The therapist could never aspire, then, to the creation of those acquired temperaments that Cabanis thought to be the goal of hygiene. In fact, Bichat concluded that if the fleeting, involuntary, sympathetic dispositions of internal organs were as influential upon animal life as were the habits of conscious sensation, we would be the "perpetual plaything of our surroundings," with our existence plummeting from that of "brute bodies" to a condition superior to our present state and thus allying the "most impressive features of intelligence with the vilest aspects of matter."[40]

In Bichat's view, the two-fold nature of man, *homo duplex*, in Buffon's words, preserved human dignity. Organic life and the merely sensitive elements of animal life were passive, while the brain was active only as a willing organ. Passive cerebral reactions to internal organic states could not generate thought, ideas, or will. While disdaining knowledge of ultimate causes, Bichat readily wrote of "spontaneous motility" and called the brain the instrument of the soul, just as the senses were instruments of the brain.[41]

More carefully than some eighteenth-century vitalist physicians, Bichat preserved a distinct place for the rational soul while he explicitly consigned organic life to the merely passive, whatever its distinctions from the laws of ordinary matter. Bichat's breach in the circle of life had ethical as well as hygienic consequences. He warned, "Let us guard against using physical principles to subvert moral principles; they are both solidly based, even if sometimes opposed."[42] A natural morality might be facilely derived from the action of a single physiological principle in man, but the only sound morality would be based on the fundamental duality of body and soul.

Maine de Biran: The Activity of Will

While Bichat carefully pursued his physiological research, a young philosopher from the region of Bergerac (Dordogne), François-Pierre Maine de Biran (1766-1824), produced one of the most extensive studies distinguishing the passive faculties of the understanding and the active faculties of the will. Even before Biran read the works of the Idéologues, he became interested in the problems of Charles Bonnet's "experimental physics of the soul." His early Journal shows his awareness of the need to revise the nonmedical psychology of Condillac and Helvétius, as well as his awareness of some works of Montpellier physicians, such as Lacaze.[43] He too wished to relate the physical and mental while retaining a moral code. A royalist who was purged from the Council of Five Hundred in the coup of Fructidor (1797), Biran devoted the next nine years to philosophy. His personal ties with the Auteuil circle began on a visit to Paris in the summer of 1802 and continued through correspondence with Cabanis (1802-1807) and, at greater length, with Destutt de Tracy (especially from 1804 to 1814).

Biran seemed every bit as determined as Tracy to relate Physiological and Rational Ideologies. We have mentioned his ambivalent reaction to Cabanis's Institute memoirs in 1798. Less than a year later, at the end of 1799, he captured Idéologue attention with his entry in the prize contest of the analysis section of the Class of Moral and Political Sciences on the "influence of habit on the faculty of thought, or the effect produced by the frequent repetition of the same operations on each intellectual faculty."

In the manuscript draft of this "first memoir," nearly identical to the final version, Biran displayed both respectful obeisance to his judges and early signs of an independent perspective. Analyzing the state of the discipline, he wrote, "If the science of man is still in its cradle, if it appears to have been stationary for centuries, the cause is lack of communication and mutual assistance of specialized scholars who have each separately studied different parts of the microcosm."[44] Determined to achieve a synthesis of the views of Bonnet and Cabanis, Biran avowed that the "author of the 'Physiological History of Sensations'," (Cabanis) had opened up new vistas for observational "metaphysics" scarcely perceived by Condillac. He called Cabanis a "profound philosopher" who had demonstrated that "feeling, movement, and thought" were all manifestations of a single principle and "purely organic results of the activity of the sensitive system." Resting on the Newtonian explanation paradigm, Biran called physical sensitivity a "general fact" or "primary faculty," like attraction—nonmechanical, but governing all phenomena and laws of intelligent beings. To him, the parallelism in state of organs and images in the mind was enough to suggest a cause and effect relationship since any such relationship was no more than "concomitant or constant succession." Because the soul was a scientifically unknowable "occult principle," the causal relationship with the body did not threaten "spiritualists." In fact, he chided "absurd theologians" for accusing Helvétius of materialism when his view of the potential equality of minds could have been used as a defense of spiritualism.[45]

Biran was far from adopting Helvétius's position. He thought Cabanis excelled in distinguishing three kinds of sense-impressions and agreed that the disposition or lesion of internal organs was particularly important in inducing images in the mind and strengthening certain passions or giving energy to certain ideas. And he felt that Cabanis's idea of partial centers of sensitivity was a great improvement on Bonnet's emphasis on brain fibers. Biran also praised Cabanis for showing that the force of passions was related to age, sex, climate, and regimen.[46] Yet even here, Biran was careful to distinguish passive from active habits. This duality would later become the basis for his divergence from the Idéologues.[47]

While no memoir won the first prize contest, Biran received an honorable mention, which encouraged him to submit a revised manuscript in 1801 for the second contest on the same subject. A commission including Tracy as spokesman and Cabanis as a member awarded him the prize in 1802. Biran, however, substantially revised the manuscript again before its publication in 1803. He removed or condensed several sections dealing with purely physiological phenomena and especially with internal impressions. While a new analytical edition of the variants remains desirable, Henri Gouhier has shown that the modifications of 1799-1803 did not necessarily reveal a philosophical conversion to the dualist spiritualism later espoused by Biran in his other prizewinning "Memoir on the Decomposition of Thought" (1805).[48] Pierre Tisserand has already argued that the changes might simply have reflected the absence of Biran's previous need to flatter his judges, and no evidence contradicts this hypothesis.

The published memoir showed a sufficient enough change in Biran's notion of physical sensitivity to overshadow his obvious debt to Cabanis and Tracy. He now stated that, like Condillac and Bonnet, he wished to "transport physics into metaphysics . . . without disturbing any hope, or attacking any of those consoling opinions which help support the fragile happiness of life, or serve to protect from vice and to encourage virtue."[49] He shared Degérando's misgivings about ignoring mental activity. Indeed, in a letter addressed to Degérando in October 1802, Biran regretted "expressions apparently too materialist" even in the final text and insisted that he would not explain intellectual life by the "action of organs," as one might in a doctrine of a single faculty or of a "sensitive property" and "transformed sensations."[50] Rather, he wished to establish morality on the activity, freedom, and responsibility of a nonorganic *moi*.

Biran acknowledged in 1802 that his doctrine resembled Bichat's ideas. He noted that his "first memoir" had been in the archives of the Institute before publication of Bichat's *Recherches*, however, and that he had at the time been ignorant "even of Bichat's name."[51] Like Bichat, Biran called internal impressions (Bichat's "organic sensitivity") and the merely "affective" component of external sensation (taste, smell, heat, cold, pain) passive.[52] Bichat, however, had explained the weakening of affective sensations by habit through comparisons with previous states. For Biran, comparison required active perception, hence it required the muscular effort of attention and the instrument of the ego.[53] Therefore, the phenomenon of weakening sensation was not active comparison, but a passive reaction of the "radical forces" (in Barthez's words) of the sensitive principle to restore the "natural tone" of a sense-organ.

For Biran, the transmission of impressions and the reaction to them were not in themselves activities. Though he admitted that internal impressions were nonmechanical and showed a "real and characteristic action of the sensitive organ," they did not result in perceived effort. They were irrevocably passive and could not merely be transformed into free, active thought.[54]

Biran's emphasis on the indispensability of muscular effort in the organs for perception of self and the world stemmed both from Barthez's separation of motive and sensitive forces and from Tracy's view (1796) of motility as the link to external reality. In fact, Biran regretted Tracy's abandonment of this role for motility (1801), because motility seemed active to him while mere sensitivity was passive.[55] The focus of the eye, the association of hearing with the voice, the mobility of the tongue in taste, the active movement of touch all required intervention of the will. Without voluntary attention and motive determination, there would be no perception, no ideas, no memory, no signs, no thought.[56]

Biran thus developed a theory of habit analogous to the views of Bichat, though more philosophically sophisticated. Habit weakened most external sensations; but natural needs and instinctive determinations, which depended on noncerebral centers of sensitivity or induced sympathetic reactions in the brain, might be "independent, up to a certain point" of the power of habit. Regardless of previous fulfillment, the "appetitive senses" would be excited by genuine need. These needs would not weaken; instinctive determinations could not improve with exercise, however, and did not comprise a perfectible faculty of the species.[57]

Another variety of passive habits that did not weaken was persistent exalted states of the brain. Images and visions might become habitual by inducing certain dispositions in internal organs and sensitive centers that in turn maintained and strengthened the original delusion. Biran was not even averse to associating habitual fear of invisible powers with superstition. He seemed to derive his notion of internal impressions originating in the brain and nervous system more from Cabanis's second category of internal impressions than from Bichat's rigid distinction of animal and organic life. Still, Biran would not attribute cerebral activity to delusions.[58] In the draft memoir on habit, Biran had already considered the imagination passive. Later, in a marginal note added after his conversion to spiritualism, Biran pointed out that the effects of imagination on internal organs were, properly speaking, "an action of the physical upon the physical," and not an example of physical-mental relations. Only the reciprocal influence of internal organs upon the willing brain was an "action relevant to the discussion of mental-physical relations."[59]

In correspondence with Tracy, Biran asserted he could no more confuse instinctive determinations with the will than the "automatic tendency" of "elective affinity" with the "true choice of a being that feels and perceives."[60] Instinctive determinations and delusions consequently offered no guides to the educator who wished to perfect intelligence by teaching the use of artificial signs. Thus, Biran clearly took his distance from

Cabanis's monist metaphysic that gave the same ontological status to internal impressions and to the highest activity of thought. In the second section of his memoir, Biran dealt with truly active habits—the operations of memory and learning and the utility of signs and their role in language.[61]

Cabanis and Tracy valued Biran's work because of his consistent aspiration to relate physical and mental. In the summer of 1802, Cabanis sent Biran a copy of the *Rapports* and, in 1803, the reeditions of *Degré de certitude* and his essays on public assistance. He also encouraged Biran to send the memoir on decomposition of thought to the Institute despite the abolition of the Second Class. In 1805 Cabanis happily sent the news that Ginguené and Joachim Le Breton (both associated with *La Décade*) on the Class of History and Ancient Literature prize commission had helped assure Biran's victory. Already in letters to Tracy in 1804, Biran had edged toward separating Physiological and Rational Ideologies.[62] From 1805, like de Bonald and de Maistre after him, he maintained that the brain was merely an instrument of a "hyperorganic force" and that only the nonmaterial ego could be the substratum of intellect.[63] Still, Cabanis could write to Biran in 1805 that "though I do not always agree with you," the memoir on the decomposition of thought was a "beautiful and rich work" needing correction in detail rather than in general conception.

At the turn of the nineteenth century, a diverse group of physicians and philosophers shared the aspiration to formulate a science of man based on the power of habit. All except Bichat had personal ties to the Auteuil circle and could, at some stage in their careers, be considered Idéologues. Their works formed a rich intellectual context for Cabanis's *Rapports* as well as for Tracy's Rational Ideology. The entire group shared two basic aspects of Cabanis's approach to psychophysiology. First, all agreed on the applicability of some form of Condillacian analytic method to medicine and to the life sciences; and second, all followed the Montpellier tradition of refusing to submerge the life sciences in physics and chemistry and refusing to reduce physiology to mechanics. The physicians also granted a privileged position to clinical observation rather than to laboratory experiment. But none could completely follow Cabanis in his assumption of unity in the Great Chain of Being or a single active force in nature. Physical, organic sensitivity could thus not be transformed into thought without the active power of the soul. Nor could organic dispositions alone provide the key to the power of habit and perfectibility.

The power of physical regimen or wisely controlled passions should in principle have been empirically testable. Then Physiological Ideology would have been able to constitute itself as a science with a shared paradigm and eventually be transmitted in institutions that would create a professional community. But while modern psychologists have also not been able to agree on fundamental metaphysical assumptions, the disagreements in the early nineteenth century on the monist-dualist issue were too sharp to allow dispassionate scientific testing of substantive questions and formation of Idéologue disciples. Religious and moral convictions intruded upon interpretation of issues concerning active powers in the living body. Thus, despite the convergence in description of phenomena by eighteenth-century mechanist and vitalist physicians—a convergence leading to a quasi-vitalist monism—nineteenth-century materialists and spiritualists once again launched their bitter verbal battle.

The views of Alibert and especially of Richerand inspire caution about any assumption of an inevitable link between empiricist philosophy and liberal politics. Cabanis's heirs did not all extend the belief in individual perfectibility to a vision of a more enlightened society. All the more reason for interpreters to be suspicious of "necessary" implications of scientific or medical thought. Yet for Cabanis himself, the implications of the science of man unmistakably required social reform. Social harmony would be achieved in a dynamic context of increasing knowledge and more widespread political participation. As a philosopher, Cabanis was ceaselessly concerned with individual mental and physical equilibrium. And as an active political figure, Cabanis developed definite views on ways that government could help achieve social equilibrium in its attitude toward the professions, toward education, and toward the constitutional mechanism itself.

CHAPTER X

In the Public Arena: Healing, Schooling, Governing

Cabanis at the Paris School of Medicine

rom 1796 to 1802, at the height of Cabanis's philosophical career, he also achieved eminence in both the medical and political worlds. A loyal adherent of the regime of the Directory and an early enthusiast for Bonaparte, he offered characteristically subtle views on the state role in regulating medicine, insuring educational opportunity, and establishing stable institutions.

Cabanis's career profited much from the patronage of friends in high places, such as Ginguené, chief of the public education division of the Interior Ministry in 1796. With the removal of hygiene from the curriculum of the central schools and the consequent cancellation of Cabanis's appointment, only the annual Institute stipend of 1,200 francs, often in arrears, provided Cabanis's salaried income.[1] After one unsuccessful candidacy, the School of Medicine nominated Cabanis a second time on a short list of three candidates (26 August 1796) for the position of "assistant professor of advanced clinical medicine." Both the military physician Desgenettes of the Val-de-Grâce hospital and the subsequently renowned surgeon Larrey outdistanced Cabanis in the balloting. Yet Ginguené and the Interior minister recommended Cabanis, "whose talents are well-known," since Desgenettes was already placed, the full professor Dubois was a surgeon, and custom dictated choice of a physician as assistant. The Directory made the appointment official only on 29 December 1796, and Cabanis began to sign the next month for his 5,000-franc annual salary.[2] Three weeks after his appointment, he wrote his cousin, the Brive official Vermeil de Conchard, that he had accepted the position because of the delay in his Institute stipend and the "ruinous condition of my affairs."[3]

According to the school prospectus, Cabanis's duties included instruction at the "hospice de perfectionnement" (not actually inaugurated until 1799) in the study of rare or nervous disorders, visits with pupils to see patients, and exact journal-keeping, including the history and progress of the disease, method of treatment, and autopsy in case of death.[4] We know that in the spring of 1797 he promised to give a course in Hippocratic medicine, with lectures on the *Aphorisms, Epidemics,* and *Acute Diseases.*[5] The surviving texts of the opening and closing lectures, first published by the editor of his works François Thurot in 1825, continued to espouse the doctrines of *Degré de certitude* and *Coup d'oeil* on the suitability of Hippocrates for lessons in modern clinical medicine. But it remains doubtful that Cabanis actually taught, since shortly after his course was to begin, he asked for a leave of absence because of an "indisposition preventing him from coming to the school."[6] The next fall, on 29 November 1797, he requested the Assembly of Professors to grant him a transfer to the vacant chair of assistant professor (to Corvisart) of "internal clinical medicine."[7] Here, he had the no less onerous responsibilities of visiting twenty acute and chronic patients at the Hospice d'Unité and compiling continuing tables of weather and the nature of disease. While Cabanis presented *Degré de certitude* to the School of Medicine in late January 1798, there is no indication that he did any clinical teaching.[8]

Indeed, after his election to the Council of Five Hundred in April 1798, Cabanis was incapable of substituting for Corvisart when the full professor asked for a summer holiday. Only nine days after the opening of the clinical hospice (29 May 1799), Cabanis requested transfer (granted on 6 August) to the position of assistant professor in "legal medicine and history of medicine." Cabanis was certainly well prepared for the history of medicine portion of this course, and he would no longer be required to make hospital visits. But legal medicine was a wide-ranging field, dealing with the legal consequences of rape, pregnancy, impotence, abortion, suicide, infanticide, insanity, and advice to health officials on death certificates and epidemic prevention. Here, too, Cabanis's diligence is doubtful.

To be fair, from September 1798 to September 1804, he did not sign for his salary; and after his appointment to a well-paid senatorial seat, he attempted in January 1800 to yield his chair to his protégé Alibert, but the Assembly of Professors deferentially rejected the proposal. On 21 December 1803, Cabanis specifically requested, this time with success, that his salary be donated, one-third to the medical library budget (later earmarked for a digest of foreign medical literature by Moreau), one-third for a scholarship to a needy and distinguished student chosen by the school, and one-third for anatomical wax models.[9] While Cabanis was thus not open to the charge of outright neglect of duties, he certainly enjoyed the prestige of a title kept more by influence than by performance.

The Paris School of Medicine nevertheless felt grateful to Cabanis for being an articulate spokesman for its interests in the Council of Five Hundred debates on the medical profession and medical schools. Cabanis's plan for organizing medicine (22 June 1798) and for attaching medical schools to higher-education lycées (19 November 1798) remained close in spirit to the Mirabeau discourses of 1791.[10] Once again, Cabanis qualified a rigorously liberal view of government with the overriding need to maintain medical standards and protect public health.

Organization of the Medical Profession

Since 1791 the professional guilds of physicians and surgeons had ceased to exist in France. Despite the establishment of three medical schools in 1795, three years later there was still no legally accredited examination for medical certification. Military health officers and others lacking degrees from the old Faculties, inactive for the most part since 1792, had no formal professional status.[11] Partially in response to Directory messages of concern, Cabanis renewed efforts in June 1798 to establish at least a new statute for medical practitioners.[12] He proposed formal licensing of all physicians and surgeons, with suitable relaxation of examination standards for competent health officers who were long removed from their studies.

These seemingly innocuous suggestions created a storm of controversy in the Council of Five Hundred. The Toulouse physician Jean-Marie Calès, in the session of 1797, had agreed to a standard medical school curriculum and examination but he opposed legal penalties against "charlatans" on the grounds that the unscrupulous would evade them anyway.[13] In the 1798 session, the Lyon physician Louis Vitet reintroduced Calès's plan and charged that Cabanis had ignored its approval by the Council commission of public instruction.[14] Neither Calès nor Vitet was a neo-Jacobin but they implied that Cabanis was the spokesman for a privileged elite that wished to deny the newly acknowledged freedom to practice any profession.[15] Cabanis was certainly not on the most liberal side of the argument.

In November 1798, the Council commission of public instruction authorized Cabanis and Antoine-François Hardy to present a medical education report that attempted to preserve high standards in medicine without closing the profession to the less wealthy.[16] Cabanis insisted that there be no right to practice medicine or surgery without success in medical examinations (in French and without fees) at existing and projected medical schools. And he would not abandon the amalgamation of medicine and surgery, a cornerstone of all medical reform proposals since 1789. But, in line with a report to the comité de salubrité of 1790 and with Daunou's higher education plan of 1797, Cabanis proposed the creation of elementary medical instruction and teaching clinics in twenty civil hospitals, to be directed by chief health officers of the hospitals.[17] Vitet argued that instruction in anatomy, chemistry, and botany would be incompetent in the civil hospitals. The lack of examinations on the spot would turn the half-educated loose on the unsuspecting populace. Vitet preferred a shorter course for surgeons to assure a sufficient supply of qualified personnel for the less prosperous rural regions.[18]

Lacking definite legislative action, the Interior Ministry authorized the Paris School of Medicine, as well as the others, to hold examinations and grant provisional certificates of capacity by the fall of 1798.[19] Only under the Consulate in March 1803 was there a final resolution of the issue. Both Dean Thouret of the Paris School of Medicine and Fourcroy supported a law establishing two categories of practitioners—physicians and surgeons holding regular degrees, and health officers certified by department juries of physicians on the basis of a shorter course of study or years of clinical experience. Arguments for the law openly avowed a kind of social discrimination with the intention to confide the "extended class" of "industrious and active people" to the less qualified health officer.

Despite the interpretations of Foucault and Salomon-Bayet, such social discrimination was never implicit in Cabanis's defeated plan of June 1798. In his June speech, Cabanis did make concessions allowing a limited period for full certification of chief military health officers and other practitioners of known clinical competence but lacking credentials. But his November plan rested on the principle that examination and certification by professors of medicine would eventually apply to all, even the students at the elementary medical schools in civil hospitals. Only such certification would provide reputable physicians and surgeons.[20]

Government regulation actually seemed to be a less sensitive political issue in this debate than the alleged will to dominate and the internal laxity in Paris. Cabanis certainly opposed government intervention to assure equality of status for all medical schools. But for three legislative sessions, Calès, another physician Jean-François Barailon, and the suspected federalist Vitet attacked the "malevolent genius" that made the departments into satellites of Paris. All three physicians insisted on parity in the number of chairs at each institution and in a uniform, government-prescribed medical curriculum.[21] Furthermore, the Interior Ministry nominated professors to Paris vacancies after Faculty submission of a short list of three rather than after competitive examination. The attack by Calès, Barailon, and Vitet on favoritism and those who enjoyed titles without teaching could have been construed in part as a personal attack on Cabanis. Cabanis and Hardy could legitimately retort, however, that the Paris School of Medicine was overflowing with medical students and required a larger staff. They both remained dedicated to the principle of centers of excellence rather than institutional parity. Yet the Council commission relented to the political pressure from at least twelve cities that petitioned the Interior Ministry for medical schools.[22] Cabanis and Hardy recommended that Dijon, Poitiers, and Toulouse receive new medical schools attached to multidisciplinary lycées. But only Paris among the three existing medical schools would be attached to a lycée, and its more numerous staff would continue to represent the natural superiority of intellectual life in the capital.[23] Once again, artificial regulation would be intended to assure the free play of cultural equilibrium.

Of course, the issue of whether there was such a thing as reputable medicine as contrasted to the dangerous nostrums of charlatans is a separate question worthy of extended discussion with all the tools that the quantitative social historian can command. Several recent articles have begun to show the relative similarity in the kinds of treatments given by accredited practitioners and by "charlatans" and to raise the problem of how those with credentials may have acquired monopolistic professional authority unjustified by superiority in therapeutic resources at their command.[24]

Here, we are only dealing with the question of freedom versus regulation. Cabanis no doubt believed that medicine had achieved a degree of certainty and was in the process of becoming more scientific with the use of analytic method and clinical journal-keeping. To that degree, he certainly was a spokesman for elitist rather than popular medicine, for a professional monopoly rather than for untutored healers. If one is to condemn this "illiberal" and regulatory position as fostering (con-

271

sciously or not) the domination of the elite, then one also must be prepared to accept the consequence that total free enterprise in health care (whatever its bourgeois liberal overtones) would have been in the better interests of the people.

Foucault has the argument both ways by seeing the double phenomenon of private individual-clinical medicine and "socialized" medicine (the concern by public and private bodies for professional and public health norms) both as part of a sinister "noso-political" design to integrate physicians into a political, administrative, and economic power structure.[25] The role of physicians in the power elite is certainly worthy of fuller discussion elsewhere. But one may discard out of hand Foucault's implication that better health care, because it includes some aspects of control and examination of individuals, is somehow a sinister conspiracy to insure the productivity of the masses. As long as health, however defined, is valued above illness, the motivations for making health care available are irrelevant so long as it is truly effective and beneficial care.

The Debate on Primary Education: The Inadequacy of the Liberalism of Smith

Cabanis's participation in the medical education debate not only followed logically from his professional status but also from his membership in the Council of Five Hundred commission for public instruction. In fact, the medical school plan was part of a comprehensive reform of public education presented by the physics teacher Roger-Martin to the Council in November 1798. As the Council minutes indicate, the plan closely corresponded to the wishes expressed in the Directory message sent two weeks earlier.[26] Cabanis explicitly associated himself with the speakers sponsoring each section. In the process, he moved far beyond the cautious innovations proposed in the Mirabeau discourses.

The history of debates on education during the radical phase of the Revolution is now an oft-told tale. Robespierre himself recommended to the Convention a plan requiring compulsory attendance at secular public boarding schools for elementary education. By the closing days of the Thermidorian Convention, there was a significant retreat not only from the principle of compulsion, which had never commanded a majority, but from the principle of free primary education, acceptable to moderates in the 1791 debate over the Talleyrand plan and in the 1793 debates over the Condorcet plan. The law of 25 October 1795 authorized creation of only about 5,000 primary schools for children aged seven to ten with a curriculum limited to reading, writing, arithmetic, and "republican morality." Teachers received only lodging indemnities, not salaries, while parents had to pay fees, though up to twenty-five percent per school could be exempted because of poverty. The Convention did protect private schools, however, in Article 300 of the Constitution of 1795, which granted any schoolmaster the right to open an institution.[27] The Convention Public Education Committee also reduced the number of chairs in the partially state-funded secondary central schools. Both popular courses—such as (1) arts and crafts, and (2) agriculture and commerce—and courses dear to the Idéologues—such as (3) hygiene, (4) logic and analysis of sensations and ideas, and (5) political economy—disappeared from the curriculum between the original decree of February 1795 and the law of October.[28]

In this atmosphere of fiscal retrenchment and political polarization, neither primary nor central schools achieved Convention objectives. At the outset, public primary schools suffered the handicap of a shortage of buildings and qualified teachers. And regional teacher selection juries struggled with the problem of appointing candidates both competent and patriotic. They excluded nonjuring priests and anyone who refused the oath of hatred to royalty. But without a fixed minimum salary, and with payment in depreciating paper currency, teachers of a strictly secular vocation were hard to attract. The boards ultimately appointed significant numbers of former nuns and constitutional priests, and high enrollment often correlated with religious instruction, despite the legal prohibition of religious indoctrination. In at least one case, armed force had to prevent irate villagers from expelling a schoolmaster who had displaced the beloved curé from his residence. Peasants who feared their children's exclusion from communion for studying with godless republican instructors sometimes destroyed government-sanctioned textbooks. Even in the Department of the Seine, an estimate of public primary school attendance gave approximately one-half to one percent of children of the eligible age group. In the same year, the number of public primary schools in the city and *faubourgs* of Paris was only fifty-six, compared to about 2,000 private establishments.[29]

In the tense atmosphere following the coup of Fructidor (September 1797), the Directory attempted to regulate by decree what the Councils refused to approve as law. In November, candidates for public office had to verify current or previous attendance by themselves or their children at public schools. In February 1798, Director François de Neufchâteau required local officials to inspect all schools for teaching of the Rights of Man, use of approved textbooks, and observance of holidays in the Revolutionary Calendar.[30] While municipalities closed a significant number of schools, surviving private institutions evaded the rules, presented a republican façade to inspectors, and retained the vast majority of pupils.

In October 1798, the Interior Ministry persisted in blaming primary school problems on royalists, negligent local officials, and the absence of regulatory power. The aforementioned Directory message to the Council of Five Hundred (24 October 1798) recommended local fixed minimum salaries for instructors, exclusion of priests from public schools, and intermediate-level schools to fill the notorious gap between primary and central schools. The post-Fructidor Directory made anticlericalism a government policy; they declared priests "unfit to educate youth in the principles of purified virtue" and stipulated that "philosophical and universal morality must be the exclusive basis of republican instruction."[31]

The subsequent debate crystallized Cabanis's concern about balancing freedom and state intervention, permitting natural, and eradicating artificial, inequality. The issues in the debate illustrated the dilemmas of Directory moderates, who in principle favored free enterprise in education. Yet an open society in a time of foreign war and latent domestic strife might be exploited by royalist or clerical enemies of the Revolution. Conversely, arbitrary regulatory measures would merely alienate some republican support and narrow the power base of the regime.

A group of moderates presented four parts of the Roger-Martin plan—reform of primary and central schools, an ambitious new level of higher-education lycées, and measures of surveillance of private schools.[32] Roger-Martin himself repudiated the ideas of Adam Smith by advocating state action to enhance educational opportunity and correct the defects of the law of 1795. On the premise that "instruction is the need of all" and "ignorance the worst enemy," he recommended creation of five times the previously authorized number of primary schools. The Republic would guarantee to all instructors, who could not be priests, a minimum salary of 100 to 400 francs, depending on local population and paid by the canton from direct tax revenues. Though the proposal envisaged enormous outlays for higher education, fully sixty percent of educational expenditures would be devoted to two levels of primary schools. To gain additional compensation for instructors, municipalities would collect fees from parents, ranging from twenty-five centimes to one franc monthly per pupil, according to income level as calculated by four classes of direct taxation. The original version had even proposed exemption from fees of all parents assessed less than two francs in direct taxes. In the final plan, twenty-five percent of the pupils would still be eligible for exemption, while parents who chose private schools would be taxed at a rate double the maximum.

An especially controversial provision envisaged about 500 (one per canton) "reinforced" primary schools, where several instructors would teach children aged eleven to thirteen. Inspired by the ideals of Condorcet, Roger-Martin would make available to children of "comfortable artisans and propertied farmers" an enriched program of basic skills, practical subjects

275

such as surveying, geography, and bookkeeping, as well as the elements of Latin, French grammar, and literature. Thus, even those who were not rich enough to attend central schools or who lived too far away would be qualified to become jurors, electors, and municipal officers. The others would be better prepared for academic secondary instruction.[33] The harshly worded plan for regulation of private schools excluded anyone who failed state examinations from state scholarships to central schools and included extensive powers, especially in the first draft, for Directory commissioners to interrogate pupils to verify their knowledge of republican principles and to write reports on the zeal of the masters. The author Dulaure saw no objection justified to a "few harmless coercive measures."[34]

Cabanis no doubt found some aspects of the Roger-Martin plan especially appealing. Although the central schools would lose their general grammar chair, they would gain the chair suppressed by the Convention in "logic and analysis of the operations of the understanding." The speaker for the reform noted the need to acknowledge the principle "long stifled by ignorance and theology" that "all reduces to the faculty of sensation."[35] The Idéologues had also long encouraged a restoration of higher education, here represented by the five lycées. Each would have thirty nonmedical chairs in the mathematical sciences, physical sciences, moral and political sciences, and belles-lettres.[36]

The general educational debate helped Cabanis to clarify his search for a middle path between state indoctrination and academic freedom.[37] At least one neo-Jacobin deputy resurrected Robespierre's principle of compulsory public boarding schools to insure egalitarian character formation. He proposed placing a public primary school in every commune (approximately twice the number proposed by Roger-Martin) and threatened a loss of civil rights to parents boycotting the schools. In his view, no cost was too great to prevent a nation "deprived of enlightenment, [from] falling under the aristocracy of the rich, the most odious of all subjections." Education in common would force children of the rich to receive the same instruction and acquire the same opinions as the poor.[38]

At the other extreme was the fiery moderate lawyer from Nancy Boulay de La Meurthe, later aligned with Siéyès and the Brumaire conspirators, who opposed the expense of primary schools in a financial crisis. Boulay thought that the great maxim that should direct the government was "laissez faire," the best protection against unnecessary taxes. The meddlesome inspection plan of Dulaure ignored the truth that "bayonets cannot destroy the power of habits." The new system would be "more intolerant than Papism."[39] Another moderate lawyer from Grenoble who opposed the curriculum of reinforced primary schools had already warned the previous year against overeducating artisans and farmers who might be tempted to abandon their work and who would slow down the proceedings of primary electoral assemblies. Only wealth and leisure, he argued, fit a man for education; and "human perfectibility" was a "vain speculation."[40]

In addition, Boulay's antipathy to the Roger-Martin plan, and the opposition of two other speakers, stemmed partly from their distrust of the radical Enlightenment. Despite the explicit references to the Supreme Being in a primary school report, they were scandalized at the thought that ethics might be taught without God. One speaker noted that the Directory message seemed to ignore that morality was a question of feeling and authority, not of reason. Implicitly attacking the Idéologues' influence in the central school reform, Pison-du-Galland, though an anticlerical, would later insist on teaching immortality of the soul to safeguard virtue and prevent "Oriental fatalism."[41]

Contrary to the assertions of textbook histories of education, then, there was no single bourgeois liberal attitude toward education, toward human perfectibility, or toward social change in the Council of Five Hundred. Moderates themselves were divided on the desirability and urgency of primary education, the justice of state regulation, and the curriculum of the central schools. The Idéologues also had internal differences on educational questions. The literary critic and *La Décade* editor François-Stanislas Andrieux thought republican festivals more useful than higher primary schools and opposed a curriculum for primary schools prescribed by the state. He even doubted the value of the Interior Minister's advisory Council of Public Instruction, which included Tracy and Garat, and which he feared would usurp legislative control over elementary textbooks. He found the plan for lycées much too grandiose. Most notably, he thought the surveillance plan would make republicans seem like a "ferocious sect," who, "having sown fear will harvest only hatred." Interrogation of instructors would make them automata promoting government doctrine rather than teachers cultivating a love of liberty.[42]

We also know the ambivalent feelings of Destutt de Tracy concerning primary education. His essay of 1801 was intended to save the central schools when the Interior Ministry of the Consulate was reorganizing education. Cabanis fully supported Tracy's efforts to establish a revised, graded, coherent curriculum for the central schools. But Tracy devoted minimal attention to the first level of schooling. Distinguishing between schools for the "working class" and those for the "learned class," he proposed two parallel educational systems—terminal primary schools for sons of workers and a multilevel system for those preparing for the professions. Tracy recommended primary schools only for those communes where parents valued education enough to pay for them. They would also be gradually established as the central schools turned out teachers qualified to staff them.[43] In light of Andrieux's and Tracy's criticisms of the Roger-Martin plan, the manuscript of the speech that Cabanis intended to deliver some time in May 1798 (after 11 Floréal VII) in the Council of Five Hundred takes on more than passing interest. It represents not only a modification of Cabanis's own views but also an Idéologue opinion favorable to enriched primary education, with all its implications for social mobility. The speech was not given because debate closed before Cabanis had his turn at the rostrum.

Cabanis agreed with Boulay's criticism saying that public education should not stipulate forced attendance at boarding schools. Analogies from this practice of ancient Greece or Rome were inapplicable, because there the "lowest class of the people, miserably enslaved, was always sacrificed to the upper classes, alone free: their pretended democracies were at bottom violent aristocracies."[44] Because the Constitution explicitly guaranteed the right of any schoolmaster to open a legally certified school, it would be unwise to obstruct exercise of this right and thus attempt to place the progress of enlightenment at the mercy of the government. Cabanis also ridiculed the emphasis of some speakers on the educational role of government-inspired national festivals. The moral influence of these events among the ancients, as well as the moderns, he pointed out, could never be realized by merely "mechanical and vulgar" means—compulsory attendance at ceremonies.

Nevertheless, as a member of the commission of public instruction, Cabanis gave his full support to all sections of the Roger-Martin plan. Referring to his own agreement with the Mirabeau discourses, Cabanis wrote, "The ideas of Smith thus modified were, I confess, mine for some time; but I declare with the same frankness, that after more mature reflection, I consider them not very solid in general . . . and especially in no way applicable to the circumstances of the French nation." We must now remove, he continued, the "overly great influence of knowledge not by trying to restrict its progress to certain channels, or to halt it, but to spread it in great waves everywhere." Knowledge must not become the exclusive privilege of "classes already favored by fortune" who sometimes oppose the national interest. As Cabanis added in somewhat florid rhetoric, "often the happiest dispositions are hidden and languish under the humble roof of the poor." He also felt that the minimum salary for primary school instructors was necessary since teachers depending exclusively on fees would be at the mercy of parents. Fathers' choices of a school for their children should not be all-powerful at this time, since present high enrollments in the private primary schools showed that republican instructors, predominant in public schools, would not necessarily be the most prosperous.[45]

At the same time, Cabanis maintained that neglecting other educational levels would only dry up the source of primary instructors without helping primary schools. Unlike Andrieux and Tracy, Cabanis defended the reinforced primary schools of the Roger-Martin plan as an important means of overcoming the influence of private schools. Perhaps Cabanis was aware that the drafting course in the central schools had the highest enrollment of sons of artisans at the secondary level. In a scientific age, argued Cabanis, craftsmen, such as tanners, bleachers, masons, and cutlers, and practical men, such as civil and military engineers and sailors, would need to study applied mathematics and the applied sciences—just the kind of subject that could be taught in the reinforced primary schools. Against the scorn of some colleagues for "demi-savants," Cabanis pointed out that educated artisans and ingenious farmers would be precisely those responsible for necessary innovation and increased productivity so vital to the nation.[46]

Aside from the need for technical education, Cabanis also added that in a republic, ignorance among potential public officials was dangerous. The government must teach the elements of ethics and politics, based on the "needs and faculties of human nature" rather than on "certain religious beliefs" that would crumble as soon as reason developed. Public supervision of the teaching of ethics would not be prejudicial to the rights of parents, according to Cabanis. As the Mirabeau discourses had already argued, there was a need to enlighten the conscience of the citizen before encouraging him to follow it. Finally, no one need fear the consequences of education for the poor. Ignorance could only mean dependence, in place of happiness or virtue. The diffusion of enlightenment would be the best defense of liberty, if for no other reason than to teach the populace to see through the blandishments of demagogues.[47]

Despite impassioned pleas from several speakers, the Council of Five Hundred once again tabled the Roger-Martin plan, and there was no further reform of the central schools and no further aid to primary education under the Directory. But despite the lukewarm attitude of the Council majority to education in a time of financial crisis, Cabanis did favor vigorous efforts in primary education to break the monopoly of the wealthy on knowledge.

To understand the difference between Cabanis's views and complacent Consulate liberalism, one need only cite the speeches of Councilors of State Fourcroy and Roederer for the public education law in the changed political atmosphere of 1802. On 14 May 1802, Roederer reminded the Tribunate that there was no use overeducating pupils who might then disdain their naturally destined condition. He also noted the uselessness of teaching the moral and political sciences at the secondary level. But the real hostility of Bonaparte to the central schools emerged in Roederer's description of the legislative sciences as immature, unfocused, and of uncertain and contradictory methods. Several weeks earlier, Fourcroy had noted that state salaries for primary instructors would encourage negligence and inertia and he explicitly cited Adam Smith's argument that education was best left to private initiative.[48]

Certainly Bonaparte showed some commitment to technical education in the lycées and in the Polytechnique as well as to improvement of some arts and crafts schools.[49] But the tenor of the 1802 educational reform and the establishment of the Imperial University (1806-1810) showed concern with the military and administrative needs of the state rather than with the diffusion of enlightenment. The religious teaching orders once more became influential in primary education, which was left to communal initiative. The Revolutionary ideal of secular universal education was postponed for several generations.

Cabanis and the Coups of Fructidor and Floréal

Cabanis's concern for educating the people did not mean that he was willing to allow untutored popular initiative to determine the public interest. Like Condorcet, he preferred enlightened decision-making and believed that the people needed time to ac-

281

quire political wisdom. Cabanis's speeches to the Council of
Five Hundred and his role in military and political coups reveal
how the traumas of the Terror made him hostile to any neo-
Jacobin views. While Cabanis remained a staunch republican,
he feared that the unpropertied and uneducated might follow
malevolent factions to undermine political and economic stability. Several times he countenanced violations of liberal principles in the name of public safety—to avoid resurgent royalism
or a renewal of Terror.

In the coup of 18 and 19 Fructidor v (4 and 5 September
1797), illegal, though bloodless use of military force in Paris assured the purge of allegedly royalist Directors and deputies, the
annulment of the election of alleged plotters, and the deportation of royalist suspects. In a letter to his cousin, Cabanis
affirmed his support for these measures:

> Be assured that the 18 Fructidor was necessary to avoid the
> most frightful civil war imaginable. The Council of 500 was
> marching resolutely toward a general upheaval. The gov-
> ernment saved the republic; tore France from the threat of
> devastation. This will be increasingly realized as the tissue of
> plots unravels; the constitution was only violated an instant
> to conserve it.[50]

Most historians admit the existence of royalist plots, bribery,
and the trend in the Councils to relax laws against émigrés' relatives and against priests. They still disagree on how great the
impending danger was from the apparently royalist parliamentary majority, however. Cabanis did not hesitate to welcome the first of the coups that would increasingly make a
mockery of oaths to the constitution. The polarized atmosphere
and the paranoia of extremists led in turn to the paranoia of the
moderates.

In Fructidor, the existence of a threat was at least debatable,
and Cabanis himself was more observer than participant. In
April and May 1798, Cabanis was directly involved in an effort
to prevent an election victory by an allegedly extremist faction.
He might have felt justified in view of royalist efforts to elimi-

nate him from the primary electoral assembly of the canton of Passy in 1797. He complained that they "spread horror stories . . . to exclude me" and accused him of being a "terrorist" and "drinker of blood."[51] The next year the Directory was bent on forestalling another embarrassing and possibly dangerous election defeat. This time, they feared the apparently effective organization of neo-Jacobin clubs and the flourishing Jacobin press.[52]

Even before the beginning of the two-stage electoral process, the Directory planned to organize reliable secessionist assemblies in cases where unacceptable candidates seemed likely to win.[53] The trustworthy slates would then be legally validated by the legislative commissions authorized to resolve electoral disputes. When police informants reported a neo-Jacobin trend in the primary assemblies, an Interior Ministry circular warned against "names which frighten peaceful citizens and vigorous patriots." Officials in the Interior Ministry also reminded Directory commissioners to departments that "majority rule cannot prevail" in troubled times—"sensible men must unite against factions."[54]

The Seine electoral assembly at the Oratory had a larger proportion of artisans and shopkeepers and relatively fewer merchants and lawyers than in previous years. Cabanis sat as one of four electors designated by the canton of Passy. In early credentials disputes, the neo-Jacobin majority excluded fifty-four of nearly 700 electors. Among the excluded was a friend of Cabanis's—the moderate ex-minister of police and a legislation teacher at a Paris central school, Lenoir-Laroche. The majority charged that royalists or proven rebels of Vendémiaire IV had been illegally admitted to the primary assembly that had elected him. The moderate faction, including Cabanis, then applied the Directory tactic of secession, and approximately 190 electors left the Oratory for the Institute chambers in the Louvre.[55] There they solemnly declared that this secession occurred because of "violence, intrigue, and cabal" and the "annihilation of operations of primary assemblies where the party of oppressors did not prevail."[56]

283

Isser Woloch's study has shown that the secessionists were of a moderately, though not significantly, higher income level as measured by tax assessment. More important, although only thirty-one percent of the total assembly went to the Institute, forty-five percent of the professionals and fifty percent of the wholesale merchants, compared to fifteen percent of the more numerous artisans and shopkeepers, joined the secessionists.[57] The electoral results did produce differences. The Oratory group elected five moderates, but also eight identifiable neo-Jacobins (even two alleged Babouvistes) and three sans-culotte personalities formerly active in Paris section committees. The Institute assembly elected only moderates, such as Cabanis and his fellow Idéologues M.-J. Chénier and F.-S. Andrieux. Cabanis was thus chosen for a three-year term to the Council of Five Hundred by the characteristically overwhelming margin of 141 out of 176 votes cast.[58]

The majority report of the five-member legislative commission investigating the Seine election favored nullification of the work of both assemblies. The Oratory had admitted seventy electors who did not meet the property qualification, while the Institute had also admitted some ineligible electors and was clearly a minority of the total number of electors. But the Directory was concerned about the general "Jacobin" trend and had staked its prestige on a victory in the Seine. Several messages to the Councils urged annulment of the Oratory's "unnatural coalition of anarchists and royalists." Council moderates feared a delegation of former apostles of Marat and Robespierre. With Directory manipulation, the Council of Five Hundred ultimately voted to accept the minority report of the commission to validate the Institute election. Several days later, in the so-called coup of 22 Floréal VI (11 May 1798), the Councils annulled contested proceedings throughout the nation regardless of whether the secessionists were in the majority or minority. In a clearly unconstitutional procedure, some partial annulments affected only individual candidates rather than the entire work of a department assembly. The election results had not brought a neo-Jacobin landslide, but eighty-three of the 113 excluded from the two councils were thought to be neo-Jacobin.[59]

Without a plot against the regime or even a clearly hostile legislative majority, the Directors violated the constitution. Though moderates had not generally been victims of violence, the mood of 1798 encouraged accusations of guilt by association. Where neo-Jacobins gained the upper hand, they were equally vindictive in their purges. The pro-Jacobin crowd outside the Paris Oratory aggravated the turbulent debates inside. Cabanis may not have been aware of Interior Ministry chicanery but he quickly reacted against any threat of a return to a regime of power in the streets, requisitions, price controls, or any resurgence of supporters of Babeuf. He willingly assumed that a minority of electors could defend the Revolution against extremists, who, in the end, would distort its ideals much more than a moderate Directory.

The Panic of 1799: Restriction of "Neo-Jacobin" Civil Liberties

The exclusions of Floréal certainly did not disarm all political opposition in the Councils, and the majority of candidates backed by the Directory lost the elections of 1799. In the face of apparent military collapse and real financial crisis, there was a strong neo-Jacobin revival in the summer of 1799. Cabanis responded with two inflammatory speeches, uncharacteristically advocating severe limits on the liberal principle of freedom of expression. In July 1799, as the Directors nervously tolerated several weeks of pro-Jacobin enthusiasm at the Manège club, Cabanis argued that there was no natural right to hold political meetings since they could be the scourge of a free government. Indeed, the government had the duty to prevent circumstances from bringing forth the evil impulse in human nature. Echoing the sentiments of Condorcet and of his own writings on public assistance, Cabanis noted that orators in large popular assemblies could stir imaginations and mask the bid for power of a few men. Turbulent meetings might further ruin public credit and prevent the revival of commerce and industry. To prevent

285

dangerous crowds, therefore, political clubs should be restricted
to a maximum of one hundred members in Paris. And to prevent the formation of a shadow government, there should be a
prohibition on electing officers, taking formal votes, or even
keeping minutes. Cabanis felt that local authorities must have
inspection rights and that the Directory should close clubs that
violated existing laws against sedition.[60]

Three weeks later, after the Directory had closed the Manège
club but had temporarily relaxed police surveillance of the
press, Cabanis appealed to national unity in a time of civil and
foreign war to prevent slander in newspapers against the Directors.[61] Indeed, the pro-Jacobin *Journal des hommes libres*
had recently attacked Cabanis's friends Siéyès and Garat for allegedly selling out the interests of France to the Coalition and
for opposing the forced loan of 1799 and the new law of hostages. Cabanis asked for a new calumny law to preserve the
moral authority of the government. In fact, the government
eventually suppressed the *Journal des hommes libres* as well as
several other Jacobin newspapers.[62]

Cabanis clearly recoiled at the neo-Jacobin proposals for
heavy taxation of the propertied, which he believed would hinder incentives to earn. In a speech printed in August 1798,
Cabanis defended an unpopular and ultimately unsuccessful Directory plan for an indirect salt tax by arguing that such a
measure would hurt the poor less than direct taxation, which
would "aggravate inequality." He reasoned that an income of
25,000 francs would more readily enable payment of a twenty
percent direct tax than an income of 100 francs.[63] Cabanis never
explained why indirect taxes would be more just for the poor,
however. Later, in August 1799, during the neo-Jacobin ascendancy, the Councils solved the problem of inequities by imposing a progressive rate on the forced loan levied on high personal and real incomes by juries of lower-income citizens. A
week after Bonaparte's coup, Cabanis urged repeal of this
measure, which, by its very existence, he claimed, discouraged
industrial enterprise, aggravated unemployment in an economic slump, and was actually ineffective without the unac-

ceptable terror of revolutionary committees and the scaffold.[64]
Given the inefficiency of collection and the economic recession,
Cabanis's charges were at least partially justified. He genuinely
believed that deflation hurt the poor the most.[65] But clearly he
thought the principle of progressive taxation, the core of the
forced loan law, an inappropriate means of lessening artificial
social inequality.

Justifying Brumaire and the Constitution of 1799

Cabanis's increasing discontent with the political and economic
situation caused him to see Bonaparte as an attractive figure. In
1797 the Institute chose the victorious general as *mécanicien*,
successor to the disgraced Lazare Carnot. After his election,
Bonaparte ingratiated himself with scholars in a famous letter
extolling the conquest of ignorance as more valuable than military triumph.[66] At the same time, he met several Idéologues in
Paris. The Institute was also duly impressed with Bonaparte's
painstaking efforts to foster research during the expedition to
Egypt, where he established both an Institute of Cairo and a *Décade égyptienne*. As the Directory floundered through the
summer and fall of 1799, Siéyès, Talleyrand, and others sought
a strong military hand to stay the swings of the political pen-
dulum. The death of General Joubert reduced the likely candidates to Bonaparte alone. For Cabanis and Garat, among others,
Bonaparte appeared to be the longed-for leader-philosophe who
would terminate the farce of the Directory and inaugurate an
era of stability for the state and glory for science and learning.
As a friend of Siéyès, an acquaintance of Joseph Bonaparte chez
Talleyrand, and a colleague of Lucien Bonaparte in the Council
of Five Hundred, Cabanis was well placed to help bring Siéyès
and the Bonapartes together. Lucien and Siéyès were occasional
Auteuil guests, and the general himself visited Mme Helvétius
after his return from Egypt. Cabanis's precise role in the coup
of Brumaire is not clear, but the public record of his speeches on
19 Brumaire is eloquent enough.

After Bonaparte's grenadiers purged the Council of Five

Hundred to a docile rump, Cabanis took the floor to advocate a provisional government with a mandate to write a new constitution.[67] Invoking threats to property, talent, and virtue, the flight of capital, and the fall in consumer spending, he called for less frequent elections to protect from factions and to avert another popular revolution. He also thought a strong executive would help end the industrial recession.[68] The same evening, he presented and may even have written the Council's *Address to the French People*, which justified the coup as a defense of liberty and as an escape from the extremes of royalism and of "revolutionary government."[69]

With Lucien, Boulay, Chénier, and Daunou, Cabanis became a member of the "organic laws of the constitution" section of the 25-member Commission of the Council of Five Hundred. During the provisional administration, he could already relish the repeal of the neo-Jacobin forced loan and law of hostages of 1799. The constitutional negotiations produced thorough discussion of Siéyès's plan for delicately balanced separation of powers, with a chief of state somewhat like an English monarch, and of Daunou's proposals for propertied electoral colleges and an executive who would be suspended if he led an army. But the First Consul's stubborn insistence on a strong executive and diluted popular sovereignty made a mockery of Idéologue republicanism.[70]

Still, Cabanis, with clear indebtedness to Siéyès's constitutional theories, produced an elaborate justification of the final draft. Its arguments showed, that despite Cabanis's support for widespread primary education, he was less committed than Condorcet to political democracy and less scrupulous than Daunou and Chénier on counterbalances to the executive. He hailed the constitution as a "new social contract," an epoch-making event in the moral and political sciences.[71] Like Siéyès, Cabanis supported the constitutional scheme of voting in which all adult males except domestic servants would form "communal" lists of candidates eligible for legislative office. Commune and department assemblies each in turn narrowed down the original list to a "national" list of one-thousandth the number of participating citizens, from which sixty life-term senators chose the 100-member Tribunate and the 300-member Legislative Body. The whole process assured, as Cabanis said, "la bonne démocratie," free from the influence of clubs and demagogues. Moreover, only those who understood the purpose of legislation would propose it and choose legislators. Cabanis held the Rousseauist tenet that pure democracy was feasible only in a small city and that a strong executive was desirable in a vast country. Now he even accepted the exclusive right of the Council of State to propose laws. As he summed up, "All is done for the people and in the name of the people; nothing by the people or under its ill-considered dictation."[72] He was also pleased that political power would be in the hands of the "middle class (*classe moyenne*) where one almost always finds the greatest talents and the most solid virtues." This class had been chiefly responsible for the growth of commerce and industry during the last three centuries and thus, in turn, for the diffusion of enlightenment and property.[73] Clearly, enlightenment and property were Cabanis's criteria of political capacity. Natural economic growth might increase the number of proprietors, while education would increase the number of the enlightened. Until then, the middle class, a dynamic force in world history, had claim to political hegemony. The ideological content, in the modern sense, of Cabanis's political thought was here unveiled.

We might ask if Cabanis's conception of government had any direct relationship to his science of man. Its premises correlated with Cabanis's physiological assumptions in at least two ways. First, there was an implicit use of the timeless body politic metaphor. When discussing the mutual relationships of the branches of government, including the strength of the executive and free discussion in the Tribunate, Cabanis remarked that flexible government was best—a "living mechanism, not an automaton." He continually advised physicians to study the living organism and not just the cadaver. Similarly, he realized that in politics the dynamic spirit of the government mattered as much as its anatomical structure. The hope that the equilibrium among organs of government would be an "ensemble in which all parts correspond" was reminiscent of the Hippocratic image of the human body in which all systems work for a common purpose. Just as a weakened organ becomes enlarged, a weak executive, lacking "unity of thought and action," would lead to usurpation rather than equitable government.[74] Even the system of election by a conservative body (the Senate) suggested the antidote to nervous disorder by achieving a satisfactory equilibrium among the centers of sensitivity in the body. Though Cabanis's politics were not directly derived from his science of man, his physiology provided a framework for his support of Siéyès's constitutional ideas. The balance among branches of government was analogous to physiological equilibrium, and the importance of the dynamic relationships rather than a merely static mechanical portrait was equally significant for understanding physiology or politics.

A more explicit relationship between Cabanis's science and his politics was his description of the constitution as an empirically developed product of historical change and therefore an example of human perfectibility, the *leitmotiv* of the science of man. Cabanis argued that all governments must satisfy both fixed and changing human needs. In fact, good governments would permit men to satisfy their own basic physical and moral needs. The social creation of government would follow, rather than disturb, nature by enabling free exercise of human faculties, including the ability to reason, to choose freely, to develop sympathetic affections, and to develop "the moral sense which provides our sweetest pleasures." But government also must be strong enough to protect individual liberty, to safeguard the means of perfectibility, to "excite the useful passions," and to "contain the harmful passions," by law if necessary. The social art, as Cabanis called it, after the Physiocrats and Condorcet, "the art of directing laws and habits," must therefore continually adjust to circumstances.[75] Like the therapist observing the clinical history of a disease, the moralist and legislator must refer to experience as well as to reason. He must know, added Cabanis, with recent events in mind, the "action of men in

290

great masses," in which there were "prejudices and extrava-
gances growing in a continually accelerated progression with
numbers themselves." Each people, and indeed the entire
human species, asserted Cabanis, had developing faculties, new
opinions, and new passions. Hence, while any social system
must satisfy universal needs, it must also adapt to the current
political situation and the current state of civilization.[76]

Cabanis followed this premise with a brief essay in political
sociology reminiscent of Adam Ferguson, Adam Smith, and
Montesquieu. He would reevaluate the historic advantages and
disadvantages of monarchic, aristocratic, and democratic governments in light of recent discoveries of the social art, representative government and the separation of powers. Just as
Cabanis had once approved Mirabeau's praise of a strong executive "in a great empire where the people are not yet enlightened," he here advocated government as strong as monarchy without the dangers of a hereditary dynasty or despotic
rule.[77] He praised the stability, talent, decency, and dignity of a
natural aristocracy as opposed to the tyranny of a hereditary
caste. Finally, he was enthusiastic about the "exaltation of all
the faculties of the human mind and the habit of acting for the
general utility" in a democracy. But he warned that one had to
avoid the "ignorant passions" destructive of order, leaving the
"wisest and most virtuous men" at the mercy of "the most absurd populace."[78]

Cabanis thus summarized the political experience he drew
from the Revolution. In his view, the new constitution was the
best adapted to assure a form of popular sovereignty without
the clubs, without disorderly crowds, without demagogues manipulating the desires of the people. The strong executive would
forestall the plots of factions, and the influence of the notables
in the Senate would assure the choice of the propertied and enlightened to the Legislative Body and the Tribunate. He
heralded a new era of political stability, confidence for proprietors and entrepreneurs, economic recovery, benevolence for the
arts and sciences, and consolation for philosophers that "all the
benefits of nature, all the creations of genius, all the fruits of

time, work, and experience will now be used to advantage . . .
the dreams of your philanthropic enthusiasm must themselves
be ultimately realized."[79]

Disaffection of the Idéologues

Certainly Cabanis must have welcomed the fulfillment of some
of his hopes in the Consulate—the currency stability, the
guarantees for property, the subsidies for scientists and inventors.[80] For his rhetorical skill and fervent support in Brumaire,
Cabanis (along with fellow Idéologues Tracy, Garat, and Volney) was among the first designated by Siéyès and Bonaparte
for a lucrative Senate appointment at an annual salary of 25,000
francs. Such an income was more than three times the sum of
his stipends as a professor at the School of Medicine and an Institute member. While he must have had some additional income from medical practice and from his property in Corrèze,
the Senate appointment assured him financial security for the
rest of his life. Cabanis did not share the early misgivings with
Bonaparte of Daunou and Chénier; indeed, he never openly
broke with the Bonaparte family. Yet in the years 1800-1802,
he witnessed the irrevocable shattering of both his scientific and
political dreams. He was hardly so cynical as to continue to
shower the regime with praise.

The Idéologue infatuation with Bonaparte did not entirely
survive the constitutional negotiations.[81] Volney sagely declined the position of Interior Minister, and Daunou, in opposition in the Tribunate in 1800, braved the wrath of the
First Consul to decline a post in the Council of State. The
government-inspired press used the term "Idéologue" deri-
sively as early as January 1800.[82] From the vantage point of the
Senate, Cabanis could observe the deterioration of the constitution of 1799. After the "infernal machine" assassination attempt on Bonaparte on 24 December 1800, the First Consul
demanded the deportation of 120 innocent neo-Jacobin political
enemies. Cabanis, Garat, and Volney joined the unsuccessful
Senate opposition to the project, and Cabanis stayed away on

the day of the vote. Daunou, Chénier, and most vehemently, Ginguené unsuccessfully opposed in the Tribunate the formation of special military tribunals for suspects.[83] Cabanis, Garat, and *La Décade* editor Le Breton continued to meet with a group weekly at a restaurant in the rue du Bac, where they brooded over the unpalatable state of the regime and forged links with the circle of Mme de Staël and Benjamin Constant. Cabanis inherited Mme Helvétius's villa after her death in August 1800, and he, in the company of Tracy, continued to preside over a salon in Auteuil where political discontent could be expressed. By the fall of 1800, Cabanis found himself in discreet opposition to the regime. When a warning from Police Minister Fouché ended the rue du Bac dinners, Idéologue opposition often gathered chez Mme Condorcet, who, by 1801, retreated for the summer season to the suburban château of La Villette.

Intent on muzzling meddlesome academics, the First Consul sought reconciliation with the Roman Catholic Church. In the process, he wished to discredit materialist philosophy and sap the sources of political opposition. In February 1801, he unleashed his wrath against "miserable metaphysicians" and "idéologues."[84] After the Tribunate balked at approving portions of the Civil Code, the First Consul wished to assure approval of the organic laws of the Concordat first signed in July 1801. When he asked the Senate to proceed with the legal election for replacement of one-fifth of the Tribunate, he unmistakably conveyed his wish that the outgoing fifth include the noisiest opposition spokesmen. Though Cabanis, Tracy, Garat, and several other senators argued in vain for a choice by lot, in January 1802, the docile Senate majority purged (effective in March) Ginguené, Chénier, Daunou, J.-B. Say, and even the quiet philosophy teacher Laromiguière from the Tribunate.[85] In April 1802, the Tribunate duly ratified the Concordat, while the Senate offered Bonaparte an extended ten-year term as Consul. Dissatisfied, Bonaparte intimidated the Senate in August 1802 into approval of a plebiscite that gave him the Consulate for life and established a new constitution further limiting the independence of the Tribunate. Cabanis was absent during this vote and also failed to respond in 1804 to the survey of senators' opinions on the desirability of an Empire. When the Senate solemnly proclaimed the Empire in 1804, Cabanis was conveniently on leave for reasons of health.[86]

Final approval of the Concordat shortly preceded Chateaubriand's vitriolic attacks on Idéologue philosophy. The regime found the Church a more effective control on wayward consciences than the pale natural morality associated with Ideology. The Concordat assured abandonment of Cabanis's ideals of secular primary education. In the Fourcroy education law of 1 May 1802, the Church was given free rein in primary education, and public lycées replaced the controversial central schools at the secondary level. While Tracy and Cabanis themselves approved restored emphasis on classical languages, the lycée curriculum offered no scope for instruction in general grammar or elements of legislation, much less a chair in analytic method or Ideology. The centralized system of school inspectors augured the tight control of teaching practices and strict loyalty to the Emperor demanded in the Imperial University.

In addition, in January 1803, Interior Minister Chaptal reorganized the Institute in the name of administrative efficiency and more meaningful elections of members by the competent Class rather than the entire membership. The same decree matter-of-factly abolished the Class of Moral and Political Sciences and divided the Idéologues between the new literary and politically conservative Second Class of French Language and Literature (Cabanis, Siéyès, Garat, Volney) and the new Third Class of History and Ancient Literature (Daunou, Ginguené). In this latter group the majority of the defunct Class found that sensitive questions of ethics, economics, and legislation could be introduced, according to the new rules, only as they related to historical problems.[87] Thus disappeared the major sources of intellectual élan for the Idéologues. Without central schools, there could be no formal propagation of Ideology to young students. Without the Class of Moral and Political Sciences, Idéologues would discuss philosophical questions meaningful to them in their books rather than in a public forum at the center of the cultural stage in France.

Cabanis silently accepted his Senate salary despite his deep disillusionment with government policy. But the apparent opportunism of Cabanis's political career should not obscure his adherence to a certain ideal of the moderate revolution that opposed the return of privilege while believing in commercial and industrial growth as the engines of general prosperity. He genuinely regretted Bonaparte's violations of civil liberties, even though his pre-Brumaire anti-Jacobin speeches showed inconsistencies with his usual defense of freedom of the press and freedom of association. Certainly his fears of popular democracy and his participation in political coups limited his notion of political liberty. His social and political thought, derived largely from Siéyès, was certainly less original than the bold syntheses of Physiological Ideology.

Like the thought of Adam Smith himself, Cabanis's liberalism was not synonymous with laissez faire. The psychophysical engineering of the applied science of man assumed that natural temperament was the necessary point of departure for producing an acquired temperament. The physician was always in the superior position of determining the best interests of individual health, though with more education in hygiene, more people would learn sound physical and moral habits. Together science and politics would enlighten fundamental self-interest and cultivate fundamental sympathy to dispose individuals toward the public good without denial of natural rights.

Thus, on all major political issues, Cabanis believed in government intervention to guide individuals to self-reliance. Public assistance wisely administered would foster independence of the poor and would attempt as far as possible to cure the sick at home in natural family surroundings. Society would thus lessen artificial inequality without harming beneficial natural inequality. Cabanis was convinced that the state could, and indeed must, regulate the medical profession and medical education without encroaching upon the rights of the individual practitioner. The lapse in licensing due to the political circumstances of the Revolution convinced Cabanis of the need to protect professional standards. Events also persuaded Cabanis more firmly of the need for public primary education to prepare everyone for citizenship and of flourishing central schools to teach Ideology for those destined for leadership. He favored widespread technical training for artisans and, unlike Tracy, saw no outright division between education for "working" and "learned" classes.

On the question of government itself, however, Cabanis's attitude was undeniably paternalistic toward the propertyless and allegedly unenlightened. He realistically recognized the danger of the conflict between rich and poor long postponing the ideal state of social harmony. He was sensitive to the need for more equitable income distribution. But he placed his confidence in education and economic growth to achieve a natural social equilibrium. In some respects, this outlook seems the forerunner of Guizot's "Enrichissez-vous," tempered with the awareness of a Saint-Simon of possible struggle between the rich and poor.

There is no simple answer to the question of whether Cabanis's political and social thought fits the Marxist image of bourgeois ideology. For some Marxists, any liberal who believed in property and free trade was automatically defending the interests of the "revolutionary bourgeoisie." In fact, if he openly defended the public interest, he could in this view be held up as an example of false consciousness or self-deception if not outright use of self-interested propaganda to foster artificial social harmony.

There is no doubt that Cabanis was a defender of the new, unprivileged commercial and industrial elite. He praised them openly, though always with the liberal assumption that their activities brought benefits and prosperity to all ranks of society. Certainly he would not have wished to provoke class struggle. And, aside from his doubts about democracy, in one medical work he did let slip the prejudice that medical treatment in hospitals and in the countryside might be less complicated than treatment of "sensitive scholars or men of affairs." If such attitudes signify bourgeois ideology, then the label is accurate.

Yet one must recall that Cabanis's use of the term "middle class" hardly fits the Marxist definition of class—a group with the same relationship to instruments of production—nor does it even fit a group with similar income levels. The middle class, as a heterogeneous group distinct only from the very rich and the poor, cannot be expected to have believed in a single ideology. Thus, the label bourgeois ideology is not in itself an invaluable aid to historical understanding.

Assuming that one could agree on definitions of "bourgeois" or, for that matter, "elite," there were still many versions of bourgeois or elite ideology. Cabanis's ideal was not a static, hierarchical society in which the rich owed nothing but private charity to the poor. He expected society itself to become more just in the distribution of wealth and realized that a purely laissez-faire approach was not enough to eliminate injustice. To some extent, the label bourgeois ideology suggests a smugness and complacency not befitting Cabanis's thought, for in his view, individual perfectibility was indissolubly linked with the therapy of society.

★ CHAPTER XI ★

The Metaphysical Twilight

*The Letter to Fauriel: The Monism
of Universal Intelligence*

abanis drowned the political sorrows of his final years in a return to intense philosophical activity. Though his creative period ended with the appearance of the *Rapports* in 1802, in 1803 he prepared a new edition of *Degré de certitude*, the essays on public assistance, the note on the guillotine, and the Mirabeau journal. The next year he published *Coup d'oeil* for the first time and helped edit Condorcet's complete works. The third edition of the *Rapports* appeared in May 1805 with Tracy's analytical index. And from 1805 to 1807 he produced two minor medical works, *Observations sur les affections catarrhales* (on the common cold among other subjects) and *Note sur un genre particulier d'apoplexie*, as well as the literary commentary *Lettre à M. T[hurot] sur les poèmes d'Homère*. These last three works were all published in Thurot's edition of Cabanis's works from 1823 to 1825. Cabanis's correspondence, on the whole not very revealing, shows an increasing attachment to Ginguené, Volney, and a businesslike as well as friendly relationship with Degérando, an Interior Ministry secretary-general. He also wrote frequently to the *littérateur* and lover of Mme Condorcet, Claude Fauriel. This latter relationship produced the strangest document in the corpus of Cabanis's works.[1]

In 1806-1807 Fauriel was at work on a history of the Stoic philosophers. Cabanis ostensibly intended to encourage him by examining his own metaphysical convictions, which in fact resembled the ancient Stoic belief that the world is one, rational, and animated by a single binding force, or pneuma.[2] In the process, Cabanis contradicted several statements in the *Rapports* and created doubts for posterity about the sincerity of his materialism. As Lehec notes, the *Letter* seems too polished for private correspondence; yet it certainly might have been altered had Cabanis intended to publish it. When the vitalist Montpellier physician and hygiene professor F.-E. Bérard published it in 1824 (Thurot also included it the next year), Cabanis's entire metaphysical significance seemed subject to reevaluation.

Though Moravia has contended that the *Letter* is an overstressed document of Cabanis's old age, we might argue, rather, that it made explicit attitudes already apparent in the *Rapports*.[3] The contradictions and the differences in tone were largely due to the abandonment of the modest agnostic reserve appropriate for a scientific work. Cabanis claimed in the *Letter* that in rigorous "philosophical discussions" dealing with the knowable, Final Causes would be "vain and sterile explanations." But in the unchartable terrain of the indemonstrable, he permitted "more or less plausible conjectures," so long as they did not betray analytic reason itself.[4]

In the *Rapports* Cabanis insisted that knowledge of the operations of physical sensitivity would be sufficient for moral science. In the *Letter*, he still shunned religious dogma and was confident that reason revealed human needs and faculties. The "constant and universal" human moral relationships were fixed even though human organization could be modified.[5] Free exercise of faculties would always be a natural right, and inalterable human sensitivity justified the expectation of a sympathetic response from fellow men.

But scientific knowledge about human organization would in itself neither satisfy human curiosity nor penetrate the deepest recesses of the human heart. Perhaps recalling the failed experiments of the Revolution, Cabanis asserted that true principles, to be influential, must "touch and agitate man rather than convince him."[6] Sympathy might be a universal need, and virtuous action might truly bring contentment, but men would seek more stirring motives for self-sacrifice. They wished to feel at home in the universe, to dissipate their "uncertainty and fright" about the mysteries transcending science, to suspect that each of their virtuous acts concurred with the order of the unknowable First Cause. The study of human nature, then, revealed an additional "need"—the irrepressible religious sentiment in the "great masses of men." Cabanis here admitted a need that the radical philosophes such as d'Holbach had vehemently denied. Yet he adamantly refused to turn to traditional religions, which misguidedly deceived men "for their own benefit." Rather, he thought that a simple, consoling religion, like that of Franklin or Turgot or the Stoics, might "direct this torrent [of feeling] instead of continuing vain efforts to dam it or dry it up."[7]

The limitations of reason could not appease the human yearning for oneness with the active forces of the universe. Eighteenth-century philosophes had often avowed "absolute ignorance" about first causes, but now Cabanis admitted the weakness of this position against the "direct, inevitable, everyday impressions" of men who cannot accept a "purely mechanical system of the universe." Why not, then, teach men plausible hypotheses about the First Cause since true knowledge was impossible? Without betraying the intellect, such speculations might meet universal needs of "imagination and sensitivity" and provide more incentives for moral behavior. Despite Cabanis's previous reservations about the effectiveness of public ceremonies, he did not hesitate here to suggest a state-sponsored cult to "satisfy the need for frequent gatherings felt by all men" and to give pomp and solemnity "never approached in our shabby modern festivals" to the call to virtue.[8] In the Catholic revival of the Empire, Cabanis's conclusion that religious sentiment is a universal need was understandable. More surprising was his continued confidence in the emotional power of a civil religion after the notorious popular indifference to the pallid *culte décadaire* and the disintegration of the intellectual circles of Theophilanthropy.[9]

Cabanis did not merely wish to invent a nonexistent First

Cause for the masses, however. He himself was willing to speculate at length about the existence of the First Cause and the persistence of the human ego after death. In the *Rapports* Cabanis seemed to banish the term "cause," even when referring to invariable natural successions. Now he believed the notion of First Cause useful in explaining the apparent unity of universal forces. In the *Rapports* he reasoned that any combination of forces would spontaneously order itself, or would show the predominance of a single force. Now he was willing to state that an external cause must have imbued matter with its properties or impressed upon it its original impulse. Providence seemed to take precedence over necessity. In a variant of ancient arguments, Cabanis invoked the observed design in the universe to postulate the existence of an ordering intelligence. Given the exquisitely refined effects of active forces, there was no probability that mechanical and physical explanations would in themselves be sufficient. On the other hand, there was some probability that there was intentional coordination of the observed effects. Final Causes, in the old Aristotelian sense, might be inadmissible as explanations of particular phenomena, but a Final Cause might be the ultimate explanation of the activity in the universe.[10]

Cabanis here expressed his belief in a cosmos—unified, rational, and animated by a single force. Already in the *Rapports*, he had developed the hypothesis of a hierarchy of forces of affinity and had speculated that gravitational attraction might well be explained as a "vague instinct" rather than sensitivity as a higher-order attraction. Now he openly preferred the primacy of sensitivity. Animal sensitivity and both animal and human intelligence were not merely attributes of organization, but emanations of universal reason. D'Holbach had assumed that the complex chemistry of life was reducible to simpler physical laws. To Cabanis, the entire hierarchy of active affinities could be reduced to a "sensitivity . . . distributed, though in different proportions, in all the particles of matter." Like the Stoics, Cabanis defended the omnipresence of "Willing Intelligence . . . everywhere in continual activity." The universe might be

301

organized so that all its parts were "mutually sympathetic." Human minds might be the "partial centers" of intelligence emanating from a "common reservoir," just as partial centers of sensitivity in the body emanated from the brain.[11]

Cabanis never forsook the eighteenth-century ideal of finding unity in nature. But he unequivocally rejected Epicurean mechanical materialism and d'Holbachian physicochemical materialism for a neo-Stoic form of animism close to that of the Montpellier physicians de Sèze and Barthez. Of course, not every animist or hylozoist studied medicine, though it is noteworthy that Maupertuis, Diderot, and Cabanis all drew inspiration from biological phenomena. The convergence of eighteenth-century vitalism and mechanism did not produce the same effect on Diderot, who never wrote the equivalent of a *Letter on First Causes*. True, Diderot believed that "latent sensitivity" might be a property of matter. But to Diderot, nature was self-sufficient and there was no hidden design in natural law. He urged men to be virtuous for the sake of reason and nature, but never because their action would concur with an intelligence and purpose immanent in nature. Cabanis's distance from d'Holbach appeared in an oblique reference in the *Letter* to spontaneous generation experiments. For d'Holbach, Needham's experiments in particular testified to the creative impulse of "blind" nature. For Cabanis, who had himself attempted spontaneous generation experiments, the constant and regular tendency of all particles of matter to form "sensitive, and therefore, intelligent organizations" indicated a higher probability for the existence of a Willing Intelligence.

Finally, Cabanis's discussion of the persistence of the ego departed even further from the philosophy of Diderot and d'Holbach. In the essay on the guillotine, Cabanis had clearly eliminated the possibility of consciousness after death. In the *Letter*, he described this position as "correct, at first glance," but actually indemonstrable. The primary reason for the change was Cabanis's altered view of the vital principle. Previously he had identified it with the sum of all conditions necessary for life, but now he called it a "real being, whose presence impresses upon the organs the movements composing their functions." Like an indestructible element, this principle emanated directly from the general active principle of the universe and might return to its source after death. Since sensitivity characterized this principle, Cabanis somewhat glibly concluded that consciousness of the ego must also be essential to it and might then also persist after death. Like a traditional moralist, Cabanis added that this latter probability would enhance the justice of the First Cause, and where rational certainty was impossible, "moral reasons" might be admitted in the argument. Still he conceded that the probability of persistence of the ego was much less than that of the existence of the First Cause. And he still denied that the persistence of the ego was necessary as a rational support of ethics.[12]

Without directly subscribing to belief in God or a soul, Cabanis was thus privately willing to make substantial concessions to conventional metaphysics. In the letter to Fauriel, he restored the congruence of cosmic purpose and human effort that marked the Providential world-view of earlier deists and natural-law theorists. If physiologically based natural law were indeed a moral law, the moralists' task of reconciling virtue and inclination might be easier. For the sake of "ennobling" moral philosophy by the "sublime idea" of human dignity and of the "great destinies to which man is called by the Supreme Orderer," Cabanis was willing to advocate the only kind of religion that, he felt, "without obscuring the natural light of reason, would present the noblest and firmest guarantee of individual virtues and of tranquillity of the social state."[13] This was a religion a philosopher could endorse, not just a narcotic for the masses. Since reason did not abdicate, there was no clean break with the view of the *Rapports*. In fact, the ambiguity appears not as a result of an intellectual or spiritual conversion in the depressing atmosphere of Idéologue failure, but rather as an optical illusion created by lack of close study of Cabanis's works.

303

"Materialism": Self-Image and the Mythology of Critics

We must thus reiterate the contention that Cabanis was a monist who believed that only one substance existed in the universe, but insist that the label "materialist" obscures his admission of the primacy of intelligence. Correspondence of Cabanis and Tracy with Mme de Staël throws further light on their reaction to the word "materialist."

In 1805 Cabanis received from Mme de Staël a manuscript, "On Materialism," written by her father, the ex-minister Necker, before his death in 1804. Necker here had labeled the Idéologues materialists. Tracy and Cabanis both disavowed the designation in letters not intended for dangerous public exposure. Though Mme de Staël was in Switzerland, we might still suspect that Tracy and Cabanis wished to disguise any obviously heretical views from the censors who might have examined the correspondence of such a notorious opposition figure. But at the same time, we must recall that both were not the least bit reticent about their anticlericalism, and in 1804 Tracy denounced traditional beliefs in the soul in the introduction to his new analysis of Dupuis's *De L'Origine des cultes*. Yet they both maintained to Mme de Staël a kind of Newtonian agnosticism on the ultimate constituents of the universe.

Tracy wrote, "All your qualities and all your enlightenment have not been able to prevent you from calling materialist men who highly profess to know what neither spirit nor matter is . . . never being concerned with determining the nature of the thinking principle because that is indifferent for all they have to say about it." The label was, in addition, "false and harmful." Three weeks later, Cabanis added:

Perhaps I could complain to find myself classed among the *materialists* in a note by your father. The fact is I am not at all one, whatever Messieurs Geoffroi and Co. say; I do not even understand the meaning of that word, any more than of the word *atheist*; and in my view one can be neither one nor the other, when one realizes the meaning of those two designations, and the motives leading to adopt them. But I see by the continuation of your father's note, that he, no more than I, knew what all that could mean; and what I must complain about would thus refute itself . . . I should have refused an imputation I do not deserve, and which is not without inconvenience at this time.[14]

Yet, with some exceptions, such as Bérard and Damiron, neither contemporaries nor posterity were willing to dissociate Cabanis from the stereotype of materialism. Long after the *Letter* to Fauriel had become public knowledge, critics of Cabanis's *Rapports* accused him of materialism or found monism equally threatening to orthodox religion and sound philosophy.

In 1842 the physician and secretary of the Academy of Medicine Frédéric Dubois d'Amiens vitriolically attacked any explanation of feeling and thought by organic movement. To him, Magendie's discovery of distinct spinal roots for sensory and motor nerves was testimony to the independence of the will. Cabanis, he claimed, had mistakenly believed that "material instruments" produced thought; and the gross stomach-brain comparison aimed definitively "to materialize the intelligence: that is how far one had come in speaking to rational men in a century of enlightenment." Even Dubois had to admit, though, that amid a "gross, amorphous, ill-digested materialism," Cabanis had introduced a "subtle vitalism," by speaking of tendencies to animalization in plant mucilage, a "vivifying faculty" in embryo formation, and the effect of attention in the brain on internal organs. But he claimed that Cabanis lacked understanding of the formative force preceding all organization, the eternal active intelligence manifest in all life. Thus, he claimed, Cabanis shared the pernicious Hobbesian moral philosophy of the supreme value of pleasure.[15]

While Dubois willfully misunderstood Cabanis's ethics and metaphysics, more careful students were equally critical. Also in 1842, the Dijon philosophy professor Joseph Tissot insisted that nervous tissue could not sense, unless sensitivity were a property of its elements. Therefore, either material impressions could not be considered sensations, or each molecule was sensitive, and there would be an infinity of egos in each man rather than a unified consciousness. On a less complicated level, material active principles would mean an infinity of souls and gods. Cabanis's materialism led to atheism, his pantheism to polytheism. Tissot also had a special aversion to Cabanis's "sensationalist materialism," because it led to a morality suitable for animals, not men. An ethic based on physiology denied human freedom and overthrew moral order.[16]

In the two following years, 1843 and 1844, the seventh and eighth editions of the *Rapports* appeared. The neurologist and hygienist L. Cérise introduced the text with his own "essay on the principles and limitations of the science of the relationship of the physical and mental." Eschewing both materialism and animism for a circumspect dualism, he favored a correlation of physical and mental without stooping to Cabanis's "reactionary materialism." Like some of the younger Idéologues, Cérise believed that Cabanis had avoided consideration of the *moral*, as if ideas themselves could not produce affective states or determine actions. According to Cérise, the *Rapports* mistakenly investigated only half the emotion-idea interaction, at the level of the ganglionic impressions. Thus, it could explain discomfort in states of indigestion, but hardly the sources of emotions or ideas. Cérise recognized Cabanis's implied belief in moral liberty but he found the result philosophically ambiguous, for Cabanis seemed to agree that certain actions were blameworthy and that the mind could exercise control, yet he thought the mental a result of the physical. Hence his physiology was one-sided, and his ethics contradictory.[17]

The physician Louis Peisse included the *Letter* to Fauriel in his 1844 edition of the *Rapports* and labeled it as an example of Germanic "universal animism." In fact, he recognized that the passage in the *Rapports* comparing attractive forces to crude sensitivity anticipated the reasoning in the *Letter*. Peisse astutely commented that, if Cabanis affirmed that mind was the guiding principle of the universe, he showed the influences of the idea of "living nature" in the medical philosophy of Stahl and of the Montpellier school. He saw insufficient development in Cabanis's metaphysics; Cabanis described the "Divine Intelligence" sometimes as transcendent and sometimes as the result of universal activity. Thus, the "Stahlianism" of Cabanis was philosophically inconclusive and deserved neither praise nor censure.

Peisse did admire Cabanis's effort to relate physiology and psychology and noted that even respectable dualists like Bonnet and Hartley had pursued the same enterprise. But even Peisse was revolted by the stomach-brain comparison. He believed that Cabanis had erred in leaving no place for the nonextended ego in the operation of sensation or for an immaterial principle in the process of thought. Thus, Cabanis confused the merely "cerebral" with the *"moral,"* according to Peisse, and foolishly tried to establish a natural morality.[18]

Cabanis's dualist editors and critics could not share his aesthetic enthusiasm for the unity in nature if such unity imperiled the acceptance of a transcendent God and an immaterial, immortal soul. They also chose to overlook Cabanis's reluctance to prematurely apply the methods of the physical sciences to medicine and his admiration for the specific properties of life and human intelligence. And even if they appreciated his refined notion of the hierarchy of forces of affinity, even if they were aware of his private attribution of all cosmic forces to a universal intelligence, they attacked spiritualist monism or pantheism as much as materialism.

Death and Persistent Influence

Cabanis did not long survive the mellowing of his metaphysical convictions. Always in frail health, he suffered an apparent cerebral hemorrhage on 22 April 1807 and thereafter spent more time at the Grouchy château of La Villette (near the Condorcet-Fauriel ménage at the château of La Maisonnette) in the village of Rueil-Seraincourt near Meulan. By the next spring, he still had difficulty exercising powers of mental concentration, but he had regained sufficient strength to have exercise in hunting, and he even gave some free consultations to poor patients in surrounding villages. His disciple Richerand supervised his convalescence but could not prevent a second cerebral hemorrhage, this time fatal, on 5 May 1808. At the time of his death, Cabanis was planning a treatise on the physical improvement of mankind as a sequel to the *Rapports* and a more solid foundation for the science of man. Despite the vicissitudes of his public career, friends never considered Cabanis an opportunist who trimmed his convictions to prevailing philosophical or political winds.

Cabanis was buried at the Pantheon, after a ceremony at Auteuil on 14 May, though his heart was enshrined in Auteuil cemetery close to the tomb of Mme Helvétius. Garat gave the eulogy at the Pantheon, and other representatives of the Institute, the School of Medicine, and the Senate all attended the funeral. The Class of French Language and Literature fittingly designated as his successor his close friend Destutt de Tracy, who was only a correspondent of the Institute since the reorganization of 1803. Tracy's reception speech, as well as his correspondence with Maine de Biran, testified to a sense of personal loss as well as a lament for the cause of the Idéologues. Ironically enough, less than three weeks before Cabanis's death, letters-patent issued to all senators proclaimed Cabanis a count in the new Imperial nobility. Such was the last honor bestowed upon an inveterate opponent of privilege. Even Cabanis's critics rarely questioned the distinction of his character. His wife Charlotte veritably worshipped the memory of her faithful husband until her death in 1844.[19]

Cabanis's ideas certainly outlived the cult by his friends and family. In the years following his death, the concepts of Physiological Ideology had a far-reaching impact despite the scarcity of direct disciples. The emphasis on nervous sensitivity, internal impressions, and the organic functioning of the brain provided a stimulus to the innovative neurophysiology of François Magendie (1783-1855) and Marie-Jean-Pierre Flourens (1794-1867). Magendie favorably cited both Cabanis and Tracy in his *Précis de physiologie élémentaire* (1816), even though his work broke away from the physiological concepts of Richerand and

Bichat. While he confidently related the brain and the intellect, his mature writings show him unwilling to discard the concept of a vital force. The physiologists, of course, revolted against the old Montpellier bias against experiment and brought closer the characteristic modern medical marriage between lab and clinic.[20]

In medicine itself, the Paris clinicians followed analytic method and developed the statistical approach. But the irascible François-Joseph-Victor Broussais (1772-1838), a student at the Paris School of Medicine in 1798-1803, shook pathology to its foundations by calling attention to local lesions rather than following the nosology of Pinel based on collections of symptoms. All the same, Broussais paid high tribute to the physiology of Cabanis and Richerand and in 1826 he was not hesitant to attribute reason, the ego, and consciousness to organic action.[21]

The hygienists, too, perpetuated the interests of Cabanis and Hallé in an increasingly influential sanitary reform and public health movement. Its theory became more sophisticated in the *Annales d'hygiène publique et de médecine légale*, founded in 1829, and in the statistical social research of physicians such as L. R. Villermé, who in 1840 published his monumental inquiry, *Tableau de l'état physique et moral des ouvriers de coton, de soie, et de laine*. The hygienists recognized the importance of the physical environment in assuring epidemic prevention and a healthy, productive labor force, in addition to the humanitarian compassion for those in squalid living conditions. They also recognized a public responsibility, over and above the individual obligation to self-help.[22]

Cabanis's works even had an impact in the realms of high-flown philosophy and social theory. Schopenhauer advised a correspondent never to discuss empirical psychophysical relations without studying Cabanis and Bichat.[23] Henri Saint-Simon openly acknowledged his indebtedness to Condorcet, the anatomist Vicq d'Azyr, Cabanis, and Bichat. A friend of the Paris physician Jean Burdin, Saint-Simon assigned privileged status to a "positive" physiology in developing his organic theory of society. His 1813 manuscript, "Memoir on the Sci-

ence of Man," paralleled Idéologue aspirations to find unity in
the sciences and laws of social behavior, while he elsewhere argued for the importance of a historical approach characteristic of
clinical medicine and for the distinctiveness of the spheres of life
and society.[24] To be sure, Idéologue social harmony was liberal,
not organic, but Saint-Simon shared the commitment to human
perfectibility and the ambition to develop guidelines for social
engineering.

Cabanis's philosophical career illuminates an important stage
in the history of monism and in the fate of the concept of the
Great Chain of Being. He attempted to synthesize a tough-
minded agnosticism on ultimate causes and a tender-minded
spiritualist monism permitting reverence for the specificity of
life and cosmic optimism on man's place in nature. He wished
to demonstrate the physiological substratum of human ideas
and passions, while at the same time understanding those inherent and environmental factors differentiating human intelligence and character. From the intellectual context of the experiments of Needham, the speculations of Buffon, the works of
Maupertuis, d'Holbach, and especially Diderot, Cabanis derived
the notion of unity of physical, mental, and moral forces. Newtonian "action at a distance," spontaneous mental activity, and
social sympathy were all affinities varying in degrees. The important point was not whether they were essentially spiritual or
material, but that there was no need to distinguish states of
mind from states of the brain and nervous system. Vital and
social forces concurred in the elemental structure of the universe. The spontaneous generation of living creatures and
variation in existing species suggested the transformation of
nonliving and living forms. If living creatures could improve
themselves by inheritance of acquired characteristics, human
perfectibility seemed all the more plausible. Men learned by experience and were malleable by the power of habit. They could
duly acquire salutary mental and moral characteristics.

The unity of knowledge through the analytic method developed by Bacon and Condillac reflected the unity of nature. But
Cabanis's medical studies and practice qualified his conviction of

unity in the Chain of Being and in the chain of truths. Sensitivity was not merely a complex chemical affinity, but an irreducible property of life. Eighteenth-century physiological mechanism and vitalism both described a property inexplicable by mechanics and unassignable to the rational soul. Like Bordeu, Cabanis attributed all to sensitivity, and in the *Letter* to Fauriel, he came close to Barthez's view of the vital principle as an emanation of higher Intelligence. Physiology and medicine could not be studied merely with anatomical and chemical apparatus. The purposiveness of the living organism was more than the resultant of the functioning of its parts.

The science of man would tailor therapy to all the variations of individual temperament. Where organic lesions or malformations produced mental illness, the therapist must understand and then attempt to heal. Physical regimen—diet, exercise, sleep, drugs, work habits—might alter the inherited dispositions of internal temperament. Thus, the physical environment would affect the "lower" centers of sensitivity, and internal impressions might change states of the brain and eventually induce an acquired temperament. The science of man would presumably collect reliably verified data on the variations of physical sensitivity according to age, sex, temperament, illness, regimen, and climate. More trustworthy than "moral treatments," physically based therapy would contribute both to individual well-being and to social harmony. Nature would not merely take its course, but the physician would intervene opportunely to help each individual and his appropriate natural equilibrium.

Critics of late eighteenth-century treatment of mental illness, such as Foucault, consider it manipulative and profoundly inhumane because it inevitably exercised a form of social control over the individual and responded to the social imperative of eliminating deviance. Cabanis's science of man did assume that there was some kind of desirable natural physical and mental equilibrium. Yet his attitude toward deviant temperaments was more tolerant than repressive, and the starting point of therapy was always the capacities and needs of the individual. The well-tempered individual was, after all, an ideal far beyond the capacity of the physician to compensate for an indefinite variety of individual idiosyncrasies.

Certainly Cabanis raised philosophical issues that transcend his era. The mind-body problem persists as a perennial, insoluble dilemma, with modern neurophysiologists gathering still more information on the functioning of the brain, which has mysteries undreamt of in Cabanis's philosophy. Yet Cabanis promoted an empirical, observational approach to psychophysiology, even though historians of psychology will be eager to point out his lack of experimentation. He raised hopes that physicians could sweep away delusions, break bonds of temperament, and cultivate habits that would promote self-realization. Behaviorist psychology and psychiatry have assembled a formidable therapeutic arsenal to help achieve these objectives. But they no longer pretend to achieve the same degree of certainty that the physical sciences do. Eighteenth-century questions about appropriate regimen for modifying temperament are not so remote in an age discussing megavitamin therapy for certain forms of schizophrenia, the lithium content and consequent antidepressant effect of mineral waters, and the proper chemical drug to administer to a hyperactive child. Universal psychological laws and infallible treatments have still proven scarce in the twentieth century.

Cabanis's concept of the social order also raises haunting questions that remain unsolved. He believed that enlightened moralists and legislators had a duty to assure salutary social equilibrium. Civil liberty and free trade would ideally complement the free exercise of individual faculties. But in a revolutionary era the state could not be an indifferent arbiter. Even to assure the free play of "natural" economic laws, the state would have to act to eliminate vestigial privilege. To allow for the benefits of natural inequality, Cabanis insisted on the preservation of individual self-reliance and incentives to work. But the state had to administer a public assistance program to lessen artificial inequality and to end the dangerous struggle between rich and poor. The difficulty of winning support for a secular, republican regime convinced Cabanis of the need for public secular schools to assure widespread literacy, technical skills, and informed political judgment. Until the realization of the grandiose goal to diffuse enlightenment, Cabanis supported a strong executive and a representative government that would assure the political power of the solid middle classes and prevent control by turbulent factions. Yet to trivialize his political thought as mere bourgeois ideology in the Marxist sense is to ignore the distinction among the several middle class viewpoints emerging from the late Enlightenment. Cabanis was certainly a political and economic liberal rather than a democrat but he expected the moral and political sciences to help guarantee the establishment of a society that was open to social mobility rather than a frozen hierarchy in which overeducation was dangerous. He also realized that in some cases the poor could not enrich themselves and that the political system would have to be flexible enough to respond to new social situations.

Society would thus be perfectible as the individual was perfectible. Cabanis recognized that, to an extent, the perfectibility of temperament was a luxury of the well-to-do and that attaining the means of perfectibility was thus a significant social problem. The other dilemmas he faced continue to puzzle both statesmen and philosophers—how much freedom and how much regulation does a healthy economy demand, how can welfare and social service programs be established without overburdening taxpayers or exhausting the resources of national and local governments, how does one preserve human rights yet achieve social justice, how does one assure educational opportunity and relate education to social mobility? We may never realize Cabanis's dream of combining ethics with science; choices may be matters of value rather than of social science. But we still rely on the present-day moral and political sciences to provide information for ethical and political decisions. The fragmented flow of such information may yet pose the greatest obstacle to Cabanis's dream of studying the whole man.

Notes

NOTES TO INTRODUCTION

1. *Oeuvres philosophiques de Cabanis* (hereafter designated *OP*), ed. Claude Lehec and Jean Cazeneuve (Paris, 1956), I, 199, 161-162.

2. Ibid., p. 142.

3. Ibid., p. 126; II, 209-210; the most thorough recent study of Cabanis's thought is in Sergio Moravia. *Il Pensiero degli idéologues* (Florence, 1974), pp. 1-290; my argument on the derivation of Cabanis's thought, independently conceived, agrees with many of Moravia's conclusions, though differences will be mentioned in the text. A summary of Cabanis's thought appeared in my article, "Cabanis and the Science of Man," *Journal of the History of the Behavioral Sciences* X (1974), 135-143.

4. Sergio Moravia's *Il Tramonto dell'illuminismo: Filosofia e politica nella società francese, 1770-1810* (Bari, 1968) is the best survey of the political and cultural impact of the Idéologues. See also the synthetic reappraisal of the Idéologues in the works of Georges Gusdorf, notably *Introduction aux sciences humaines* (Paris, 1960), pt. IV, ch. 3; and *Dieu, la nature, l'homme au siècle des lumières* (Paris, 1972), ch. 5. I completed this study before reading Gusdorf's *La Conscience révolutionnaire, les idéologues* (Paris, 1978), but I have commented on it briefly in the Preface. Older studies, now largely superseded, are François Picavet, *Les Idéologues* (Paris, 1891); Charles Van Duzer, *The Contribution of the Idéologues to French Revolutionary Thought* (Baltimore, 1935); Emile Cailliet, *La Tradition littéraire des idéologues* (Philadelphia, 1943), and Jay Stein, *The Mind and the Sword* (New York, 1961).

5. *OP*, I, 121; "Génie du christianisme," *Oeuvres complètes de Chateaubriand* (Paris: Garnier, n.d.), II, 85-86, 91, 130-132, 304-309.

6. *Oeuvres complètes de J.-H. Bernardin de Saint-Pierre*, ed. L. Aimé-Martin (Paris, 1818), I, 243-245.

7. François Furet and Denis Richet, *La Révolution du 9 thermidor au 18 brumaire* (Paris, 1966), p. 277; Heinrich Haeser, ed., *Lehrbuch der Geschichte der Medicin und epidemischen Krankheiten* (Jena, 1881), II, 476.

315

8. *Lettre (posthume et inédite) de Cabanis à M. F . . . sur les causes premières,* ed. F.-E. Bérard, (Paris and Montpellier, 1824), pp. 104, 180, 163; Jean-Philibert Damiron, *Essai sur l'histoire de la philosophie en France au xixe siècle* ([1828] Paris, 1834) i, 89-92.

9. See Chapter XI below.

10. Jules M. Guardia, *Histoire de la médecine d'Hippocrate à Broussais et ses successeurs* (Paris, 1884); Guardia, *La Médecine à travers les siècles* (Paris, 1865); the most intelligent assessments by historians of medicine have been, Paul Delaunay, "L'Evolution philosophique et médicale du biomécanicisme: De Descartes à Boerhaave, de Leibnitz à Cabanis," *Le Progrès médical* (1927), cols. 1290-1293, 1338-1343, 1368-1384; and George Rosen, "The Philosophy of Ideology and the Emergence of Modern Medicine in France," *Bulletin of the History of Medicine* xx (1946), 328-339.

11. Moravia, *Tramonto,* pp. 25-26; on letter to Fauriel, see Moravia, *La Scienza dell'uomo nel settecento* (Bari, 1970), p. 70; cf. Moravia, *Il Pensiero,* pp. 30, 118-119.

12. For the older view, see Leonora C. Rosenfield, *From Beast-Machine to Man-Machine* (1940; 2d ed., New York, 1968); protests appear in Julien Offray de La Mettrie, *Lamettrie's "L'Homme Machine": A Study in the Origins of an Idea,* ed. Aram Vartanian (Princeton, 1960), p. 20; Jacques Roger, *Les Sciences de la vie dans la pensée française du XVIIIe siècle* (Paris, 1963); R. M. Young, "Animal Soul," *Encyclopedia of Philosophy* (New York, 1967), ii, 122-127; and Roger Smith, "The Background of Physiological Psychology in Natural Philosophy," *History of Science* xi (1973), 75-123. Cf. Karl Figlio, "Theories of Perception and the Physiology of Mind in the Late Eighteenth Century," *History of Science* xii (1975), 201.

13. See Chapter VII below.

14. On the term "ideology," see Emmet Kennedy, "'Ideology' from Destutt de Tracy to Marx," *Journal of the History of Ideas* xl (1979), 353-368.

15. On professionals versus charlatans, see the articles by Jean-Pierre Goubert, Toby Gelfand, and Matthew Ramsey cited in Chapter X; on health care as a means of exercising power (implicitly unjustified), see Michel Foucault et al., *Les Machines à guérir (aux origines de l'hôpital moderne)* (Paris, 1976), pp. 11-21.

16. The best printed sources for biography of Cabanis are *OP* i, v-xxi; Antoine Guillois, *Le Salon de Mme Helvétius. Cabanis et les idéologues* (Paris, 1894); P.-L. Ginguené, "Cabanis," *Biographie uni-*

verselle [Michaud] VI (1843), 298-303; and J.-L. Moreau de La Sarthe, "Moral," *Encyclopédie méthodique* CLXXIII, *Partie médicale* X (1821), 250-276; adequate summaries in Georges Canguilhem, "Cabanis," *Dictionary of Scientific Biography* (New York, 1971), III, 1-3; and Lester Crocker, "Cabanis," *Encyclopedia of Philosophy* (New York, 1967), II, 3-4; for confirmation of details, I have consulted manuscript dossiers in the Bibliothèque historique de la ville de Paris; the Parent de Rosan collection (Mairie du XVIᵉ arrondissement, Paris); Archives Nationales (hereafter designated AN); and Archives départementales de la Corrèze (Tulle), (hereafter designated AD Corrèze).

17. For family name and history, see J.-B. Champeval, *Dictionnaire généalogique des familles nobles et notables de la Corrèze* (Tulle, 1913), II, 61-63; abbé J.-B. Poulbrière, *Dictionnaire historique et archéologique des paroisses du diocèse de Tulle* (1890; 2d ed., Brive, 1964), I, 362-363; AD Corrèze, paroisse de Cosnac, B.M.S. 1747; and AD Corrèze, E. 35; C. 178.

18. See Louis de Nussac, "La 'Venue' de Georges Cabanis: Son Nom et sa famille, son père et son berceau," *Bulletin de la Société scientifique, historique, et archéologique de la Corrèze* XLIV-XLV (1923), 243-270; AN, H. 1503, Registres de la Société d'agriculture de Brive; and Musée Ernest Rupin, Brive, Records of the Société d'agriculture de Brive, 1743-1774; on the agronomic movement, see A.-J. Bourde, *Agronomie et agronomes en France au XVIIIᵉ siècle*, 3 vols. (Paris, 1967).

19. See Antoine Guillois, *Pendant la Terreur, le poète Roucher* (Paris, 1890), pp. 19-20.

20. AD Corrèze, 1.E.6, letter of Treilhard to de Puymarets, 2 July 1772; Guillois, *Pendant la Terreur*, pp. 23-24.

21. See bibliography of Iliad MSS, *OP* II, 541-543.

22. P. Astruc, "Sur Dubreuil, maître de Cabanis," *Le Progrès médical*, supplément illustré (24 January 1945), 45; Jean Meyer, "Le Personnel médical en Bretagne à la fin du XVIIIᵉ siècle," in J.-P. Desaive et al., *Médecins, climat, et epidémies à la fin du XVIIIᵉ siècle* (Paris, 1972), p. 177.

23. *OP* I, 24; Anatole Feugère, "Raynal, Diderot, et quelques autres 'historiens' des deux indes," *Revue d'histoire littéraire de la France* XX (1914), 343-378.

24. Guillois, *Le Salon*, p. 46; Cabanis, *Cabanis, choix de textes et introduction*, ed. Georges Poyer (Paris, n.d. [1910]), p. 222; Alan Kors, *D'Holbach's Coterie: An Enlightenment in Paris* (Princeton, 1976), p. 106.

25. See Bibliothèque de l'Institut, MS 2222, papiers présumés de l'abbé Martin Lefebvre de La Roche; on verification of name, see Parent de Rosan collection XI, 60 (*not* Pierre-Louis Lefebvre de La Roche); Bibliothèque historique de la ville de Paris, dossier of Cabanis.

26. Louis Amiable, *Une Loge maçonnique d'avant 1789: Les Neuf Soeurs* (Paris, 1897), pp. 17-18, 28, 31-32, 66, 357, 389-393; see also Moravia, *Tramonto*, pp. 55-61; Nicholas A. Hans, "UNESCO of the 18th Century: La loge des Neuf Soeurs and its venerable master Benjamin Franklin," *Proceedings of the American Philosophical Society* XCVII (1953), 513-524; Alain Le Bihan, *Franc-maçons parisiens du Grand Orient de France (fin du 18ᵉ siècle)*, 2 vols. (Paris, 1967).

NOTES TO CHAPTER I

1. Frances Yates, *Giordano Bruno and the Hermetic Tradition* (Chicago, 1964); Yates, *The Rosicrucian Enlightenment* (London, 1972); Arthur Koestler, *The Sleepwalkers* (London, 1959); and Betty Jo Dobbs, *The Foundations of Newton's Alchemy: "The Hunting of the Greene Lyon"* (Cambridge, 1976).

2. "Principes de la philosophie" (orig. ed. Latin 1644), *Oeuvres de Descartes*, ed. Charles Adam and Paul Tannéry (Paris, 1897-1913) IX, pt. II, 64, 75.

3. See Richard Westfall, "The Role of Alchemy in Newton's Career," in M. L. Righini Bonelli and William R. Shea, eds., *Reason, Experiment, and Mysticism in the Scientific Revolution* (New York, 1975), pp. 189-232.

4. See also Alexandre Koyré, *Newtonian Studies* (Cambridge, Mass., 1965); Henry Guerlac, *Newton et Epicure* (Paris, 1963); *The Leibniz-Clarke Correspondence*, ed. H. G. Alexander, (Manchester, 1956); P. M. Heimann and J. E. McGuire, "Newtonian Forces and Lockean Powers: Concepts of Matter in Eighteenth-Century Thought," *Historical Studies in the Physical Sciences* III (1971), 233-306; J. E. McGuire, "Force, Active Principles, and Newton's Invisible Realm," *Ambix* XV (1968), 154-208; Roger Smith, "The Background of Physiological Psychology in Natural Philosophy," *History of Science* XI (1973), 76-77, 102-103; and Richard Westfall, *Force in Newton's Physics* (London, 1971).

5. See fuller discussion in my article, "Newton and Voltaire: Constructive Sceptics," *Studies on Voltaire and the Eighteenth Century* LII (1968), 29-56; and P. M. Heimann, "Voluntarism and Immanence:

Conceptions of Nature in Eighteenth-Century Thought," *Journal of the History of Ideas* xxxix, 2 (1978), 271-283.

6. On eighteenth-century Newtonianism, see the informative, though occasionally confusing Robert Schofield, *Mechanism and Materialism: British Natural Philosophy in an Age of Reason* (Princeton, 1970); and Arnold Thackray, *Atoms and Powers: An Essay on Newtonian Matter-Theory and the Development of Chemistry* (Cambridge, Mass., 1970); see also Thomas Steele Hall, "On Biological Analogs of Newtonian Paradigms," *Philosophy of Science* xxxv (1968), 6-25; Georges Gusdorf, "La Géneralisation du paradigme newtonien," *Les Principes de la pensée au siècle des lumières* (Paris, 1971), pp. 180-192.

7. John Locke, *An Essay Concerning Human Understanding* (1690), ed. A. C. Fraser (Oxford, 1894), ii, 192-193; i, 413; René Pomeau, *La Religion de Voltaire* (Paris, 1956), p. 219 n.2.

8. Arthur Lovejoy, *The Great Chain of Being: A Study of the History of an Idea* (Cambridge, 1936); Charles Bonnet, *Contemplation de la Nature* (1764).

9. Lovejoy, *The Great Chain*, pp. 242-287.

10. Forerunners of transformism are a main theme of Jacques Roger, *Les Sciences de la vie dans la pensée française du XVIIIe siècle* (Paris, 1963); the following sections draw amply on Roger in discussions of Needham, Buffon, Maupertuis, and Diderot.

11. John Turbervill Needham, *Mémoires pour servir à l'histoire d'un polype d'eau douce* (Leyden, 1744); J. R. Baker, *Abraham Trembley of Geneva: Scientist and Philosopher, 1710-1784* (London, 1952); Joseph Schiller, "Queries, Answers, and Unsolved Problems in Eighteenth-Century Biology," *History of Science* xii (1974), 184-199; Aram Vartanian, "Trembley's Polyp, La Mettrie, and Eighteenth-Century French Materialism," *Journal of the History of Ideas* xi (1950), 259-286.

12. Needham, "A Summary of Some Late Observations upon the Generation, Composition, and Decomposition of Animal and Vegetable Substances," *Philosophical Transactions* xlv, no. 490 (December 1748), 615-666 cited in revised French translation, *Nouvelles Observations microscopiques* (1750), in Roger, *Les Sciences*, pp. 501-512; see *OP* i, 520.

13. Paul Farber, "Buffon and Daubenton: Divergent Traditions within the *Histoire naturelle*," *Isis* lxvi (1975), 67; Buffon, *Oeuvres philosophiques*, ed. Jean Piveteau (Paris, 1954), p. 247A-B; Roger, *Les*

Sciences, pp. 547, 556; see also Roger, "Buffon," *Dictionary of Scientific Biography* (New York, 1970), II, 579.

14. Robert Wohl, "Buffon and His Project for a New Science," *Isis* LI (1960), 194-199; Buffon, *Oeuvres*, pp. 39A-B, 238B; see Roger, *Les Sciences*, p. 549; and Sergio Moravia, *Il Pensiero degli idéologues* (Florence, 1974), pp. 139n., 23, 78, 135-139.

15. Buffon, *Oeuvres*, pp. 239A, 240B, 248B, 37A-B, 38A, 175A; see Roger, *Les Sciences*, pp. 537, 544, 548, 568, 580.

16. Buffon, *Oeuvres*, pp. 233A, 294, 323, 325, 337.

17. Ibid., p. 313; see Paul Farber, "Buffon and the Concept of Species," *Journal of the History of Biology* v (1972), 259-284; Buffon, *Oeuvres*, pp. 394-414; *OP* I, 410-411, 474-475, 515-518.

18. See Bentley Glass, "Maupertuis, Pioneer of Genetics and Evolution," *Forerunners of Darwin: 1745-1859*, ed. Glass, Temkin, and Straus (Baltimore, 1959), pp. 51-83, esp. 78; on Maupertuis, see also Pierre Brunet, *Maupertuis*, 2 vols. (Paris, 1929); *Actes de la journée Maupertuis, Créteil, 1-12-73* (Paris, 1975).

19. Emile Callot, "Maupertuis," *La Philosophie de la vie au XVIIIe siècle* (Paris, 1965), pp. 149-194, esp. 189; Anne Fagot, "Le 'Transformisme' de Maupertuis," in *Actes de la journée Maupertuis*, pp. 163-182; Maupertuis, *Oeuvres* (Lyon, 1768; reprint ed., Hildesheim, 1965), II, 88-89.

20. Maupertuis, *Oeuvres* II, 146-149, 152, 158-159; Callot, "Maupertuis," p. 185.

21. Maupertuis, *Oeuvres* II, 164; see Fagot, "Le 'Transformisme'," pp. 167-168, for critiques of Maupertuis as a "precursor."

22. Maupertuis, *Oeuvres* II, 160, 174; cf. Glass, "Maupertuis," p. 65.

23. "Pensées sur l'interprétation de la nature," *Oeuvres complètes de Diderot*, ed. J. Assézat and M. Tourneux (Paris, 1875), II, 49-50; Callot, "Maupertuis," pp. 176-177; Moravia, *Il Pensiero*, p. 121.

24. Aram Vartanian, "From Deist to Atheist: Diderot's Philosophical Orientation: 1746-1749," *Diderot Studies* I (1949), 46-63; Diderot, *Lettre sur les aveugles*, ed. Niklaus (Geneva, 1951); Roger, *Les Sciences*, pp. 599-600, 608-611; Lester Crocker, "Diderot and Eighteenth-Century French Transformism," in *Forerunners*, ed. Glass, Temkin, and Straus, pp. 114-143, esp. 120-121, 130-131, 134-135; Jean Mayer, *Diderot, homme de science* (Rennes, 1959).

25. *Oeuvres complètes de Diderot*, II, 15-16; Diderot, *Le Rêve de d'Alembert*, ed. Paul Vernière (Paris, 1951), pp. 55-56, 69-71; see also Roger, *Les Sciences*, pp. 661-664.

26. Moravia, *Il Pensiero*, p. 104; cf. "Discours de M. le comte de Tracy," *Recueil des discours . . . lus dans les séances publiques et particulières de l'Académie française, 1803-1819*, 1re partie (Paris, 1850), p. 305.

27. Moravia, *Il Pensiero*, pp. 99-100; *Oeuvres complètes de Diderot* II, 64-70; for another contrary view, see Jean-Claude Guédon, "Chimie et matérialisme: la stratégie anti-newtonienne de Diderot," *Dix-huitième siècle* XI (1979), 185-200.

28. See Crocker, "Diderot," p. 132; Callot, "Diderot," in *La Philosophie*, pp. 275, 282; Arthur Wilson, *Diderot* (New York, 1972), pp. 557-570; Diderot, *Correspondance*, ed. G. Roth, letter to Sophie Volland, 10 October 1765 (Paris, 1960), V, 140-141, cited in Roger, *Les Sciences*, p. 618.

29. Diderot, *Rêve*, pp. 13-14, 67, 141.

30. Alan Kors, *D'Holbach's Coterie: An Enlightenment in Paris* (Princeton, 1976), p. 12; "Discours de M. le comte de Tracy," p. 305.

31. On d'Holbach, see Pierre Naville, *D'Holbach et la philosophie scientifique du XVIIIe siècle* (1943; reprint ed., Paris, 1967); and Callot, *La Philosophie*, pp. 317-368.

32. D'Holbach, *Système de la nature, par Mirabaud* (London [Paris], 1774), I, 24n., 49-52; cf. Callot, *La Philosophie*, p. 334.

33. D'Holbach, *Système* I, 2; cf. *OP* I, 121.

34. D'Holbach, *Systéme* I, 135, 111, 114.

35. Ibid., pp. 129-133, 81, 206-207.

36. Ibid., p. 345; see also Roland Mortier, "D'Holbach et Diderot: affinités et divergences," *Revue de l'Université de Bruxelles* (Brussels, 1972), pp. 223-237.

37. D'Holbach, *Systéme* I, 133-135.

38. Ibid., p. 161.

39. On Bonnet, see Raymond Savioz, *La Philosophie de Charles Bonnet de Genève* (Paris, 1948); *OP* I, 141.

40. Bonnet, "Palingénésie philosophique" (1769; rev. ed. 1783), *Oeuvres complètes* XV, 218-220, 236, 238, cited in Lorin Anderson, "Charles Bonnet's Taxonomy and Chain of Being," *Journal of the History of Ideas* XXXVII (1976), 51, 52 n. 26, 57; see also Bentley Glass, "Heredity and Variation in the Eighteenth-Century Concept of Species," in *Forerunners*, ed. Glass, Temkin, and Straus, esp. pp. 164-170.

41. Savioz, *La Philosophie*, pp. 37-38, points out the fears of the dualist physician and correspondent of Bonnet, Jerome Gaub, that Bonnet's hypotheses would be interpreted as materialistic.

42. Savioz, *La Philosophie*, pp. 137-139, 188; Bonnet, "Essai de psychologie," *Oeuvres d'histoire naturelle et de philosophie* VIII (Neuchatel, 1782), 73; Bonnet, "Essai analytique," *Oeuvres* VI, xxii, xxiv.

43. Bonnet, "Essai analytique," pp. 66-67, 16n.

44. Savioz, *La Philosophie*, p. 193; Bonnet, "Essai analytique," 40n.

45. Bonnet, "Essai analytique," p. 415; Bonnet, "Essai de psychologie," p. 104.

46. D'Alembert, *Preliminary Discourse to the Encyclopedia of Diderot (1751)*, ed. Richard Schwab (Indianapolis, 1963), p. 5; see also Keith Baker, *Condorcet: From Natural Philosophy to Social Mathematics* (Chicago, 1975), pp. 197-202.

47. J. H. Randall, "The Development of the Scientific Method in the School of Padua," *Journal of the History of Ideas* I (1940), 177-206, esp. 196-199; Galileo, *Opere*, ed. Nazionale, IV, 520; VII, 75; XVII, 90, 160 cited by Randall in "The Development," 199n., 206n.; Henry Guerlac, "Newton and the Method of Analysis," *Dictionary of the History of Ideas* III (1973), 378-391.

48. *The Works of Francis Bacon*, ed. James Spedding and Robert Ellis (London, 1868), IV, 97, 127-145, 154-155 (*Novum Organum*, bk. I, CIV; bks. II, IX, XI-XIII); on Baconian method, see among others Margery Purver, *The Royal Society: Concept and Creation* (London, 1967).

49. Just as Bacon never completed his rules of method for "Physics," so Descartes failed to complete the third section of the *Regulae ad Directionem Ingenii*, intended to deal with physical questions "not perfectly understood"; see Descartes, *Oeuvres philosophiques*, ed. Ferdinand Alquié (Paris, 1963), I, 156 n. 2.

50. Descartes, *Regulae ad Directionem Ingenii*, ed. Ferdinand Alquié, I, 100-102, 154. See also *Oeuvres de Descartes*, ed. Charles Adam and Paul Tannéry, X, 279-381, 427. Further discussion of analysis and synthesis appears in Descartes, *Replies to the Second Objections of Mersenne*, ed. Ferdinand Alquié, II, 581-584; and in *Oeuvres de Descartes*, ed. Adam and Tannéry, VII, 380.

51. Sir Isaac Newton, *Mathematical Principles of Natural Philosophy* (1687), ed. Florian Cajori, trans. Andrew Motte (Berkeley, 1962), I, xx-xxi.

52. See Georges Le Roy, *La Psychologie de Condillac* (Paris, 1937); and Isabel Knight, *The Geometric Spirit: The Abbé de Condillac and the French Enlightenment* (New Haven, 1968). The latter volume is

stimulating and comprehensive though the author overplays the thesis of a contradiction between Condillac's idealism and empiricism.

53. Condillac, "Essai" (1746), in *Oeuvres philosophiques*, ed. Georges Le Roy (Paris, 1951), I, 3A-B.

54. Condillac, "Logique" (1780), in *Oeuvres* II, 405.

55. Condillac, "Traité des systèmes" (1749), in *Oeuvres* I, 213n.; "Logique," pp. 374-375.

56. Condillac, "Art de penser" (1775), in *Oeuvres* I, 773.

57. Condillac, "Traité des systèmes," p. 213; "Logique," p. 379; "Cours d'études—Grammaire" (1775), in *Oeuvres* I, 435.

58. Condillac, "Traité des systèmes," p. 215; "Cours d'études—Discours préliminaire," in *Oeuvres* I, 407B; "Traité des systèmes," p. 121A.

59. Condillac, "Art de raisonner" (1775), in *Oeuvres* I, 637, 628A-630B.

60. Condillac, "Art de penser," p. 770A; "Essai," p. 7.

61. Condillac, "Logique," p. 392.

62. Condillac, "Traité des sensations" (1754), in *Oeuvres* I, 239. See Mayer, *Diderot*, p. 310 for a discussion of the emergence of the statue-myth in the 1740s after André-François Boureau-Deslandes' *Pigmalion, ou la statue animée* (London [Paris], 1741). Condillac, "Traité des sensations" p. 255A.

63. Condillac, "Essai," pp. 13B, 48, 31.

64. Condillac, "Traité des animaux" (1755), in *Oeuvres* I, 362-364.

65. Condillac, "Dissertation sur la liberté," appended to "Traité des sensations," p. 317.

66. On Helvétius, see Albert Keim, *Helvétius: Sa Vie et son oeuvre* (Paris, 1907); D. W. Smith, *Helvétius: A Study in Persecution* (Oxford, 1965); Ian Cumming, *Helvétius: His Life and Place in the History of Educational Thought* (London, 1955); *OP* I, 112.

67. Helvétius, *Oeuvres complètes* (Paris, 1795), II, 253n.; III, 176, 105n., 173, 170n. Citations from the first two volumes refer to *De L'Esprit*; from the last two, to *De L'Homme*.

68. Ibid., III, 106; I, 184; II, 57; III, 384.

69. *Oeuvres complètes de Diderot* II, 379, 283, 320, 344.

70. But see Harry G. Payne, *The Philosophes and the People* (New Haven, 1976), pp. 164-165.

71. *Oeuvres complètes de Diderot* II, 304, 316, 357.

72. Helvétius, *Oeuvres complètes*, I, 160; III, 122-124n.; IV, 415n.; III, 113; I, 125-126.

73. Ibid., III, 431-432n.; I, 283; 317.

NOTES TO CHAPTER II

1. See Owsei Temkin, *Galenism: The Rise and Decline of a Medical Philosophy* (Ithaca, 1973), esp. pp. 175-182; see also Sergio Moravia, "Philosophie et médecine en France à la fin du XVIIIᵉ siècle," *Studies on Voltaire and the Eighteenth Century*, LXXXIX (1972), 1098-1105.

2. *OP* II, 303-340, see 312 for this critique of the Hippocratic *Corpus*; on medical education, see René Taton, ed., *Enseignement et diffusion des sciences en France au XVIIIᵉ siècle* (Paris, 1964), ch. 2, pp. 169-258; Paul Delaunay, *Le Monde médical parisien au XVIIIᵉ siècle* (Paris, 1906).

3. Introductions to the study of Hippocrates are to be found in Hippocrates, *Hippocrate: Médecine grecque*, ed. Robert Joly (Paris, 1964); Louis Bourgey, *Observation et expérience chez les médecins de la collection hippocratique* (Paris, 1953); *OP* II, 65; *The Works of Hippocrates*, ed. W.H.S. Jones (London, 1940), II, 287.

4. *OP* II, 99-100; "Decorum," par. 5, in *The Works of Hippocrates* II, 287; in context, *sophien* could be better translated as "wisdom" (modesty, reserve, fairness) than as "philosophy," but eighteenth-century commentators commonly interpreted this aphorism as a statement of method; see Daniel LeClerc, *Histoire de la médecine* (The Hague, 1729; reprint ed., Amsterdam, 1967), p. 114.

5. *OP* I, 74, 137; "Precepts," par. 1, in *The Works of Hippocrates* I, 313; *OP* II, 312.

6. "The Art," pars. 7-13, in *The Works of Hippocrates* II, 201-217; "Tradition in Medicine," pars. 1, 3, and 13, in *The Medical Works of Hippocrates*, ed. John Chadwick and W. N. Mann (Oxford, 1950), pp. 15, 19.

7. "On the Nature of Man," par. 4, in *The Medical Works of Hippocrates*, p. 204; and in *The Works of Hippocrates* IV, 11-12; the four humors relate to Empedocles' four "elements", and to a series of corresponding tetralogies; see Erich Schöner, *Das Vierschema in der Antiken Humoralpathologie. Sudhoffs Archiv für Geschichte der Medizin und der Naturwissenschaften*, supplement 4 (Wiesbaden, 1964); Appendix A gives a summary chart.

8. "Ancient Medicine," par. 19, in *The Works of Hippocrates* I, 51.

9. "Prognostic," par. 20 in *The Works of Hippocrates* II, 43.

10. "Epidemics," bk. VI, pt. 5, par. 1, in *Oeuvres complètes d'Hippocrate*, ed. Emile Littré (Paris, 1846), V, 315.

11. "The Art," par. 6, cited in *OP* I, 89n.; "On the Nature of Man,"

par. 9, in *The Medical Works of Hippocrates*, p. 208; and in *The Works of Hippocrates*, IV, 25-29.

12. *OP* I, 21, 40-41, and II, 149.

13. "On the Nature of Man," par. 9.

14. "Airs, Waters, Places," pars. 13, 24, in *The Works of Hippocrates* I, 109-111, 133-137.

15. Ibid., pars. 19-23, in *The Works of Hippocrates* I, 121-131; see *OP* I, 462, 511-512.

16. "On Nutriment," par. 23, in *The Works of Hippocrates* I, 351; "Places in Man," par. 1, cited in *OP* I, 189, 255, and II, 209.

17. *OP* II, 116; see Owsei Temkin, "On Galen's Pneumatology," *Gesnerus* VIII (1951), 180-189; Leonard G. Wilson, "Erasistratus, Galen, and the *Pneuma*," *Bulletin of the History of Medicine* XXXIII (1959), 293-314; and Galen, *De Usu Partium*, ed. Margaret May (Ithaca, 1968), I, 44-67.

18. Galen, *Oeuvres anatomiques, physiologiques, et médicales de Galien*, ed. Charles Daremberg (Paris, 1856), II, 63; Temkin, *Galenism*, pp. 44-45, 103-104.

19. Galen, "Ars Medica," in *Claudii Galeni Opera Omnia*, ed. C. G. Kühn (Leipzig, 1821), I, 305-412; see L. J. Rather's discussion in "The 'Six Things Non-Natural': A Note on the Origins and Fate of a Doctrine and a Phrase," *Clio medica* III (1968), 337-347; Peter H. Niebyl, "The Non-Naturals," *Bulletin of the History of Medicine* XLV (1971), 486-492; S. Jarcho, "Galen's Non-Naturals," *Bulletin of the History of Medicine* XLIV (1970), 372-377, Galen, *Oeuvres* II, 77, 84.

20. See Walter Pagel, *The Religious and Philosophical Aspects of Van Helmont's Science and Medicine* (Baltimore, 1944); and the numerous works of Allen Debus on the English Paracelsians and Helmontians.

21. Auguste-Georges Berthier, "Le Mécanisme cartésien et la physiologie au XVIIe siècle," *Isis* III (1920), 21-58; Leonora Rosenfield, *From Beast-Machine to Man-Machine* (New York, 1940; 2d ed., 1968); Heiki Kirkinen, *Les Origines de la conception moderne de l'homme-machine: Le Problème de l'âme en France à la fin du règne de Louis XIV (1670-1715)* (Helsinki, 1960); see also Sergio Moravia, "Dall' 'homme machine' all' 'homme sensible'," *Belfagor* XXIX (1974), 633-648, (translated in *Journal of the History of Ideas* XXXIX (1978), 45-60); on differences between Italian and Cartesian mechanism, see François Duchesneau, "Malpighi, Descartes, and the Epistemological Problems of Iatromechanism," in M. L. Righini Bonelli and William

R. Shea, eds. *Reason, Experiment, and Mysticism in the Scientific Revolution* (New York, 1975), 111-130; see also M. D. Grmek, "A Survey of the Mechanical Interpretations of Life," in Allen D. Breck and Wolfgang Yourgrau, eds. *Biology, History, and Natural Philosophy* (New York, 1972).

22. See *OP* I, 140; cf. Sergio Moravia, *Il Pensiero degli idéologues* (Florence, 1974), pp. 37-38, 43, 47.

23. Descartes, *Treatise of Man*, ed. Thomas Steele Hall (Cambridge, Mass., 1972), pp. 81, 85-86; T. S. Hall, "Descartes's Physiological Method," *Journal of the History of Biology* III (1970), 53-79; Descartes, *Traité sur les passions de l'âme*, ed. Geneviève Rodis-Lewis (Paris, 1955), par. 13; Georges Canguilhem, *La Formation du concept de réflexe aux XVIIe et XVIIIe siècles* (Paris, 1955), 27-56 for discussion of the asymmetrical nature of Descartes's reflex mechanism.

24. Descartes, *Treatise*, p. 68, n. 113; Descartes, *Discours de la méthode* (1637), ed. Etienne Gilson (Paris, 1930), p. 62.

25. Hermann Boerhaave, *Institutiones Medicae* (ed. 1746), pp. 9, 361-362, cited in L. J. Rather, *Mind and Body in Eighteenth-Century Medicine: A Study Based on Jerome Gaub's "De Regimine Mentis"* (London, 1965), p. 119.

26. *OP* II, 140-142; on Boerhaave, see Lester Snow King, *The Medical World of the Eighteenth Century* (Chicago, 1958), 63-68; and King, "Some Problems of Causality in Eighteenth-Century Medicine," *Bulletin of the History of Medicine* XXXVII (1963), 19; G.-A. Lindeboom, *Hermann Boerhaave: The Man and His Work* (London, 1968), pp. 265-266, 272, 276.

27. Boerhaave, *Sermo Academicus de Honore Medici Servitate* (1731), p. 8, cited in Lindeboom, *Hermann Boerhaave*, p. 275; Boerhaave, *Praelectiones de Morbis Nervorum* (1730-1735), reprinted in G.-A. Lindeboom, ed., *Analecta Boerhaaviana* (Leiden, 1959), II, 256-257, cited in Karl Figlio, "Theories of Perception and the Physiology of Mind in the Late Eighteenth Century," *History of Science* XII (1975), 181; the term *hormen* or *enormon* originated in Hippocrates' "Epidemics," bk. VI, in *Oeuvres* V, 347, and has been transformed into the modern "hormone."

28. On Gaub, see L. J. Rather's masterful critical edition of the lectures, *Mind and Body*; T. S. Hall, *Ideas of Life and Matter* (Chicago, 1969), II, 77-81, who classes Gaub among those making a "transition to vitalism"; cf. Moravia, *Il Pensiero*, pp. 51-58.

29. *OP* II, 143, 215.

30. Rather, *Mind and Body*, pp. 34-55, esp. 37, 48-49, 54-55.

31. Ibid., pp. 60-65; J. B. Winslow's *Exposition anatomique du corps humain* (Paris, 1732) discusses ganglia of the "great sympathetic nerves" as "miniature brains."

32. Rather, *Mind and Body*, pp. 75, 78-79, 86-91, 110-111.

33. Ibid., p. 117.

34. Ibid., pp. 156-161, 173, 179-181.

35. André Joussain, "Le Spiritualisme de Cabanis," *Archives de philosophie* xxi, no. 3 (1958), 386-409.

36. Diderot, *Eléments de physiologie*, ed. Jean Mayer (Paris, 1964), pp. xiii-xv.

37. Antoine Le Camus, *Médecine de l'esprit* (Paris, 1769), pp. viii-ix, 2-3, 8-10, 14, 18, 20, 35-39, 232-233.

38. Ibid., pp. 118-143, 149-150, 158, 211-212.

39. Ibid., pp. 218-224, 269-279, 291-292, 307-311, 333.

40. William Coleman, "Health and Hygiene in the *Encyclopédie*: A Medical Doctrine for the Bourgeoisie," *Journal of the History of Medicine* xxix (1974), 411-414.

41. Owsei Temkin, "The Classical Roots of Glisson's Doctrine of Irritation," *Bulletin of the History of Medicine* xxxviii (1964), 297-328; E.B.M. Bastholm, "The History of Muscle Physiology," *Acta Historia Scientiarum Naturalium et Medicinalium* (Copenhagen) vii (1950), 219-225.

42. Boerhaave, *Praelectiones Academicae Proprias Institutiones rei Medicae, edidit et notas addidit*, ed. Albrecht von Haller (Göttingen, 1740), ii, 664, note f.

43. On Haller biography, see S. d'Irsay, *Albrecht von Haller. Eine Studie zur Geistesgeschichte der Aufklärung*, 2 vols. (Leipzig, 1930), esp. i, 46-56; Richard Toellner, *A. von Haller, über die Einheit im Denken des letzten Universalgelehrten. Sudhoffs Archiv*, supplement 10 (Wiesbaden, 1971), esp. pp. 171-182; and, more specifically, see G. Rudolph, "Hallers Lehre von der Irritabilität und Sensibilität," in Karl Rothschuh, ed., *Von Boerhaave bis Berger. Die Entwicklung der Kontinentalen Physiologie im 18. und 19. Jahrhundert* (Stuttgart, 1964), pp. 14-34; Figlio, "Theories of Perception," pp. 185-191, 197-200; T. S. Hall, *Ideas of Life and Matter* i, 391-408; and Moravia, *Il Pensiero*, pp. 191-216.

44. Albrecht von Haller, "On the Sensible and Irritable Parts of Animals," ed. Owsei Temkin, *Bulletin of the Institute of the History of Medicine*, iv (1936), 651-699, esp. 658-659, 676-677, 682-687, 690

(edition based on a French translation by the physician S. A. Tissot of a revised enlarged version of Haller, "Mémoires sur la nature sensible et irritable des parties du corps animal" [Lausanne, 1756], i); Haller's notion of irritability was at once too modest and too comprehensive for the modern biologist. Some level of irritability is now considered a property of all living cells, not merely of muscle fibers. Yet muscular contractility, or, irritability, is commonly dependent on the nervous system, unlike Haller's hypothesis of independent muscular motion or independent movement of excised tissue.

45. Ibid., p. 692; for translation, see also Hall, *Ideas of Life and Matter* i, 401-404.

46. *Goettingsche gelehrte Anzeigen* (1747) (hereafter designated *GGA*), p. 907, cited in Richard Toellner, "Anima et Irritabilitas: Hallers Abwehr von Animismus und Materialismus," *Sudhoffs Archiv* li, no. 2 (1967), 137 n. 28, 142 n. 43; see also R. K. French, *Robert Whytt, The Soul, and Medicine* (London, 1969), pp. 68-70.

47. French, *Robert Whytt*, pp. 63-76.

48. Haller, "On the Sensible and Irritable Parts of Animals," pp. 678, 695-696; *GGA* (1752), p. 459, cited in Toellner, "Anima et Irritabilitas," p. 141 n. 36.

49. Stanley W. Jackson, "Force and Kindred Notions in Eighteenth-Century Nerve Physiology," *Bulletin of the History of Medicine* xliv (1970), 397-410, 539-554; Eric T. Carlson and Meribeth Simpson, "Models of the Nervous System in Eighteenth-Century Neurophysiology and Medical Psychology," *Bulletin of the History of Medicine* xliv (1969), 101-115.

50. Haller, "On the Sensible and Irritable Parts of Animals," p. 695.

51. Erich Hintzsche, "A. V. Hallers Korrespondenz mit Johann Stephan Bernard," *Clio medica* i (1966), 324-343.

52. Albrecht von Haller, *First Lines of Physiology* ([1747] Edinburgh, 1786 translation) ed. Lester Snow King (New York, 1966), preface, p. xliii.

53. La Mettrie, *L'Homme machine*, ed. Aram Vartanian (Princeton, 1960), pp. 58, 154; see Pierre Lemee, *Julien Offray de La Mettrie* (Saint-Malo, 1954); Emile Callot, *La Philosophie de la vie au XVIIIe siècle* (Paris, 1965), pp. 195-244; Moravia, *Il Pensiero*, pp. 63-74; and Ann Thomson, "Quatre lettres . . . de La Mettrie," *Dix-huitième Siècle* vii (1975), 5-19.

54. La Mettrie, *L'Homme machine*, pp. 21-22, 151, 181-182, 183, 189, 287; besides Gaub, Abraham Kaau-Boerhaave, a nephew of Her-

mann, discussed the *enormon* in *Impetum Faciens Dictum Hippocrati per Corpus Consentiens, Philologice, et Physiologice Illustratum* (1745).

55. La Mettrie, *L'Homme machine*, pp. 186, 192, 178.

56. Ibid., pp. 152-164, 173-175, 189, 195-196.

57. Callot, *La Philosophie*, p. 196; cf. Jean Perkins, "Diderot and La Mettrie," *Studies on Voltaire and the Eighteenth Century* x (1959), 49-100; Aram Vartanian, "Cabanis and La Mettrie," *Studies on Voltaire and the Eighteenth Century* CLV (1976), 2149-2166. Vartanian's discussion on the reasons for not acknowledging La Mettrie is cogent enough, though he mistakenly places the *Rapports* preface in 1796, rather than in 1802. I cannot, however, accept his explanation of the various functions of mechanism in Cabanis's thought. Attacks at the Institute by Cambacérès in 1798 and Mercier in October and November 1801 against La Mettrie may also have motivated Cabanis's silence. See *Mémoires de l'Institut . . . Classe des sciences morales et politiques* III, no. 13; and Bibliothèque de l'Arsénal, Papers of Mercier, MS 15087 (c), fol. 108n., "Extrait de mémoires sur Kant."

58. *OP* (London [Berlin], 1751), "Discours préliminaire," cited in Callot, *La Philosophie*, p. 221.

NOTES TO CHAPTER III

1. On the origins of Stahl's views, see B. J. Gottlieb, "Bedeutungen und Auswirkungen des hallischen Professors und Kgl. Preussischen Leibarztes Georg Ernst Stahl auf den Vitalismus des XVIII. Jahrhunderts, insbesondere auf die Schule von Montpellier," *Nova Acta Leopoldina* (Halle), n.s. (1943), esp. pp. 444-452; for studies of Stahl, see François Duchesneau, "G. E. Stahl: Antimécanisme et physiologie," *Archives internationales d'histoire des sciences* XXVI (1976), 3-26; L. J. Rather, "G. E. Stahl's Psychological Physiology," *Bulletin of the History of Medicine* XXXIV (1961), 37-49; Lester Snow King, "Stahl and Hoffmann: A Study in Eighteenth-Century Animism," *Journal of the History of Medicine* XIX (1964), 118-130; J.-E. Chancerel, *Recherches sur la pensée biologique de Stahl* (Paris, 1934); Thomas Steele Hall, *Ideas of Life and Matter* (Chicago, 1969), I, 351-366; and Sergio Moravia, "Dall' 'homme machine' all' 'homme sensible'," *Belfagor* XXIX (1974), 637-638 (translated in *Journal of the History of Ideas* XXXIX [1978], 45-60).

2. Michel Foucault, *Les Mots et les choses* (Paris, 1966), p. 139

(trans. *The Order of Things*, New York, 1970); Duchesneau, "G. E. Stahl," pp. 3, 26.

3. Georg Ernst Stahl, "Paraenesis," *Oeuvres médico-philosophiques et pratiques de G.-E. Stahl*, ed. Théodore Blondin (Paris, 1863), II, 157, 172; Stahl, "Ars Sanandi," p. 26, cited in Albert Lemoine, *Le Vitalisme et l'animisme de Stahl* (Paris, 1864), p. 101.

4. *OP* II, 131.

5. Stahl, "Demonstratio de Mixti et Vivi Corporis Vera Diversitate," (Halle, 1707), in *Oeuvres* II, 261-262, 265; Stahl, "Disquisitio de Mechanismi et Organismi Diversitate," (Halle, 1706), in *Oeuvres* II, 199-205, 213, 218, 224-228; Stahl, *Theoria Medica Vera* (Halle, 1708), in *Oeuvres* III, 43; Duchesneau, "G. E. Stahl," pp. 13-15, 20, 34.

6. Stahl, "Disquisitio," p. 245; Stahl, "Paraenesis," p. 36; Duchesneau, "G. E. Stahl," pp. 7, 9, 23; *OP* II, 133.

7. Stahl, "Paraenesis," pp. 173-174; Stahl, "Disquisitio," p. 354.

8. Stahl, "Disquisitio," p. 228; Stahl, *Theoria*, pp. 52, 422-423, 431; cf. Duchesneau, "G. E. Stahl," pp. 5-7.

9. Stahl, "Disquisitio," pp. 242, 326; Stahl, *Theoria*, pp. 104-105, 120, 303-307, 324, 363.

10. Stahl, "Disquisitio," pp. 239-240; cf. Duchesneau, "G. E. Stahl," p. 22.

11. *OP* II, 132, 143, 206, 499; I, 87, 304, 368.

12. Robert Whytt, *Observations on the Nature, Causes, and Cure of those Disorders Which Have Been Commonly Called Nervous, Hypochondriac, or Hysteric . . .* (Edinburgh, 1764).

13. Herbel E. Hoff and Peter Kellaway, "The Early History of the Reflex," *Journal of the History of Medicine* VII (1952), 211-249; on Whytt, see Hall, *Ideas of Life and Matter* II, 68-73; and R. K. French, *Robert Whytt, The Soul, and Medicine* (London, 1969).

14. Whytt, *Essay* (1763), pp. 242ff., cited in Hoff and Kellaway, "Early History of the Reflex," pp. 224-225; Whytt, *Observations* I, 42; Whytt, *Essay* (1751), p. 270, cited in Georges Canguilhem, *La Formation du concept de réflexe aux XVIIe et XVIIIe siècles* (Paris, 1955), p. 205; see also Canguilhem, *La Formation*, pp. 98-101, for discussion of the dissertation published by Haller (1749) of the French physician Jean Astruc (1684-1766), *An Sympathia Partium a Certa Nervorum Positura in Interno Sensorio* (1736). See also French, *Whytt*, pp. 56-59, 66, 76, 138.

15. French, *Whytt*, pp. 64-65, 104, 152; Canguilhem, *La Formation*, p. 106.

16. Hoff and Kellaway, "Early History of the Reflex," pp. 231-234; (Whytt, *Observations* I, 30-31, 50-51; Sympathies would now be classified as sympathetic nervous phenomena, nonautonomic reflexes, and hormonal phenomena (see French, *Whytt*, p. 36).

17. Whytt, *Physiological Essays* (1755), pt. II, "Observations on the Sensibility and Irritability of the Parts of Men and Other Animals; Occasioned by Dr. Haller's Latest Treatise on These Subjects," pp. 161, 176; see also Hoff and Kellaway, "Early History of the Reflex," pp. 227-228.

18. Whytt, *Observations* I, 74; Whytt, *Essay* (1751), p. 291; cf. Hoff and Kellaway, "Early History of the Reflex," p. 226.

19. French, *Whytt*, p. 118.

20. Ronald Tobey, "The Medical Speculations of William Cullen," (unpublished master's thesis, Cornell University, 1966), pp. 46-48; the moral sense theory, succeeded by concepts of innate sympathy, appeared in works of the third earl of Shaftesbury and in works of the Scottish philosophers Francis Hutcheson and Adam Smith, most recently in Smith's *Theory of Moral Sentiments* (1759).

21. On the foundation and history of the Faculty of Medicine, see A.-C. Germain, *L'Ecole de médecine de Montpellier: Ses Origines, sa constitution, son enseignement* (Montpellier, 1880), esp. pp. 9-10; on intellectual history, F.-E. Bérard, *Doctrine médicale de l'école de Montpellier* (Montpellier, 1819); Louis Dulieu, "Le Mouvement scientifique montpelliérain au XVIIIe siècle," *Revue d'histoire des sciences* XI (1958), 227-249; see also Sergio Moravia, "Filosofia e 'sciences de la vie' nel secolo XVIII," *Giornale critica della filosofia italiana* XXI (1966), 83-84, 103, 106-109; Moravia, *La Scienza dell'uomo nel settecento* (Bari, 1970), pp. 18, 55-60, 66 n. 15; and Moravia, "Philosophie et médecine en France à la fin du XVIIIe siècle," *Studies on Voltaire and the Eighteenth Century* LXXXIX (1972), 1090-1093, 1123.

22. Jacques Proust, *L'Encyclopédisme dans le Bas-Languedoc au XVIIIe siècle* (Montpellier, 1968), pp. 10-12; on Bordeu and Diderot, see Herbert Dieckmann, "Théophile Bordeu und Diderots 'Rêve de d'Alembert'," *Romanische Forschungen* LII, no. 1 (1938), 55-122; Jacques Roger, *Les Sciences de la vie dans la pensée française du XVIIIe siècle* (Paris, 1963), pp. 618-630; Arthur Wilson, *Diderot* (New York, 1972), pp. 557-570, 828-834; for Cabanis on Montpellier, see *OP* I, 46; II, 143-144.

23. Boissier de Sauvages, *Nosologie méthodique* (1763) (Lyon, 1771), II, 9, 14-15; on Sauvages, see Bérard, *Doctrine médicale*, pp.

44-53; Hall, *Ideas of Life and Matter* II, pp. 68-76; R. K. French, "Sauvages, Whytt, and the Motion of the Heart: Aspects of Eighteenth-Century Animism," *Clio medica* VII (1972), 35-54; Lester Snow King, "Boissier de Sauvages and 18th-Century Nosology," *Bulletin of the History of Medicine* XI (1966), 43-51.

24. Sauvages, *Nosologie* I, 49-50, 53 (par. 242), cited in Bérard, *Doctrine médicale*, 49n.; cf. Sauvages, *Nosologie* I, 75-78, and Bérard, *Doctrine médicale*, p. 45.

25. For Cabanis on Sydenham, see *OP* II, 138; on Sydenham, see also Kenneth Dewhurst, *Dr. Thomas Sydenham (1624-1689): His Life and Original Writings* (London, 1966); on classification, see Henri Daudin, *De Linné à Jussieu: Méthodes de classification et idée de série en botanique et en zoologie (1740-1790)* (Paris, 1926); Michel Foucault, *Naissance de la clinique* (Paris, 1963), pp. 3-8; Foucault, *Les Mots et les choses*, p. 150.

26. *The Works of Thomas Sydenham*, ed. Greenhill, trans. P. G. Latham (London, 1848), I, 12-14, based on London, 1676 ed. of Sydenham, *Observationes Medicae circa Morborum Acutorum Historiam*.

27. Sauvages, *Nosologie* (1771), II 12-13, 26-27; *OP* I, 69; II, 214.

28. Proust, *L'Encyclopédisme*, pp. 35-43; L. Cornet, "Théophile de Bordeu, le biologiste," *Bulletin de la Société des sciences, lettres, et arts de Pau*, 4ᵉ série, I (1966), 123-125; Paul Hoffmann, "L'Idée de liberté dans la philosophie médicale de Théophile de Bordeu," *Studies on Voltaire and the Eighteenth Century* LXXXVIII (1972), 769-787; see also Roger, *Les Sciences*, pp. 618-630; Moravia, *Il Pensiero*, pp. 222-226; and Moravia, "Dall' 'homme machine' all' 'homme sensible'," pp. 640-648.

29. *OP* I, 152; II, 83, 89, 101, 116, 122.

30. Bordeu, "Recherches sur les maladies chroniques" (1775), (hereafter designated "Maladies chroniques"), *Oeuvres complètes de Bordeu*, ed. B.-A. Richerand (Paris, 1818), II, 924.

31. Bordeu, "Recherches sur le pouls" (1754), *Oeuvres* I, 420-421; cf. Bordeu, "Recherches sur quelques points d'histoire de la médecine" (1764), (hereafter designated "Histoire de la médecine"), *Oeuvres* II, 667-668.

32. Bordeu, "De sensu" (1742), *Oeuvres* I, 9-13, 37-45; cf. Bordeu, "Recherches anatomiques sur la position des glandes et leur action" (1752), (hereafter designated "Glandes"), *Oeuvres* I, 163n.; for Bordeu's early conversion to Newtonianism, see letter to his father, 2 July

1740, in *Correspondance*, ed. Martha Fletcher, I (Montpellier, 1977), 43-44.

33. Bordeu, "Glandes," p. 50; Bordeu, "Recherches sur le tissu muqueux" (1767), *Oeuvres* II, 738-739, 752.

34. Bordeu, "Maladies chroniques," p. 800; Bordeu, "Analyse médicinale du sang" (1775), (hereafter designated "Sang"), *Oeuvres* II, 937, 1010; cf. Dieckmann, "Théophile Bordeu," p. 77.

35. Bordeu, "Glandes," 193n.; Bordeu, "Histoire de la médecine," pp. 679, 801, 831.

36. Bordeu, "Glandes," pp. 189, 202, 137, 198; Bordeu, "Sang," p. 955; Bordeu, "Histoire de la médecine," p. 676; cf. Dieckmann, "Théophile Bordeu," pp. 109, 117.

37. Bordeu, "Glandes," p. 187; Diderot used this image in his *Pensées sur l'interprétation de la nature* (1753) and *Le Rêve de d'Alembert*.

38. Bordeu, "Maladies chroniques," pp. 829-830.

39. Bordeu, "Glandes," pp. 123-125, 130-131, 158, 163-166, 201; Bordeu, "Sang," p. 940; on this subject, see the excellent paper by Elizabeth Haigh, "Vitalism, the Soul, and Sensibility: The Physiology of Théophile Bordeu." *Journal of the History of Medicine* XXXI (1976), 30-41.

40. Bordeu, "Glandes," 163n.

41. Bordeu, "Sang," pp. 1001-1006, 931-936.

42. Ibid., p. 989; Bordeu, "Crises" (1754), in *Oeuvres* I, 249.

43. L. Cornet, "Un Protecteur de Théophile de Bordeu: Le Médecin Louis Lacaze (1703-1765)," *Bulletin de la Société des sciences, lettres, et arts de Pau*, 3ᵉ série, XXVI (1966), 55-63; Jacques Roger, "Méthodes et modèles dans la préhistoire du vitalisme français: Lacaze, Fouquet, Ménuret de Chambaud," *XIIᵉ Congrès international d'histoire des sciences, Actes, IIIB* (Paris, 1971), pp. 101-108; Louis Lacaze, *Idée de l'homme physique et moral* (Paris, 1755), pp. 222-225, 382-383, 395-398, 434-435.

44. Lacaze, *Idée*, pp. 8-9; see Roger, *Les Sciences*, p. 632, on Ménuret's Encyclopedia article, "Observation."

45. Henri Fouquet, "Sensibilité, Sentiment," *Encyclopédie, ou Dictionnaire raisonné des sciences et des arts* XV (1765), 38A, 50A, 51A-B, 52A; Roger, *Les Sciences*, p. 103; L. Dulieu, "Les Articles d'Henri Fouquet dans l'*Encyclopédie*," *Revue d'histoire des sciences* V (1952), pp. 18-25; *OP* II, 206.

46. Victor de Sèze, *Recherches* (Paris, 1786), pp. 58, 5-12; cf. Sergio

Moravia, "Philosophie et médecine," pp. 1092-1093; on the Dupatys and Grouchys, see Antoine Guillois, *La Marquise de Condorcet: Sa Famille, son salon, ses amis 1764-1822* (Paris, 1897), ch. 1, pp. 79-90.

47. De Sèze, *Recherches*, pp. 31, 73, 275, 64, 75, 88, 284-285, 299.

48. Paul-Joseph Barthez, *Nouveaux Eléments de la science de l'homme* (Montpellier, 1806), ii, notes (separate pagination), 24, 99; see Jacques Lordat, *Exposition de la doctrine de P.-J. Barthez* (Paris, 1818); L. Dulieu, "Paul-Joseph Barthez," *Revue d'histoire des sciences* xxiv, no. 2 (1971), 149-176; *OP* ii, 169-170; for more background, see Paul Delaunay, *Le Monde médical parisien au XVIIIe siècle* (Paris, 1906), pp. 155-156.

49. Barthez, *Nouveaux Elémens* (Montpellier, 1778), pp. i-vii, x, xii, xviii; see also Barthez's perceptive, if somewhat unfair critique of Condillac's broad definition of analysis in the 1806 edition of the "Preliminary Discourse." Barthez's definitions of analytic and synthetic methods resembled that in Roger Cotes's preface to Newton's *Principia* (1713 ed.).

50. Ibid., pp. 30, 39, xiv, 6, 348, 2 (cf. 1806 edition, i, 49).

51. Ibid., 1806 edition, i, 186-187; Notes, ii, 99-100; 1778 edition, pp. 4, xviii-xix, 348.

52. Ibid., 1778 edition, 52, 58-62.

53. Ibid., pp. 210, 43, 69, 77, 82, 85-86; ed. 1806, i, 179-180.

54. Ibid., 1778 edition, pp. 142, 149, 153-154, 182, 227-228.

55. Ibid., pp. 285-286, 289-292.

56. "Letter from Diderot to Duclos, 10 October 1765," cited in Diderot, *Oeuvres philosophiques*, ed. Paul Vernière (Paris, 1964), p. 249; cf. Diderot "Entretien de d'Alembert," in *Oeuvres philosophiques*, pp. 260-261.

57. See Arthur Wilson, *Diderot* (New York, 1972), pp. 698-699; Jean Mayer, *Diderot, homme de science* (Rennes, 1959); Diderot, *Eléments de physiologie*, ed. Jean Mayer (Paris, 1964), pp. xiii-xvi; see also Y. François and T. François, "Quelques Remarques sur les 'Eléments de physiologie' de Diderot," *Revue d'histoire des sciences* v (1952), 77-82; Aram Vartanian, "The Enigma of Diderot's *Eléments de physiologie*," *Diderot Studies* x (1968), 285-301.

58. Diderot, *Eléments*, pp. 53-54, 59, 301, 306; 20, 35, 31, 73; 64, 265.

59. Ibid., pp. 284-289; cf. Diderot, *Le Rêve de d'Alembert*, ed. Paul Vernière, pp. 271-272, 293, 320-321.

60. Diderot, *Eléments*, pp. 84-87, 238; cf. Diderot, "Rêve," 330,

335, 356-357, 360; see an excellent parallel discussion of Diderot's *Eléments* in Moravia, *Il Pensiero*, pp. 157-164.

61. For ample discussion of Diderot's materialism and his ethics, see Wilson, *Diderot*, pp. 55-58, 97-102, 187-198, 380-381, 448, 488, 580-581, 665-668, 673, as well as bibliography in Wilson's notes; on the history of the concept of the brain as gland, see the paper by Elizabeth Haigh, "Glandular Secretion, Sensibility, and the Soul in the Work of Théophile de Bordeu," Canadian Learned Societies Conference, Edmonton, 1975, p. 13 n. 5; on Cabanis's opinions, see Chapter VII below.

NOTES TO CHAPTER IV

1. *OP* I, 24, 100n.

2. Dossier of Cabanis (no longer numbered) Bibliothèque historique de la ville de Paris (hereafter designated BHVP). See Appendix B for medical reading notes attributed to Cabanis.

3. *Biographie universelle ancienne et moderne* (Michaud), "Bosquillon," v (Paris, 1843), 121-122; "Leroux," XXIV, 253-255; see also AN (Archives Nationales) 0¹* 499, fol. 73, cited in Louis Greenbaum, "Jean-Sylvain Bailly, the baron de Breteuil, and the 'Four New Hospitals' of Paris," *Clio medica* VIII (1973), 268.

4. Henry Ingrand, *Le Comité de salubrité de l'Assemblée nationale constituante (1790-1791)* (Paris, M.D. Thesis 1934), pp. 13-15; Pierre Huard, "L'Enseignement médico-chirurgical," in René Taton, ed. *Enseignement et diffusion des sciences en France au XVIIIe siècle* (Paris, 1964), pp. 169-258, esp. pp. 172-177; A. Corlieu, *L'Ancienne Faculté de médecine de Paris* (Paris, 1877); Paul Delaunay, *Le Monde médical parisien au XVIIIe siècle* (Paris, 1906), ch. 1.

5. Antoine Guillois, *Le Salon de Mme Helvétius* (Paris, 1894), appendices, 297-299; Delaunay, *Le Monde médical*, pp. 331-356; *Commentaires de la Faculté de médecine de Paris, 1777-1786*, ed. Steinheil (Paris, 1903), I, 1153-1154, 1247-1288 (1784); on Mesmerism, see Robert Darnton, *Mesmerism and the End of the Enlightenment in France* (Cambridge, Mass., 1968).

6. Dossier of Cabanis, BHVP; O. Guelliot, "Cabanis à la Faculté de médecine de Reims," *Bulletin de la Société française d'histoire de la médecine* (1908), 186-192.

7. Printed licentiate thesis *An a pastu quies?* ; "Serment d'un médecin," *Feuille hebdomadaire de la Généralité de Limoges*, 10e année,

no. 11, 27 April 1785; printed titles give the erroneous date of 1783 for the "reception," contradicted by the manuscript dossier and the printed thesis.

8. *OP* ii, 300-302.

9. Dossier of Cabanis, BHVP.

10. "Statuts," *Commentaires*, ed. Steinheil, ii, 319 (art. 28).

11. Delaunay, *Le Monde médical*, pp. 166-207, 301-330; Owsei Temkin, "The Role of Surgery in the Rise of Modern Medical Thought," *Bulletin of the History of Medicine* xxv (1951), 250, 255-257; on the surgical profession, see Toby Gelfand, "The Training of Surgeons in Eighteenth-Century Paris and Its Influence on Medical Education," Ph.D. dissertation at Johns Hopkins University, 1973.

12. Huard, "L'Enseignement;" on G.-F. Rouelle, see J.-P. Contant, *L'Enseignement de la chimie au Jardin royal des plantes* (Cahors, 1952); and the articles by Rhoda Rappaport in *Chymia* vi (1960), 68-101, and vii (1961), 73-102; see Appendix D for description of a manuscript attributed to Cabanis, "Leçons de Chimie," which is in fact a transcription, though not identifiably by Cabanis, of chemistry lectures by Hilaire-Marin Rouelle at the Jardin des plantes.

13. Delaunay, *Le Monde médical*, pp. 37-39.

14. Caroline C. Hannaway, "The Société Royale de Médecine and Epidemics in the Ancien Régime," *Bulletin of the History of Medicine* xlvi (1972), 257-273; Delaunay, *Le Monde médical*, pp. 310-328.

15. See essays by J.-P. Desaive, Jean Meyer, Jean-Pierre Peter, J.-B. Goubert, et al., *Médecins, climat, et epidémies à la fin du XVIIIe siècle* (Paris, 1972).

16. See *Commentaires*, ed. Steinheil, i, xviii-xxi.

17. Vicq d'Azyr, "Nouveau Plan de constitution pour la médecine en France, . . ." *Histoire et mémoires de la Société royale de médecine, années 1787-1788* (Paris, 1790), ix, 1-170, esp. 60; Dora Weiner, "Le Droit de l'homme à la santé—Une Belle Idée devant l'Assemblée constituante: 1790-1791," *Clio medica* v (1970), 209-223, esp. 215.

18. See Sergio Moravia, "Philosophie et médecine en France à la fin du XVIIIe siècle," *Studies on Voltaire and the Eighteenth Century* lxxxix (1972), 1089-1092, 1095.

19. Vicq d'Azyr, "Nouveau Plan," *Histoire et mémoires* ix, 1-290; David Vess, *Medical Revolution in France 1789-1796* (Gainesville, Fla., 1975), 23-39; Toby Gelfand, "The Hospice of the Paris College of Surgery (1774-1793): 'A Unique and Invaluable Institution'," *Bulletin of the History of Medicine* xxvii (1972), 375-393.

20. On Fourcroy, see William A. Smeaton, *Fourcroy, Chemist and Revolutionary (1755-1809)* (London, 1962); and G. Kersaint, *Antoine-François de Fourcroy (1755-1809) Sa Vie et son oeuvre* (Paris, 1966).

21. See Antoine-François de Fourcroy, "Recherches pour servir à l'histoire du gaz-azote ou de la mofète, comme principe des matières animales," *Histoire et mémoires, année 1786* (Paris, 1790), VIII, 346-355; cf. *Annales de chimie* XXVII, 71; other statements appear in *Encyclopédie méthodique* (CLXIV) (*Médecine*) Fourcroy, "Action des médicaments," X (1787), 133-175.

22. See Fourcroy, "Prospectus," *La Médecine éclairée par les sciences physiques*, pp. 1, 3; I, 4-5; cf. Smeaton, *Fourcroy*, p. 204.

23. AN, AJ¹⁶ Aᴾ¹. Procès-verbaux de l'assemblée des professeurs, Faculté de médecine, 29 Nivôse VI (19 January 1798), reviewed by Goulin and Dubois 9 Pluviôse VI (28 January 1798); *OP* I, 35, 37; *Degré de certitude* was also sent to the Second Class of the Institute 17 Pluviôse VI (5 February 1798); (Archives de l'Académie des sciences morales et politiques, fol. 117, Procès-verbaux de la Classe des sciences morales et politiques.

24. *OP* I, 41-47.

25. "Discours prononcé dans l'Académie française, le jeudi 21 février 1782, à la réception de M. de Marquis de Condorcet," in *Oeuvres complètes de Condorcet*, ed. A. Condorcet O'Connor and M. F. Arago, I (Paris, 1847), 392, cited in Keith Baker, *Condorcet* (Chicago, 1975), p. 86, see also pp. 170-171, 181-182.

26. *OP* I, 102-103n.; cf. II, 173n.

27. *OP* I, 40-41; Constantin Hillemand, "*Du Degré de certitude de la médecine* d'après Cabanis," *Le Progrès médical* (1932), no. 2, cols. 66-77, no. 7, cols. 294-301, no. 19, cols. 823-832.

28. *OP* I, 50-53, 56, 91.

29. Ibid., pp. 82-84, 77. Erna Lesky, "Cabanis und die Gewissheit der Heilkunde," *Gesnerus* XI (1954), 152-182, cleverly paralleled Cabanis's responses to critics and Hippocratic replies (*The Art, Diet,* etc.) to Greek detractors of medicine.

30. *OP* I, 69-72; cf. II, 214-218; on Cabanis's attitudes to nosology, see Moravia, "Philosophie et médecine," pp. 1129-1131.

31. *OP* I, 58-64; cf. Condillac, *Traité des systèmes* (1749); Voltaire, *Eléments de la philosophie de Newton* (1738).

32. Fourcroy, "Mémoire sur l'application de la chimie pneumatique à l'art de guérir," *Annales de chimie* XXVIII, 256.

33. *OP* I, 73-74.

34. Ibid., nn. 99-101.

35. Camille Bloch, *L'Assistance et l'état en France à la veille de la Révolution* (Paris, 1908), pp. 47-48, 191, 219; see also Michel Foucault, *Naissance de la clinique* (Paris, 1963), pp. 38-43; George Rosen, "Hospitals, Medical Care, and Social Policy in the French Revolution," *Bulletin of the History of Medicine* xxx (1956), 124-149. The excellent articles in Michel Foucault, Blandine Kriegel, et al., *Les Machines à guérir (aux origines de l'hôpital moderne)* arrived too late for assimilation into the discussion in this chapter but they do not seem to change the basic nature of the issues. Foucault's introduction on the politics of health care would require a separate essay and will only be mentioned briefly in Chapter X.

36. On hospital reform and the Academy of Sciences commission, see the excellent series of studies by Louis Greenbaum, " 'The Commercial Treaty of Humanity': La Tournée des hôpitaux anglais par Jacques Tenon en 1787," *Revue d'histoire des sciences* xxiv (1971), 317-350, "Jean-Sylvain Bailly," cited above; and "Tempest in the Academy: Jean-Baptiste Le Roy, the Paris Academy of Sciences, and the Project of a New Hôtel-Dieu," *Archives internationales d'histoire des sciences* xxiv (1974), 122-140; see also P.N.A. Richmond, "The Hôtel-Dieu of Paris on the Eve of the Revolution," *Journal of the History of Medicine* xvi (1961), 335-353; Marcel Candille, "Les Projets de translation de l'Hôtel-Dieu de Paris hors de la cité," *Revue de l'Assistance publique à Paris* vii (1956), 743-752; and viii (1957), 239-263, 343-359, 433-449.

37. Louis Greenbaum, " 'Measure of Civilization': The Hospital Thought of Jacques Tenon on the Eve of the French Revolution," *Bulletin of the History of Medicine* xlix (1975), 43-56.

38. *Extrait des registres de l'Académie royale des sciences du 22 novembre 1786. Rapport des commissaires chargés, par l'Académie, de l'examen d'un Projet d'un nouvel Hôtel-Dieu* (2d ed., Paris, 1787), pp. 6-7, 18-21, 104-134; [Jean-Sylvain Bailly], *Discours et Mémoires, par l'auteur de l'Histoire de l'Astronomie* ii (Paris, 1790), 321-340, 341-391, for reports of 20 June 1787 and 12 March 1788.

39. See Louis Greenbaum, "Health Care and Hospital-Building in Eighteenth-Century France: Reform Proposals of Du Pont de Nemours and Condorcet," *Studies on Voltaire and the Eighteenth Century* clii (1976), 895-930; on the image in question, see Bloch, *L'Assistance et l'Etat*, p. 188 and Weiner, *Le Droit de l'homme*, p. 210.

40. Du Pont de Nemours, *Idées* (Philadelphia and Paris, 1786).

41. *Extrait*, pp. 104-116.

42. Camille Bloch and Alexandre Tuetey, eds., *Procès-verbaux et rapports du comité de mendicité* (Paris, 1911), pp. 7, 65.

43. *OP* I, 7-27. For a recent perspective on clinical journal-keeping in the small hospital by a contemporary, see the memoir of October 1789 by Chambon de Montaux discussed in Toby Gelfand, "A Clinical Ideal: Paris 1789," *Bulletin of the History of Medicine* LI (1977), 397-411.

44. Bloch and Tuetey, eds. *Procès-verbaux*, pp. 391; on Cabanis's writings on public assistance, see also Sergio Moravia, *Il Tramonto dell'illuminismo* (Bari, 1968), pp. 97-107.

45. L. Duguit and H. Monnier, *Les Constitutions . . . depuis 1789* (Paris 1923), pp. 1-2.

46. *OP* I, 6.

47. On the depots, see Camille Bloch, *L'Assistance et l'Etat en France à la veille de la Révolution* (Paris, 1908), as well as Christian Paultre, *De La Répression de la mendicité et du vagabondage en France sous l'ancien régime* (Paris 1906); Jean-Pierre Gutton, *L'Etat et la mendicité. . . .* (Lyon 1973); Thomas Adams, "Mendicity and Moral Alchemy: Work as Rehabilitation," *Studies on Voltaire and the Eighteenth Century* CLI (1976), 47-76.

48. Leclerc de Montlinot, *Etat actuel du dépôt de Soissons, précédé d'un essai sur la mendicité* (Soissons 1789), pp. 2-7, 15-25.

49. See *OP* I, 567-574, 576, 578.

50. Ibid., pp. 28-30.

51. Ibid., pp. 6, n. 6, 29; cf. II, 17.

52. Ibid., I, 29.

53. Ibid., II, 10-11.

54. Ibid., I, 29-31.

55. Ibid., p. 5.

NOTES TO CHAPTER V

1. See Sergio Moravia, *Il Tramonto dell'illuminismo* (Bari, 1968), pp. 109-113, 122-139.

2. Cabanis, *Journal de la maladie et de la mort de Mirabeau* (Paris, 1791), pp. 4-5.

3. Victor de Seilhac, *Scènes et portraits de la Révolution en Bas-Limousin* (Paris, 1878), pp. 117-150; on other disturbances in 1790,

see Samuel F. Scott, "Problems of Law and Order during 1790, the 'Peaceful' Year of the French Revolution," *American Historical Review* LXXX (1975), 859-888.

4. Lucien Picqué and Louis Dubousquet, "L'Incident du salon de Mme Helvétius (Cabanis et l'abbé Morellet)," *Bulletin de la Société française d'histoire de la médecine* XVII (1914), 281-296.

5. Sigismond Lacroix, ed. *Actes de la Commune de Paris* (Paris, 1894), IV, 301-302, 322, 334-341, 508.

6. AD Correze (Tulle), 6.F.239, letter of Cabanis to J.-B.-H. Serre, 17 April 1790; Parent de Rosan collection (Mairie du XVIᵉ arrondissement), "Copie des Archives de la Préfecture de la Seine; contributions d'Auteuil," vol. 28, fol. 292v.

7. Keith Baker, *Condorcet* (Chicago, 1975), pp. 272-285, esp. 281; see also Moravia, *Tramonto*, pp. 152-161; Augustin Challamel, *Les Clubs contre-révolutionnaires* (Paris, 1895), pp. 391-443.

8. F.-A. Aulard, ed., *La Société des Jacobins* (Paris, 1889), I, xl.

9. On the general topic, see J. Bénétruy, *L'Atelier de Mirabeau* (Geneva, 1962).

10. Ibid., pp. 315-317, 330, 466-479; text of discourses in *Oeuvres complètes de Cabanis* (hereafter designated *OC*), ed. François Thurot (Paris, 1823), II, 363-581; see E. Dreyfus-Brisac, "Petits Problèmes de bibliographie pédagogique," *Revue internationale de l'enseignement* (1892), pp. 273-300; *OP* II, 546-547; H. Monin, "Le Discours de Mirabeau sur les fêtes publiques," *La Révolution française* XXV (1893), 214-231; see also Mona Ozouf, *La Fête révolutionnaire, 1789-1799* (Paris, 1976), n. 76.

11. Ozouf, *La Fête*, pp. 76-81.

12. *OC* II, 445, 451, 476; cf. *OP* II, 261, 265.

13. Parent de Rosan Collection, "Registres des délibérations du conseil municipal d'Auteuil (1790-1859) à l'hôtel de ville," vol. 28, fol. 69r.; "Auteuil, documents administratifs, copies separées, 1790-1859," vol. 28, pp. 250-251.

14. The following titles are a selection from the vast literature on education during the Revolution: Félix Ponteil, *Histoire de l'enseignement en France* (Paris, 1966); Maurice Gontard, *L'Enseignement primaire en France de la Révolution à la loi Guizot (1789-1833)* (Paris, 1959); Célestin Hippeau, *L'Instruction publique en France pendant la Révolution*, 2 vols. (Paris, 1881-1883); Albert Duruy, *L'Instruction publique et la Révolution* (Paris, 1882); Louis Liard, *L'Enseignement supérieur en France 1789-1889*, 2 vols. (Paris, 1888-1894); H. C. Barnard, *Education and the French Revolution* (Cambridge,

1969); James Leith, "Modernization, Mass Education, and Social Mobility in French Thought, 1750-1789," *Studies in the Eighteenth Century* (Canberra, 1973), II, 223-238.

15. *OC* II, 371, 384-386 (cf. *OP* I, 76-77), 482-486.

16. Adam Smith, *Wealth of Nations* (1776), bk. v, pt. III, art. 2.

17. *OC* II, 437, 481, 490-492, 549.

18. Ibid., pp. 390-393, 437, 382, 492-493.

19. Ibid., pp. 505, 509-520, 527-536.

20. Ibid., pp. 392-398, 422-431.

21. Ibid., pp. 399-401, 488.

22. Ibid., pp. 408-411.

23. Cabanis, *Journal*, p. 70; cf. Moravia, *Tramonto*, p. 161; *Discours de Cabanis en offrant au Conseil des cinq-cents la gravure du portrait de Mirabeau*, 13 Thermidor VI.

24. *Le Républicain, ou le défenseur du gouvernement représentatif; par une société des républicains* (July 1791), 4 nos.

25. On Duchâstelet, see *Bulletin de la Societé historique d'Auteuil et de Passy* II (1895-1897), 229-230; Parent de Rosan collection, "Copie des Archives de la Préfecture de la Seine. Conseil général d'Auteuil. 1793," vol. 28, fol. 38v.

26. *Opinion de Cabanis sur les Réunions s'occupant d'objets politiques* (Paris, n.d.), 6 Thermidor V, 3n., 4n. Moravia, *Tramonto*, pp. 162-163, also cites this pamphlet, though the date given in the works of Cabanis should be changed to an VII, because Cabanis was not yet in the Council of Five Hundred in an V and the topic concerned Jourdan's motion to proclaim the *patrie en danger*, debated in an VII.

27. For further details, see Moravia, *Tramonto*, p. 173.

28. Dossier of Cabanis, Bibliothèque historique de la ville de Paris.

29. Michel Bouchet, *L'Assistance publique en France pendant la Révolution* (Paris, 1908), pp. 252-257.

30. Camille Bloch and Alexandre Tuetey, eds., *Procès-verbaux et rapports du comité de mendicité* (Paris, 1911), p. 65.

31. Alexandre Tuetey, ed., "Procès-verbaux du comité des hôpitaux, 15 avril-3 octobre 1791," *Bulletin d'histoire économique de la Révolution* (Paris, 1916), pp. 67-153; Germain Garnier, *Rapport fait au conseil du département de Paris, à l'ouverture de la session du 15 Novembre 1791 . . . par M. Garnier . . . contenant l'exposé des travaux du Directoire, et le compte de sa gestion*.

32. "Procès-verbaux du comité des hôpitaux," pp. 97, 115-116, 126-127, 130-131, 139, 147; Garnier, *Rapports*, pp. 27-28, 31-33.

33. Toby Gelfand, "A Confrontation over Clinical Instruction at the

Hôtel-Dieu of Paris during the French Revolution," *Journal of the History of Medicine* xxviii (1973), 268-282.

34. *OP* ii, 57-58.

35. AD Seine 6 AZ 52 (printed), *Rapport sur la nouvelle distribution des secours proposés dans le Département de Paris par le comité de mendicité* (Paris, 1791), p. 9.

36. *OP* ii, 413.

37. M. Brièle, ed., *Collection des documents pour servir à l'histoire des hôpitaux de Paris* ii (Paris, 1883), 284-286.

38. Archives de l'Académie des sciences morales et politiques, Procès-verbaux de la Classe des sciences morales et politiques (hereafter designated CSMP), 17 Vendémiaire v, in i, fol. 39, 27 Brumaire vii, in ii, fol. 21; *Recueil de mémoires sur les établissements d'humanité*, ed. Adrien Duquesnoy, 17 vols., ans vii-xii (1798-1803).

39. *OP* ii, 44-45.

40. Ibid., pp. 48-59, esp. 57-58.

41. Procès-verbaux de la CSMP, 7 Vendémiaire v, in i, fol. 38; Claude Delasselle, "Les Enfants abandonnés à Paris au XVIIIe siècle," *Annales* xxx (1975), 187-218.

42. *OP* ii, 37-43.

43. Procès-verbaux de la CSMP, 7 Thermidor iv, in i, fol. 23; *OP* ii, 34-36; see Michel Foucault, *Surveiller et punir: Naissance de la prison* (Paris, 1975), pp. 125-127, who cited Jonas Hanway, *The Defects of Police* (1775) for another English precedent; see also François Doublet, *Mémoire sur la nécessité d'établir une réforme dans les prisons . . .* (Paris, 1791), by a physician active in the Hospitals and Prisons Department and in the Royal Society of Medicine.

44. *OP* ii, 3-5, 11-14, 17-18, 20.

45. Ibid., pp. 11, 18-19, 29; cf., 391, 481.

46. Ibid., pp. 6, 12-14.

47. Ibid., pp. 7-8, 15-17, 63.

48. Morton Eden's publication appeared in London in 1797; see *Dictionary of National Biography* vi, 356-357; for attribution of review to Cabanis, see *Recueil de mémoires*, ed. Duquesnoy, vii, 5 n. 1; see also AN F17A 1014, Interior Ministry files, for sponsorship of the series; Cabanis's review of Eden in *Mercure français*, 20 Messidor vi (8 July 1798), xxix, 257-272, 30 Messidor vi (18 July 1798), xxx, 321-330, 20 Thermidor vi (7 August 1798), xxxii, 65-72.

49. *Mercure* xxxii, 70-71; and xxix, 272; *OP* ii, 27.

50. *Mercure* xxx, 332; cf. *OP* ii, 16-17.

51. Garnier, *Rapports*, p. 44; see Yvonne Forado-Cunéo, *Les Ateliers de charité de Paris pendant la Révolution française (1789-1791)* (Paris, 1934); Michel Bouchet, *L'Assistance publique*, pp. 212-240.

52. Bloch and Tuetey, *Procès-verbaux*, pp. 331, 427.

53. *Mercure* xxx, 328-330.

54. Ibid., p. 324; *OP* ii, 8-9, 25-30.

55. *OP* ii, 5, 22, 63; Law of 19 March 1793, in *Réimpression de l'ancien moniteur*, (21 March 1793), xv, 748-749.

56. *OP* ii, 59-60.

57. *La Décade philosophique, littéraire, et politique* (10 Frimaire xii), p. 398n.; cf. Joanna Kitchin, *"La Décade" (1794-1807): Un journal 'philosophique'* (Paris, 1965), p. 196.

NOTES TO CHAPTER VI

1. *Réimpression de l'ancien moniteur* (23 August 1792), xiii, 496.

2. AN BB³⁰ 25, letters of Cabanis to Minister of Justice Gohier, 23 March, 26 March, 30 March, undated (2 April?), and 23 April [1793]; see James Logan Godfrey, *Revolutionary Justice* (Chapel Hill, 1951), pp. 4-15, 29-31; *Réimpression de l'ancien moniteur* xvi, 147, 150, 213, 220-221.

3. See Sergio Moravia, *Il Tramonto dell'illuminismo* (Bari, 1968), pp. 197-213, 225.

4. Vermeil de Conchard, *Trois Etudes sur Cabanis d'après des documents inédits* (Brive, 1914), pp. 12, 15-16.

5. Parent de Rosan collection, "Registres des déliberations du conseil municipal d'Auteuil (1790-1859) à l'hôtel de ville," vol. 28, fol. 74v.; Antoine Guillois, *Le Salon de Mme Helvétius* (Paris, 1894), pp. 83-84.

6. Sophie Condorcet, *Théorie des sentimens moraux . . . Lettres à Cabanis, sur la théorie des sentimens moraux* (Paris, an vi [1798]), ii, 311-442; Franck Alengry, *Condorcet* (Paris, 1904), p. 734.

7. Parent de Rosan collection, vol. 28, fols. 9v., 19v., 32r., 84v., 88v., 90v., 95v.; Richard Cobb, *Les Armées révolutionnaires: Instrument de terreur dans les départements, avril 1793-floréal an II* (Paris, 1961), ii, 480, 502 n. 129.

8. Guillois, *Le Salon*, pp. 81-102; Kitchin, *"La Décade"*; see also Marc Régaldo, *"La Décade* et les philosophes du XVIIIe siècle," *Dix-huitième Siècle* ii (1970), 113-130.

9. David Vess, *Medical Revolution in France 1789-1796* (Gainesville, Fla., 1975), pp. 71-92, 117-136, 162, 170.

10. James Guillaume, ed., *Procès-verbaux du comité d'instruction publique de la Convention Nationale* iv (Paris, 1901), 980; v (1904), 282, 316, 323-324.

11. Guillaume, ed., *Procès-verbaux d'instruction publique* vi (1907), 389, 708, 757.

12. *OP* ii, 66-67; see also Constantin Hillemand, "*Coup d'oeil* de Cabanis *sur les révolutions et sur la réforme de la médecine*," *Le Progrès médical* (1932), no. 39, cols. 1626-1639, no. 40, cols. 1658-1673.

13. *OP* ii, 70-75, 312-315; cf. Sergio Moravia, "Philosophie et médecine," *Studies on Voltaire and the Eighteenth Century* lxxxix (1972), 1092, 1097-1098.

14. D'Alembert, *Preliminary Discourse to the Encyclopedia of Diderot* (1751), trans. Richard Schwab (New York, 1963), p. 29; see d'Alembert's caution on hasty application of mathematics to medicine, pp. 24-25.

15. *OP* i, 124-125; ii, 82, 423.

16. *OP* i, 240-241, 329-331.

17. *OP* ii, 204-208, 230-231, 248.

18. Ibid., p. 169; cf. p. 315. See also Moravia, "Philosophie et médecine," pp. 1095, 1101.

19. *OP* ii, 174-175. The medical history derived largely from Daniel Le Clerc, *Histoire de la médecine* ([The Hague, 1729] Amsterdam, 1967) and Théophile de Bordeu, *Recherches sur quelques points d'histoire de la médecine* (Liège, 1764). Cabanis was less erudite than either source, though he contributed remarkable psychological insight into the charisma of early priest-healers (modeled, no doubt, on contemporary works on religion like that of the Idéologues' friend Charles Dupuis's *Origines de tous les cultes, ou religion universelle, . . .* 4 vols. [Paris, an iii]).

20. *OP* ii, 100, 151; *Le Conservateur, journal politique, philosophique, et littéraire*, ed. Garat, Daunou, and Chénier 9 Vendémiaire vi (30 September 1797), p. 237. Cabanis contributed this fascinating statement under the rubric "Sciences, Philosophie," which he sometimes used for book reviews. His tolerance for system-builders exceeded that of d'Alembert in his *Preliminary Discourse*, who warned that the spirit of conjecture was now obsolete. Cabanis's scheme was also similar to passages in Condorcet's manuscripts, to which he might have had access (see Keith Baker, *Condorcet* [Chicago, 1975], p. 118).

21. See Frank Manuel, *The Prophets of Paris* (Cambridge, Mass., 1962); Thomas Kuhn, *The Structure of Scientific Revolutions* (2d ed., Chicago, 1969).

22. *OP* ii, 307-308, 153, 97-98.

23. *OP* i, 122 n. 1; *Séances des écoles normales* . . . (2ᵉ ed., Paris, an ix), i, 157-158; cf. definition of "analyse" by Laromiguière in his Institute memoir, "Analyse des sensations" (27 Germinal iv), which closely paralleled Condillac; cf. Moravia, *Tramonto*, pp. 380-391, and "Philosophie et médecine," p. 1124.

24. *OP* ii, 160.

25. *OP* ii, 154-166; cf. Moravia, "Philosophie et médecine," pp. 1139, 1146, 1149-1151.

26. *OP* ii, 185-192; see Condillac, "Logique," in *Oeuvres philosophiques*, ed. Georges Le Roy (Paris, 1951), ii, 374-376.

27. *OP* ii, 195-197.

28. See Célestin Hippeau, *L'instruction publique en France* (Paris, 1883), ii, 416-417, passage cited in Moravia, *Tramonto*, pp. 383-384.

29. *OP* ii, 248-249.

30. Philippe Pinel, *Nosographie philosophique, ou la méthode de l'analyse appliquée à la médecine* (Paris, an vi [1798]), i, xi-xii, xvi-xvii, xxxix, 4; ii, 333, 374, 383-385; Philippe Pinel, *Traité médico-philosophique sur l'aliénation mentale, ou la manie* (Paris, an ix [1801]), p. xxxv; Walther Riese, *The Legacy of Philippe Pinel: An Inquiry into Thought on Mental Alienation* (New York, 1969), pp. 85-102; and Riese, "La Méthode analytique de Condillac et ses rapports avec l'oeuvre de Philippe Pinel," *Revue philosophique* clviii (1968), 321-336.

31. *OP* ii, 176-177.

32. Ibid., p. 77; cf. *OP* i, 126. Because of the late publication date of *Coup d'oeil* and the 1802 publication of the *Rapports* preface, one must note the priority in use of the term "anthropology" by Cabanis's colleague J.-L. Moreau de La Sarthe in 1801 (in *La Décade* [20 Prairial ix], pp. 458-459), as well as by Cabanis's student François Péron, *Observations sur l'Anthropologie* . . . (1800). On the latter, see Sergio Moravia, *Il Pensiero degli idéologues*, (Florence, 1974) 578; Georges Gusdorf, *Dieu, la nature, l'homme au siècle des lumières* (Paris, 1972), pp. 405-408, 417-423 has noted the sixteenth-century use of the term in Latin, its occurrence in French in a translation from the Italian in 1755, and its use in German by Wilhelm von Humboldt and others from 1785-1797; see also Sergio Moravia, *La Scienza dell'uomo*

nel settecento (Bari, 1970), pp. 75-80, 214-215 on Péron and others.

33. *OP* II, 209-213, 247-249, 225, 77-78.

34. On the central schools, see L. Pearce Williams, "Science, Education, and the French Revolution," *Isis* XLIV (1953), 311-330; the bibliography of regional studies in H. C. Barnard, *Education and the French Revolution* (Cambridge, 1969); documents in Guillaume, ed., *Procès-verbaux du comité d'instruction publique* v (1904), 298, 550; VI (1907), 338, 553, 573-575, 879.

35. AN F^{17} 1344^{27}, and F^{17} 1344^{28} Ecoles centrales—Seine; Guillaume, *Procès-verbaux du comité d'instruction publique* (1907) VI, 553, 575.

36. AN F^{17A} 1011, documents of Conseil d'instruction publique; Destutt de Tracy, *Observations sur le système actuel de l'instruction publique* (Paris, an IX [1801]).

NOTES TO CHAPTER VII

1. For Condorcet's usage, see Keith Baker, *Condorcet* (Chicago, 1975), pp. 388-395; on foundation of the Institute, Léon Aucoc, *L'Institut de France: Lois, statuts, règlements* (Paris, 1889); Jules Simon, *Une Académie sous le Directoire* (Paris, 1885), pp. 39-83; James Guillaume, ed., *Procès-verbaux du comité d'instruction publique de la Convention Nationale* VI (Paris, 1907), 335-341, 576, 644-645, 789-798, 833-839, 861, 869-873.

2. Simon, *Une Académie*, pp. 216-218.

3. Archives de l'Académie des sciences morales et politiques, Registre de procès-verbaux de la Classe des sciences morales et politiques, I; *OP* I, 161-162n.

4. In a note of 1805 (*OP* I, 126n., 1), Cabanis baptized this combination of disciplines "anthropologie" in imitation of German usage; cf. *Coup d'oeil* (1804); and *OP* II, 77. The anthropology of Ernst Platner and Kant defined the field of physiological psychology much more than that of physical or cultural anthropology in the modern sense. These latter disciplines were developed by the Société des observateurs de l'homme, including Jauffret, Péron, and Degérando as active members, on which see Sergio Moravia, *La Scienza dell'uomo nel settecento* (Bari, 1970). In 1859 Paul Broca founded the Société d'anthropologie de Paris, in which the usage of the term "anthropology" to mean physiological psychology was still evident (*Revue d'anthropologie* I).

5. Baker, *Condorcet*, pp. 219-225, based primarily on Condorcet, "De L'Influence de la Révolution" (1786), in *Oeuvres* VIII, ed. M. F. Arago, 5-6; see also Keith Baker, "Condorcet's notes for a revised edition of his reception speech to the Académie française," *Studies on Voltaire and the Eighteenth Century* CLIX (1977), 44-45.

6. On Volney see Jean Gaulmier, *Volney: Un Grand Témoin de la Révolution et de l'Empire* (Paris, 1959); Cabanis to printer Saltier, 22 June, and 6 July 1793, cited in *OP* II, 527, only the second letter is located in the Parent de Rosan Collection XX, fols. 46-47; *OP* I, 119n.

7. Volney, *La Loi naturelle*, ed. Gaston-Martin (Paris, 1934), pp. 105, 108-109, 111, 115, 119, 141, 146-147.

8. Ibid., pp. 134-136, 153; 121-131, 143-144.

9. Ibid., pp. 148-150; for a precedent, see Siéyès, *Reconnaissance et exposition raisonnée des droits de l'homme et du citoyen* (Versailles, 1789).

10. *Séances des écoles normales recueillies par des stenographes et revues par les professeurs* ([an III] Paris, an IX); *Débats* I, 217-219, 221; III, 14, 23-24, 43-47, 72-76, 85, 110-111, 115; see also several passages cited in Sergio Moravia, *Il Tramonto dell'illuminismo* (Bari, 1968), p. 395, where he interprets the debate differently. On Saint-Martin, see bibliography in Moravia, *Tramonto*, and A. Becque and N. Chuquin, "Un Philosophe toujours inconnu: L. Cl. de Saint-Martin," *Dix-huitième Siècle* IV (1972), 169-190.

11. Thomas Kuhn, *The Structure of Scientific Revolutions* (2d ed., Chicago, 1969).

12. *Mémoires de l'Institut national des sciences et arts. Classe des sciences morales et politiques*. "Mémoire sur la faculté de penser," read on (2 Messidor IV [20 June 1796]), published (Paris, Thermidor VI), I, 344-345.

13. "Pinel, Traité médico-philosophique sur l'aliénation mentale, ou la manie," extrait, *La Décade philosophique* (20 Prairial IX [9 June 1801]), 458-459n.

14. B.-A. Richerand, *Nouveaux élémens de physiologie* (Paris, an IX), was already hailed by Cabanis in 1801 and went through ten editions by 1833. On Alibert's "Discours sur les rapports de la médecine avec les sciences physiques et morales," *Mémoires de la Société médicale d'émulation* II (Paris, an VII), see Sergio Moravia, "Philosophie et médecine," *Studies on Voltaire and the Eighteenth Century* (1972), pp. 1092-1096, 1100, 1110, 1118-1119, 1123, 1133.

15. Destutt de Tracy, *Projet d'élémens d'idéologie* (Paris, 1801), p.

1; see the more accessible reprint of the 1817 edition, *Eléments d'idéologie: Idéologie proprement dite*, ed. Henri Gouhier (Paris, 1970), xiii.

16. Maine de Biran, *Influence de l'habitude sur la faculté de penser* (Paris, an xi-1803), and "Mémoire sur la décomposition de la pensée," (an xiii) in *Oeuvres de Maine de Biran*, ed. Pierre Tisserand (Paris, 1920-1949); see Chap. 9 for bibliography.

17. See J.-M. Degérando, *Des Signes, et de l'art de penser considérés dans leurs rapports mutuels*, 4 vols. (Paris, an viii); Degérando, *Considérations sur les diverses méthodes à suivre dans l'observation des peuples sauvages* (Paris, n.d. [1800]); Degérando, *De La Génération des connaissances humaines* (Berlin, 1802); on Degérando, see Sergio Moravia, *Il Pensiero degli idéologues* (Florence, 1974), pp. 417-456; Laromiguière was the author of a *Projet d'élémens de métaphysique* (1794) as well as Institute memoirs published in 1798, "Sur la Détermination de ces mots, Analyse des Sensations," and "Extrait d'un mémoire sur la détermination du mot Idée;" Cabanis also cited P.-F. Lancelin, author of a three-volume *Introduction à l'analyse des sciences, ou de la Génération, des fondemens, et des instruments des nos connaissances*, an ix (1801)- an xi (1802). Jacquemont prepared a work on "Les Essences réelles." See *OP* i, 112-113n.

18. Destutt de Tracy, "Sur un Système méthodique de bibliographie," *Moniteur* (8 and 9 Brumaire vi [29 and 30 October 1797]) Emmet Kennedy, "Destutt de Tracy and the Unity of the Sciences," *Studies on Voltaire and the Eighteenth Century* clxxi (1977), 223-239, esp. 231-232.

19. The dates in *OP* ii, 548 have been verified in the *Registres* of the Archives de l'Académie des sciences morales et politiques.

20. Georges Gusdorf, *Naissance de la conscience romantique au siècle des lumières* (Paris, 1976).

21. *OP* i, 118-120, 361.

22. Ibid., pp. 159-161.

23. Ibid., p. 142; cf. Moravia, *Il Pensiero*, pp. 32-33, 60-61.

24. *OP* i, 197-198.

25. Ibid., pp. 327-331; see notes on the experiments of Alexander von Humboldt in 1797 and on the Institute commission headed by the physician J.-N. Hallé. See also Karl Rothschuh, *Alexander von Humboldt et l'histoire de la découverte de l'électricité animale* (Paris, 1960).

26. *OP* I, 121, 539-540.

27. Ibid., pp. 531-532; Moravia does not hesitate to use the designation "materialist," but I would argue that he overstates the case; see *Il Pensiero*, pp. 28-29, 77, 87-90, 190, and Chapter XI below.

28. *OP* I, 360-361, 600-601; Pierre-Simon de Laplace, *Exposition du système du monde* (Paris, 1796 [an IV]), I, 302, 306.

29. *OP* I, 236, 528-531; see Guyton de Morveau, "Affinité," *Encyclopédie méthodique. Chimie, pharmacie, métallurgie* I (Paris, 1786), 535-539, 570; cf. Moravia, *Il Pensiero*, pp. 108-113, who gives, I believe, an incorrect interpretation of Guyton's position.

30. On the older idea of affinity, see Henry Guerlac, "The Background to Dalton's Atomic Theory," in *John Dalton and the Progress of Science*, ed. D.S.L. Caldwell (New York, 1968), pp. 74-80.

31. Berthollet, "Essai de statique chimique," extrait, *La Décade philosophique* (10 Messidor XI [June 29, 1803]), pp. 10-18, esp. pp. 14-17; for attribution to Cabanis, see Joanna Kitchin, *"La Décade" (1794-1807): Un Journal "philosophique"* (Paris, 1965), p. 134.

32. *OP* I, 528.

33. Ibid., pp. 529, 527.

34. Ibid., p. 550; J. E. McGuire, "Force, Active Principles, and Newton's Invisible Realm," *Ambix* XV (1968), 154-208.

35. *OP* I, 236n., 241-242; Jan Ingenhousz, *Experiments upon Vegetables, discovering their Great Power of Purifying the Common Air in Sunshine, but Injuring it in the Shade or Night* (London, 1779; Fr. trans., 1787-1789); Jean Senebier, *Recherches sur l'influence de la lumière solaire pour métamorphoser l'air fixe en air pur, par la végétation* (Geneva, 1785).

36. *OP* I, 236-239, 516.

37. Jan Ingenhousz, *Nouvelles expériences et observations sur divers objets de physique* (Paris, 1789), II, 8, 60.

38. *OP*, I, 121.

39. Ibid., pp. 517-519, 525-526.

40. J.-B. Fray, *Essai sur l'origine des corps organisés, et sur quelques phénomènes de physiologie animale et végétale* (Paris, 1817); *Institut de France. Académie des Sciences. Procès-verbaux des séances de l'Académie tenues depuis la fondation de l'Institut jusqu'au mois d'août 1835* ([1816-1819] Hendaye, 1915), VI, 242, 373-374, 462.

41. Fray, *Essai*, pp. 52-53, 191n., 197, 213.

42. Ibid., pp. 96-97, 107.

43. On Lamarck, see Marcel Landrieu, "Lamarck, le fondateur du transformisme: Sa Vie, son oeuvre, *Mémoires de la Société zoologique de France* xxi (Paris, 1909); Leslie Burlingame, "Lamarck," *Dictionary of Scientific Biography*, vii (New York, 1973), 584-593; Richard W. Burkhardt, Jr., "Lamarck, Evolution, and the Politics of Science," *Journal of the History of Biology* iii (1970), 275-298; "The Inspiration of Lamarck's Belief in Evolution," *Journal of the History of Biology* v (1972), 413-438; M.J.S. Hodge, "Lamarck's Science of Living Bodies," *British Journal for the History of Science* v (1971), 323-352.

44. Moravia, *La Scienza dell'uomo*.

45. Burkhardt, "Lamarck," pp. 280-283.

46. *OP* i, 461.

47. Lamarck, *Système des animaux sans vertèbres* (Paris, an ix [1801]), p. 13.

48. Ibid., pp. 15-16.

49. Burkhardt, "The Inspiration," p. 428; Burlingame, "Lamarck," pp. 589-590.

50. "Discours sur la durée des espèces," *Histoire naturelle des poissons* ii (an viii), in *Oeuvres du comte de Lacépède*, ed. M.A.G. Desmarest (Paris, 1826), i, 453-495, esp. 464-466, 489, 471; see Louis Roule, *Lacépède . . . et la sociologie humanitaire de la nature* (Paris, 1932); Lacépède sent his discourse to the Paris School of Medicine by the summer of 1800 (see AN AJ[16] A[P1], ii, 40).

51. *OP* i, 168 n. 1.

52. Ibid., pp. 521-523.

53. Ibid., p. 524 n. 1.

54. Ibid., p. 535.

55. Ibid., pp. 567, 569-574.

56. See review of Mme Condorcet's book by François Thurot in his *Mélanges de feu François Thurot* (Paris, 1880), pp. 246-251. Corrections in Cabanis's hand to Thurot's manuscript (never published in his lifetime) are evident in ms 2958 at the Bibliothèque de l'Institut. The only significant change is in a passage where Thurot described the effort that virtue required to overcome "our inclinations or our interests." Cabanis inserted "at least apparent and momentary" before "interests." For Cabanis, there was always only an apparent conflict between self-interest and virtue.

57. *OP* i, 575-576, 568, 578.

58. Ibid., pp. 576, 578.

59. Ibid., pp. 551-558, 586-588; see Moravia, *Il Pensiero*, pp. 276-288 for an excellent discussion of this topic.

60. *OP* I, 165, 113.

61. Descartes, *Treatise of Man*, ed. Thomas Steele Hall (Cambridge, Mass., 1972), p. 68; Antoine Le Camus, *Médecine de l'esprit* (Paris, 1753), pp. 18, 20.

62. Turgot, *Oeuvres*, ed. Schelle, I (1913), 820; and d'Alembert, "Essai sur les éléments de philosophie" (1759) in *Oeuvres* (ed. 1805), pp. 259-260, both cited in Gusdorf, *Naissance de la conscience*, pp. 300-302.

63. *OP* I, 492-504; cf. Moravia, *Il Pensiero*, pp. 197-201.

64. *OP* I, 169-172, 166-167; on Cabanis's critique of Haller, see Moravia, *Il Pensiero*, pp. 204-205.

65. *OP* I, 537n.; cf. Moravia, *Il Pensiero*, p. 202.

66. See Moravia, *Il Pensiero*, pp. 210-216.

67. See Appendix C on this subject.

68. *OP* I, 219-220.

69. Ibid., pp. 174-177, 539.

70. Ibid., p. 175; see Gusdorf, *Naissance de la conscience*, pp. 167, 210-212 for discussion of this subject, with citation of passages from the work by Paul Hoffmann, *La Femme dans la pensée des lumières* (Paris, 1976).

71. *OP* I, 363-364, 205, 538n.

72. Ibid., pp. 197, 562, 189.

73. Ibid., pp. 543-549.

74. Ibid., pp. 371-372.

75. Ibid., p. 178.

76. Ibid., pp. 213-214.

77. Ibid., pp. 191-193.

78. Ibid., pp. 209-210, 447-448, 589-591.

79. Ibid., pp. 205-208, 593-595, 578-580.

80. Ibid., pp. 154-155, 583-585, 595.

81. Ibid., pp. 586-587.

82. Ibid., pp. 597-598.

83. Destutt de Tracy, "Mémoire sur la faculté de penser," pp. 362-365, 368, 393; see Emmet Kennedy, *A Philosophe in the Age of Revolution: Destutt de Tracy and the Origins of "Ideology"* (Philadelphia, 1978), pp. 60-61.

84. Destutt de Tracy, *Eléments d'idéologie*, ed. Henri Gouhier (Paris, 1970), pp. 67-70, 242, 246-247, 249-250; see also Kennedy, *A Philosophe*, pp. 114-116, 145-146, 151-152.

85. *OP* I, 233-234.

86. Destutt de Tracy, *Traité de la volonté* (Paris, 1815), pp. 526-527.

87. Ibid., pp. 538-539, 544, 547-548, 551-552, 567; see also Kennedy, *A Philosophe*, pp. 217-218..

88. "Influence de l'habitude sur la faculté de penser," *Oeuvres de Maine de Biran* II (Paris, 1922), 20-21, 45, 47; see the Biran-Tracy correspondence (1804-1814) in *Oeuvres de Maine de Biran* VI (Paris, 1930), 227-366.

89. *OP* I, 195-196; cf. Moravia, *Il Pensiero*, pp. 255-257.

90. *Magasin encyclopédique* XLV (an XI [1802]), 153; Cabanis, "Essai sur les principes et les limites de la science des rapports du physique et du moral," in his *Rapports du physique et du moral* (Paris, 1843), pp. xxxiii-xxxiv.

91. Heinrich Haeser, ed., *Lehrbuch der Geschichte der Medicin und der epidemischen Krankheiten* (Jena, 1881), II, 476.

92. William Cullen, *Physiologie de M. Cullen*, trans. Bosquillon (Paris, 1785), pp. 22, 78-80, 83, 92, 198-199; citation in English taken from Cullen, *First Lines of the Practice of Physick* (Edinburgh, 1784), IV, 122-123; cf. Cullen, *Médecine pratique*, trans. Bosquillon (Paris, 1785), II, 717-718.

93. *OP* I, 197-198.

94. Cabanis, *Oeuvres complètes de Cabanis*, ed. François Thurot (Paris, 1824), IV, 466.

95. Frédéric Dubois d'Amiens, *Examen des doctrines de Cabanis, Gall, et Broussais* (Paris, 1842), p. 48.

96. An analogous case occurred in the edition of Newton's *Opticks* apparently used by Leibniz. In the original imprint, the word "tanquam" was omitted in the comparison of space and the sensorium of God in "Query" xx of the *Optice* (1706). The result was a lively polemic and, more recently, an article by Alexandre Koyré and I. B. Cohen, "The Case of the Missing 'Tanquam': Leibniz, Newton, and Clarke," *Isis* LII (1961), 555-566.

97. Aside from the review of Pinel cited above, see also Moreau de La Sarthe, "Encore des réflexions et des observations relatives à l'influence du moral sur le physique, et à l'emploi médical des passions, des affections, et des émotions," *La Décade philosophique* (10 Nivôse IX [31 December 1800]), pp. 70-71.

98. *OP* II, 337.
99. *OP* I, 601-602, 616.
100. Ibid., p. 612.
101. Cabanis, *Rapports*, ed. Louis Peisse (Paris, 1844), 596-597n.
102. *OP* I, 586-587.

NOTES TO CHAPTER VIII

1. *OP* I, 239-240, 217-218n.
2. Ibid., 510n.
3. "Discours prononcé dans l'Académie française le jeudi 21 février 1782 à la réception de M. le Marquis de Condorcet," *Oeuvres de Condorcet*, ed. A. Condorcet O'Connor and François Arago (Paris, 1847), I, 392; Keith Baker, "Condorcet's notes for a revised edition of his reception speech to the Académie française," *Studies on Voltaire and the Eighteenth Century* CLXIX (1977), 44-45.
4. "Discours lus à l'Académie des sciences lorsque la comtesse et le comte du nord (depuis Paul Ire) y vinrent prendre séance, le 6 juin 1782," *Oeuvres de Condorcet* I, 422.
5. "Tableau général de la science qui a pour objet l'application du calcul aux sciences politiques et morales," *Journal de l'instruction sociale*, ed. Condorcet, Siéyès, and Duhamel (22 June and 6 July 1793), in *Oeuvres de Condorcet* I, 544, 552; for correct dating, see Keith Baker, *Condorcet* (Chicago, 1975), pp. 472 and 337; for classification methods, see pp. 122-125, 372; and Frank Manuel, *The Prophets of Paris* (Cambridge, Mass., 1962), pp. 91-95.
6. *Oeuvres de Condorcet* VI, 617-619, 623-625.
7. Long citation as translated in Condorcet, *Sketch for a Historical Picture of the Progress of the Human Mind*, ed. and trans. June Barraclough (London, 1955), pp. 199-201, see also pp. 185-186, 192, 197; and see *Oeuvres de Condorcet* VI, 176, 183-186; citations in Baker, *Condorcet*, pp. 214-217, 223-224.
8. *Oeuvres de Condorcet* VI, 628-629, cited in Baker, *Condorcet*, pp. 214-215.
9. *Oeuvres de Condorcet* VI, 628; for other interpretations of Condorcet, see Sergio Moravia, *Il Tramonto dell'illuminismo* (Bari, 1968), pp. 216-221, 331-341; and *Il Pensiero degli idéologues* (Florence, 1974), pp. 675-716.
10. *OP* II, 513.
11. *Séances des écoles normales recueillies par des sténographes et*

revues par les professeurs . . . Leçons (an III; 2d ed., Paris, an IX), II, 446-447.

12. *OP* II, 519.

13. Ibid., pp. 240-241, 214n.

14. Ibid., p. 251.

15. Philippe Ariès, *Centuries of Childhood: A Social History of Family Life*, trans. Robert Baldick (New York, 1962), chaps. 1 and 2; cf. *Jean-Jacques Rousseau, Emile*, bks. II and v.

16. *OP* II, 441.

17. *OP* I, 260, 265-266, 267, 270.

18. Cf. *OP* II, 29-30.

19. Georges Gusdorf, *Naissance de la conscience romantique au siècle des lumières* (Paris, 1976), pp. 163-172; see Paul Hoffmann, *La femme dans la pensée des lumières* (Paris, 1976).

20. *OP* I, 281-282.

21. Ibid., pp. 273, 614, 495.

22. Ibid., pp. 257, 304-307.

23. Ibid., p. 310.

24. Ibid., pp. 278-279, 348, 284.

25. Ibid., pp. 291-293, 297; cf. I, 16.

26. Letter of Cabanis to Mme de Staël concerning *Delphine*, 28 Frimaire XI, Collection Labrousse, Musée Ernest Rupin, Brive.

27. *OP* I, 293, 297-299.

28. Jane Abray, "Feminism in the French Revolution," *American Historical Review* LXXX (1975), 43-62.

29. Antoine Guillois, *Le Salon de Mme Helvétius* (Paris, 1894), pp. 4-47, 191-192; and *La Marquise de Condorcet: Sa Famille, son salon, ses amis, 1764-1822* (Paris, 1897).

30. *OP* I, 313-315; see Emmet Kennedy, *A Philosophe in the Age of Revolution: Destutt de Tracy and the Origins of "Ideology"* (Philadelphia, 1978), pp. 259-87; for attacks by Chateaubriand and Rivarol on the arid analysis of the Idéologues, see Joanna Kitchin, *"La Décade" (1794-1807): Un Journal "philosophique"* (Paris, 1965), pp. 118, 129.

31. *OP* I, 319-320.

32. Ibid., pp. 151-152, 321-322, 364.

33. Ibid., pp. 335-346.

34. Ibid., pp. 346-349, 351.

35. The eminent hygienist of the Paris School of Medicine and member of the First Class of the Institute Jean-Noël Hallé, who had high praise for Cabanis, developed a revised temperament classification

in "Sur Les Observations fondamentales d'après lesquelles peut être établie la distinction des tempéraments," *Mémoires de la Société médicale d'émulation* III (an VIII [1800]), 342-394. Hallé stressed the importance of the lymphatic as well as the circulatory system. He refined the analysis of the nervous system to differentiate *susceptibilité* (strength of sensation), *successibilité* (facility in association), and *durabilité* (memory), all of which varied with age, sex, climate, and even social status. Hallé called the bilious and pituitous (phlegmatic) temperaments of the ancients only "partial dispositions" of particular organs.

36. *OP* I, 324-325. See E. N. Harvey, *A History of Luminescence* (Philadelphia, 1957), pp. 185, 493-494.

37. *OP* I, 326, 330 n. 1.

38. Ibid., pp. 328-331.

39. Ibid., pp. 620-624, esp. p. 621.

40. Ibid., pp. 369-371, 362, 391; see Montesquieu, *Esprit des lois*, bk. XIV, par. 2 in *Oeuvres complètes*, ed. Daniel Oster (Paris, 1964), pp. 613-614.

41. For an ample discussion of eighteenth-century travel literature, see Moravia, *Il Pensiero*, pp. 533-584, followed by a discussion of Volney, pp. 585-671, which supplants Moravia's previous work on the same topic in *La Scienza dell'uomo nel settecento* (Bari, 1970).

42. [Volney], *Questions de statistique à l'usage des voyageurs* (Paris, 1813); see also Volney, *Voyage en Egypte et en Syrie* (1787), ed. Jean Gaulmier (Paris, 1959), 6n.

43. Volney, *Voyage*, pp. 11, 56, 401-405; see also Moravia, *Il Pensiero*, pp. 614-619.

44. Volney, *Voyage*, pp. 371-398; Volney, "Tableau," in *Oeuvres complètes*, ed. A. Bossange (Paris, 1821), VII, 358-382 on Canadians, and 383-481 on Indians; cf. Moravia, *Il Pensiero*, pp. 637-638.

45. *Séances des écoles normales . . . Leçons* III, 412-416; see Jean Gaulmier, "Volney et ses Leçons d'historie," *History and Theory* II (1962), 52-65.

46. *Séances des écoles normales . . . Leçons* II, 228, 440-441, 219; III, 436.

47. *OP* I, 464-466.

48. Ibid., pp. 511-512.

49. Ibid., p. 629; *OP* II, 260.

50. *OP* I, 511.

51. Ibid., p. 472.

52. Ibid., pp. 467-468.

53. Ibid., p. 474, 474-475 n. 1.

54. Ibid., pp. 402-403; see a refutation of the effect of climate on puberty age in J. M. Tanner, "Earlier Maturation in Man," *Scientific American* CCXVIII (January 1968), 21-27. Cabanis used a wide variety of travellers' reports, including Jean-Frédéric Gmelin, *Voyage en Sibérie* (Fr. trans. 1767); John Meares, *Voyages made in the Years 1788 and 1789 from China to the North West Coast of America* (1790, Fr. trans. 1795); George Dixon, *A Voyage Round the World . . . in 1785, 1786, 1787, and 1788* (1789); George Vancouver, *A Voyage of Discovery* (1798, Fr. trans. 1799); Pierre-Simon Pallas, *Voyages à travers plusieurs provinces de l'empire russe* (trans. 1788-1793); as well as physicians' reports from French Guiana, Santo Domingo, and from South Carolina.

55. *OP* I, 404-408, 412; Cabanis believed that air was a compound not a mixture, of gases, possibly because of the works of the geologist de Saussure. I owe this interpretation to Seymour Mauskopf of Duke University.

56. Ibid., pp. 482-495.

57. Ibid., pp. 500-504, esp. p. 503.

58. Ernest Labrousse et al., *Histoire économique et sociale de France* II (1660-1789) (Paris, 1970).

59. *OP* I, 476, 478-479, 484.

60. Ibid., pp. 510n., 498.

61. William Coleman, "Health and Hygiene in the *Encyclopédie*: A Medical Doctrine for the Bourgeoisie," *Journal of the History of Medicine* XXIX (1974), 414; see also Coleman's citations of Hallé's articles in Fourcroy, ed., *La Médecine éclairée par les sciences physiques* IV (1792), 225-235; and Fourcroy, "Hygiène," *Encyclopédie méthodique (Médecine)* VII, 373-437.

62. *OP* I, 393, 395, 397; cf. Coleman, "Health and Hygiene," p. 407, who argues that Encyclopedist hygienists saw health as a merely individual problem, with few ramifications for the species or for public policy.

63. *OP* I, 416, 418, 420-421, 423.

64. Ibid., pp. 427, 429, 433, 435, 438.

65. Ibid., pp. 440-443, 446-447.

66. Ibid., pp. 393, 449; Bernardino Ramazzini, *De Morbis Artificum Diatriba*, Mutinae (Modena), 1700.

67. *OP* I, 452-454, 630; cf. Adam Smith, *An Inquiry into the Nature and Causes of the Wealth of Nations* (1776), ed. E. Cannan (London, 1904), bk. I, chap. 10, pt. 2.

68. *OP* I, 456.

69. George Rudé, *The Crowd in the French Revolution* (Oxford, 1959), pp. 246-248 gives an occupational analysis of Revolutionary crowds.

70. *OP* I, 451-452; on hospital ventilation, see Du Pont de Nemours, *Idées sur les secours à donner aux pauvres malades dans une grande ville* (Philadelphia and Paris, 1786).

71. *OP* I, 355.

72. Ibid., pp. 356-358.

73. Cf. remarks of Boissy d'Anglas on diversity justifying political inequality in the debate on the Constitution of an III, cited in Moravia, *Tramonto*, p. 242; Daunou and Siéyès held comparable positions.

74. François Thurot, "Rapports du physique et du moral," *La Décade* XXV (20 Floréal, 20 and 30 Prairial VIII), 262-270, 462-468, 521-528 (citation on 528).

75. "R.," "Rapports du physique et du moral de l'homme," *La Décade* XXXIV (20 Fructidor x), 455-464.

76. Moreau de La Sarthe, "Rapports du physique et du moral de l'homme," *Revue philosophique, littéraire, et politique* XLVI (successor to *La Décade*) (29 July and 8 and 18 August 1805), 193-202, 257-263, 321-328.

77. Balthasar-Anthelme Richerand, *Nouveaux Elémens de physiologie* (Paris, 1801 [an IX], revised ed. 1802 [an x]); Charles Dumas, *Principes de physiologie, ou Introduction à la science expérimentale, philosophique, et médicale de l'Homme vivant*, 4 vols. (Paris, 1800-1803).

78. *Oeuvres de Maine de Biran* VI, ed. Pierre Tisserand (Paris, 1930), 344.

79. See citations in Moravia, *Tramonto*, pp. 434-435.

80. "Opinion de Pison-du-Galland," reprinted in *Le Moniteur universel* XXIII (14, 15, and 16 Germinal VII), 794-796.

81. *Oeuvres complètes de Chateaubriand* II (Paris, Garnier, n.d.), 85-86, 91, 130-132, 304-309; see also Moravia, *Tramonto*, pp. 526-548.

82. Louis de Bonald, "Recherches philosophiques sur les premiers objets des connaissances morales" (1818), *Oeuvres complètes de M. de*

Bonald III, ed. Migne (Paris, 1859), cols. 147-150, 208-215, 233-242.

83. Maine de Biran to De Feletz, in *Oeuvres de Maine de Biran* VI, 139-140.

84. Destutt de Tracy, *Projet d'élémens d'ideologie* (Paris, 1801 [an IX]), p. 14; Destutt de Tracy, *Eléments d'ideologie*, ed. Henri Gouhier (Paris, 1970), I, xxxi.

85. Destutt de Tracy, *Elémens d'idéologie*, pt. 3. *Logique* (Paris, 1805), pp. vii-viii.

86. Destutt de Tracy, "Sur La Décomposition de la faculté de penser," *Mémoires de l'Institut. Classe des sciences morales et politiques* II (1799), 349.

87. Tracy, *Elémens d'idéologie*, ed. Gouhier, I, 34-37.

88. Ibid., p. 234; cf. pp. 28-29, 262; for a different interpretation, see Moravia, *Il Pensiero*, pp. 381-382.

89. Tracy, "Sur La Décomposition," p. 301; on Tracy's opinions, see Emmet Kennedy, *A Philosophe in the Age of Revolution* (Philadelphia, 1978), pp. 114-115; for Cabanis's opinions, see *OP* I, 180-183, 546-549.

90. Tracy, *Elémens d'idéologie*, ed. Gouhier, I, 299-300n.

91. Tracy, *Logique*, pp. 312-320.

92. In letters to Biran and Fauriel in 1811, Tracy cited other authors for his views, including Cuvier's summaries of physiological work from 1789 to 1808, Jean Itard, the physician who attempted to "educate" the "wild boy" from the Aveyron, the phrenologist Gall, and the physiologist César-Julien-Jean Le Gallois; see Kennedy, *A Philosophe*, p. 217.

93. Destutt de Tracy, *Traité sur la volonté . . . Morale.* "Idées préliminaires" (Paris, 1815), v, 556-564; for Xavier Bichat's physiology, see his *Recherches physiologiques sur la vie et la mort* (Paris, 1800).

NOTES TO CHAPTER IX

1. Philippe Pinel, *Traité médico-philosophique sur l'aliénation mentale, ou la manie* (Paris, 1801 [an IX]), p. 81. The book was available at least by 11 October 1800, since the School of Medicine received a copy on 19 Vendémiaire IX (AN AJ[16] AP[2], II, 47).

2. See *Mémoires de la Société médicale d'émulation* (hereafter designated *MSME*), I, an V (Paris, an VI); on the Société médicale d'émulation, see Sergio Moravia, "Philosophie et médecine," *Studies on Voltaire and the Eighteenth Century* LXXXIX (1972), 1089-1090, *passim*.

3. Pinel, *Traité*, pp. xxxv, xxvii, li-lii, 14, 150, 136; *MSME* iii (an viii), 9, 17.

4. Pinel, *Traité*, pp. 81-82, 137-148, 156, 160-161, 166.

5. Ibid., pp. 89, 106, 122-135.

6. Ibid., pp. 196, 208, 210.

7. Ibid., pp. 40-42, 46-47, 82-84, 232-233, 250, 266.

8. Ibid., pp. 57, 72, 75.

9. Ibid., pp. 104, 58, 78, 99, 238.

10. Jean-Louis Alibert, "Discours sur les rapports de la médecine avec les sciences physiques et morales," *MSME* ii, an vi (Paris, an vii), lxvi, lxix, lxxix-lxxx; cf. Moravia, "Philosophie et médecine."

11. Alibert, "Du pouvoir de l'habitude dans l'état de santé et de maladie," *MSME* i, 396-415.

12. See Pierre Roussel, "Note sur les sympathies," *MSME* i, 512.

13. Alibert, "Discours," *MSME* ii, xciii.

14. Alibert, *Physiologie des passions, ou nouvelle doctrine des sentiments moraux* (Paris, 1825), p. i.

15. See AN AJ¹⁶ Aᴾ³, Assemblée générale des professeurs, iii (23 June 1807).

16. B.-A. Richerand, *Nouveaux Eléments de physiologie* (Paris, 1802 [an x]), i, lxi, lxxix; ii, 155, 467, 149, 151-153, 165n.

17. Richerand, *Nouveaux Eléments de physiologie* (Paris, 1833), ii, 409, 413, 429.

18. Richerand, *De La Population* (Paris, 1837), pp. 5-6, 16n.

19. Charles Dejob, *De L'Etablissement connu sous le nom de Lycée et d'Athénée et de quelques établissements analogues* (Paris, 1889). For a full bibliography of Moreau's works, see Paul Delaunay, "La Médecine et les idéologues: L.-J. Moreau de La Sarthe," *Bulletin de la Société française d'histoire de la médecine* xiv (1920), 61-70; on the lycées, see in the same article, pp. 33-35 n. 2, 36.

20. Jacques-Louis Moreau de La Sarthe, "Quelques Réflexions philosophiques et médicales sur l'Emile communiquées à l'une des séances littéraires du Lycée Républicain," *La Décade philosophique* (20 Prairial viii), p. 460; Moreau, "Esquisse d'un cours d'hygiène ou de médecine appliquée à l'art d'user la vie et de conserver la santé," extrait par Sédillot, *Recueil périodique de la Société de médecine de Paris* viii, 75.

21. "Pinel, Traité médico-philosophique sur l'aliénation mentale, ou la manie," extrait par J.-L. Moreau de La Sarthe, *La Décade philosophique* (20 Prairial ix), p. 458, 458-459n.

22. Moreau, "Encore Des Réflexions et des observations relatives à l'influence du moral sur le physique, et à l'emploi médical des passions, des affections, et des émotions," *La Décade philosophique* (10 Nivôse IX), 70-71, 73.

23. Moreau, "Moral," *Encyclopedie méthodique* CLXXIII *(Médecine)*, x (1821), 250-276.

24. Moreau, "Encore Des Réflexions," 71 n. 4

25. Moreau, "Sur Plusieurs Maladies à la guérison desquelles les ressources pharmaceutiques n'ont pas concouru," *Recueil périodique de la Société de médecine* VI (Paris, an VII), 389-390.

26. François Picavet, *Les Idéologues* (Paris, 1891), pp. 434-437.

27. On Bichat, see, among others, F. Colonna d'Istria, "La Psychologie de Bichat," *Revue de métaphysique et de morale* XXXIII (1926), 1-38; "Bichat et la biologie contemporaine," *Revue de métaphysique et de morale* XVI (1908), 261-280.

28. Frank Manuel, *The Prophets of Paris* (Cambridge, Mass., 1962), pp. 121-123.

29. Auguste Comte, *Système de politique positive* IV (Paris, 1854), 402 (Insert B), "calendrier positiviste," treizième mois. Bichat is the patron of the month honoring "modern science."

30. Xavier Bichat, *Recherches physiologiques sur la vie et la mort* ([1800] Paris, 1805), pp. 1, 136, 80-84.

31. Claude Bernard, "Définition de la vie" (1875), cited in G. J. Goodfield, *The Growth of Scientific Physiology* (London, 1960), p. 68.

32. Bichat, *Recherches*, pp. 85-90 (arts. 8-9).

33. Ibid., p. 125.

34. *OP* I, 115-116.

35. Bichat, *Recherches*, pp. 60, 140-143, 133.

36. Ibid., pp. 64, 67-68, 77-78.

37. Ibid., pp. 40-46.

38. Ibid., pp. 48-49.

39. Ibid., pp. 150-152.

40. Ibid., p. 33.

41. Ibid., pp. 5, 197, 23.

42. Ibid., p. 45.

43. For the most comprehensive account see Henri Gouhier, *Les Conversions de Maine de Biran* (Paris, 1948), esp. pp. 108, 111-112, 116 n. 2; more recent studies in D. Voutsinas, *La Psychologie de Maine de Biran* (Paris, 1964); and F.C.T. Moore, *The Psychology of Maine de Biran* (Oxford, 1970); the sections in Moravia, *Il Pensiero*

degli idéologues (Florence, 1974), pp. 462-464, 470, 484-485 review literature on Biran's background.

44. Bibliothèque de l'Institut, MS 2128, Maine de Biran, "Mémoire sur l'habitude," p. 23; cf. *Oeuvres de Maine de Biran*, ed. Pierre Tisserand (Paris, 1922), II; and Moravia, *Il Pensiero*, pp. 485-486.

45. Biran, "Mémoire sur l'habitude," pp. 6-7, 21, 39-40; see *Oeuvres de Maine de Biran* II, 225-230, 232, 348-350, 359-360. Tisserand published pp. 12-32 and 33-34 of the manuscript in the appendix to vol. II.

46. Biran, "Mémoire sur l'habitude," pp. 14, 16-17, 35, 37; cf. *Oeuvres de Maine de Biran* II, 229-230; and Gouhier, *Les Conversions*, p. 103. See also Emmet Kennedy, *A Philosophe in the Age of Revolution* (Philadelphia, 1978), pp. 120-123.

47. Biran, "Mémoire sur l'habitude, pp. 46, 63, 69, 82-83.

48. Gouhier, *Les Conversions*, p. 122.

49. *Oeuvres de Maine de Biran* II, 17.

50. Letter to Degérando, 26 Vendémiaire XI, in *Oeuvres de Maine de Biran* VI (1930), 148-149; cf. Gouhier, *Les Conversions*, p. 163, and Moravia, *Il Pensiero*, p. 508.

51. See Moravia, *Il Pensiero*, p. 486.

52. *Oeuvres de Maine de Biran* II, 14-15; cf. Moravia, *Il Pensiero*, pp. 490-494.

53. "Note de Maine de Biran au Citoyen B," *Oeuvres de Maine de Biran* VI, 197-207.

54. *Oeuvres de Maine de Biran* II, 20-21, 45, 47; cf. Moravia, *Il Pensiero*, p. 488.

55. Letter to Tracy (1804), *Oeuvres de Maine de Biran* VI, 231-233.

56. *Oeuvres de Maine de Biran* II, xx, 76, 22n., 52-53, 34; cf. Moravia, *Il Pensiero*, p. 491.

57. *Oeuvres de Maine de Biran* II, 171, 93-94.

58. Ibid., pp. 157, 165, 172-173.

59. Ibid., p. 170 n. 1.

60. Ibid., VI, 268.

61. Ibid., II, 179-297.

62. Ibid., VI, 209, 213-214, 220, for letters to and from Cabanis; for more on the Biran-Tracy relationship, see Moravia, *Il Pensiero*, pp. 399-400, 405-406.

63. *Oeuvres de Maine de Biran* VI, 148-149, shows that in a letter to Degérando in 1802, Biran disavowed the "dangerous and desolate system" of materialism and vowed to base morality on an "ego endowed

with a force, a power of reaction to modify itself." Moravia, *Il Pensiero*, p. 508, also discusses this letter.

NOTES TO CHAPTER X

1. Léon Aucoc, *L'Institut de France: Lois, statuts, et règlements* (Paris, 1889), p. 39; Archives de l'Institut. Comptabilité. Registre indicatif des présences, ans v-xi. Cabanis's attendance at Institute meetings could have earned him up to 300 francs more each year, but his "assiduity" at meetings averaged less than 25% in an v, less than 15% in an vi, and his attendance was rare indeed in subsequent years.

2. A. Debidour, ed. *Recueil des actes du Directoire exécutif* iv (Paris, 1917), 544-545; AN, AJ[16] A[P1], Procès-verbaux de l'assemblée des professeurs, i, 143-144, 236; AJ[16] A[P2], ii, 238; Table des matières, fol. 40.

3. Letters of Cabanis to Vermeil, 24 and 25 Nivôse v, cited in Col. Vermeil de Conchard, *Trois Etudes sur Cabanis d'après des documents inédits* (Brive, 1914), p. 30.

4. *Plan général de l'enseignement de l'Ecole de santé de Paris* (Paris, an iii), pp. 40-43.

5. AN, AJ[16] A[P1], i, 271.

6. AN, AJ[16] (numbering incomplete) Procès-verbaux des séances du comité d'administration 13 May 1796-18 August 1800, fol. 51v.

7. AN, AJ[16] A[P1], i, 346.

8. *Ibid.*, pp. 179, 386-387; *Plan général de l'enseignement*, pp. 46-49.

9. AN, AJ[16] A[P2], ii, 247.

10. *OP* ii, 388-401, 405-424.

11. David Vess, *Medical Revolution in France 1789-1796* (Gainesville, Fla., 1975), pp. 71-92, 117-136, 162, 170.

12. *Rapport fait . . . sur un mode provisoire de police médicale présenté par Cabanis* (4 Messidor vi); *OP* ii, 388-401.

13. *Projet de résolution de Calès* (12 Prairial v); citations from originals, but medical education debates also available in A. de Beauchamp, ed., *Enquêtes et documents relatifs à l'enseignement supérieur*. t. xxviii, *Médecine et Pharmacie. Projets de lois, 1789-1803* (Paris, 1888).

14. *Projet de résolution de Vitet* (17 Ventôse vi), p. 13, 29-31n.; *Motion d'ordre de Vitet* (4 Messidor vi).

15. Michel Foucault, *Naissance de la clinique* (Paris, 1963), pp. 69-86, also discusses this controversy and gives, I believe, an erroneous interpretation of the social implications of Cabanis's 1798 reports.

16. Cabanis, *Rapport fait . . . sur l'organisation des écoles de médecine* (29 Brumaire VII); *Rapport fait par Hardy. . . .* (1 Frimaire VII).

17. *OP* II, 417-418.

18. *Opinion de Vitet* (23 Nivôse VII), pp. 9-10; see also *Opinion de [Jean-François] Barailon* (17 Germinal VI), p. 9.

19. AN, AJ¹⁶ AP¹, I, 344, 352; AN, AJ¹⁶ Procès-verbaux des séances du comité d'administration, fols. 100-101.

20. *Tribunat. Rapport fait . . . par Thouret sur le projet de loi relatif à l'exercice de la médecine* (16 Ventôse XI), pp. 13-14; cf. *OP* II, 388-400; and Claire Salomon-Bayet, "L'Institution de la science: Un Exemple au XVIIIᵉ siècle," *Annales ECS* xxx (1975), 1028-1044, esp. 1035-1037.

21. See *Projet de résolution de Calès*, p. 14; *Projet de résolution de Vitet*, p. 11; *Opinion de Barailon*, pp. 7-8; and *Opinion de Vitet*, p. 2; see also *Procès-verbaux des séances du Conseil des cinq-cents*, 23 Nivôse VII (Paris, ans VI-VIII), p. 473.

22. AN, F¹⁷ 2273. Petitions to Interior Ministry on establishment of medical schools.

23. *OP* II, 409; cf. Condorcet, "Rapport . . . sur l'organisation générale de l'instruction publique," in *Oeuvres de Condorcet* VII, 449-573; and Daunou report to the Council of Five Hundred on higher education in 1797.

24. On professionals and charlatans, see Toby Gelfand, "Medical Professionals and Charlatans. The *comité de salubrité enquête* of 1790-91," *Histoire sociale–Social History* (May 1978), pp. 62-97; Matthew Ramsey, "Medical Power and Popular Medicine: Illegal Healers in Nineteenth-Century France," *Journal of Social History* x (1977), 560-587; Jean-Pierre Goubert, "L'Art de guérir. Médecine savante et médecine populaire dans la France de 1790," *Annales ESC* xxxii (1977), 908-926.

25. Michel Foucault et al., *Les Machines à guérir (aux origines de l'hôpital moderne)* (Paris, 1976), pp. 11-21.

26. *Procès-verbaux des séances du Conseil des cinq-cents* (3 Brumaire VII), pp. 111-141; *Rapport général fait par Roger-Martin sur l'organisation de l'instruction publique* (19 Brumaire VII) (Le⁴³ 2438; redraft, Le⁴³ 2801, Pluviôse VII). Cabanis's name also appears in the Council minutes as a member of a commission on *brevets d'invention*, Prairial VI (p. 37); a special commission on the election of a judge to the civil tribunal of Creuse (p. 107); a commission for cassation court replacements, 4 Messidor VI (p. 60); and a commission for secessionist

assemblies in the Gard, 18 Messidor (pp. 271-272). He is also mentioned with regard to the Liancourt school, 24 Messidor (p. 377); and currency, 28 Messidor. On 26 Messidor, he made a rousing speech in tribute to the United Irishmen; he spoke in Thermidor VI on the law against calumny (pp. 131-132); he was a member of a special commission on a uniform for public officials (p. 243); and a member of another on an indemnity for lead oxide producers, 22 Thermidor (p. 355). On 21 Fructidor VI (p. 318), he served on a commission on the primary assembly of Basses-Pyrénées; on 28 Brumaire VII, on a special commission on the entrepreneurs of the land survey of Corsica; on 16 Germinal VII (p. 257), on a special commission on the electoral assembly for Loiret; on 26 Germinal, on a special commission on collection fraud in the *octroi* for charities in Paris; and on 6ᵉ jour comp. VII, (p. 493), on the weights and measures commission; finally, on 5 Brumaire VIII (p. 79), he spoke on the need for secrecy in Council debates. None of these activities has been listed elsewhere by students of Cabanis.

27. See especially Robert J. Vignery, *The French Revolution and the Schools: Educational Policies of the Mountain, 1792-1794* (Madison, Wis., 1965); and J. Guillaume, ed. *Procès-verbaux du comité d'instruction publique de la Convention nationale*, 6 vols. (Paris, 1891-1907).

28. For staff and Interior Ministry policy on central schools, see AN, F¹⁷ 1344²⁷ and F¹⁷ 2274; for documents, see Guillaume, ed., *Procès-verbaux* VI, 553, 575, 869-873; on the central schools, there are many regional studies and the overall summaries in L. Pearce Williams, "Science, Education, and the French Revolution," *Isis* XLIV (1953), 311-330; Charles Van Duzer, *The Contribution of the Idéologues to French Revolutionary Thought* (Baltimore, 1935), despite many inaccuracies; and more recently, Sergio Moravia, *Il Tramonto dell'illuminismo* (Bari, 1968), pp., 352-370.

29. Jonathan Helmreich, "The Establishment of Primary Schools in France Under the Directory," *French Historical Studies* II (1961), 189-208; see also "Les Manuels de l'enseignement primaire de la Révolution et les idées révolutionnaires," in J. Morange and J.-F. Chassaing, *Le Mouvement de réforme de l'enseignement en France, 1760-1798* (Paris, 1974), pt. II, pp. 97-193.

30. AN, F¹⁷ᴬ 1014, Interior Ministry files on translations of public assistance memoirs.

31. See also Ernest Allain, *L'Oeuvre scolaire de la Révolution* (Paris, 1891), p. 272; Célestin Hippeau, *L'Instruction publique en France*

pendant la Révolution II (Paris, 1883), 293; *Procès-verbaux des séances du Conseil des cinq-cents* (3 Brumaire VII), p. 125.

32. The sponsors were Heurtault-Lamerville (22 Brumaire VII, Le[43] 2440) on primary education, Bonnaire (23 Brumaire VII, Le[43] 2444) on central schools, Briot (27 Brumaire VII) on lycées, and Dulaure (2 and 7 Frimaire VII, Le[43] 2456) on surveillance measures applying to public and private schools.

33. *Rapport général fait par Roger-Martin*, pp. 10-11, 22, 25-35.

34. Dulaure, *Sur La Surveillance et la police des écoles* . . . (Le[43] 2456), pp. 18-32.

35. *Rapport de Bonnaire* (Le[43] 2444), p. 9.

36. *Rapport général fait par Roger-Martin*, pp. 4-6, 13-17; the text of the Daunou plan of 1797 appears in Louis Liard, *L'Enseignement supérieur en France, 1789-1889* II (1894), 419-471.

37. Of thirteen speakers whose opinions were printed, seven favored more primary schools than called for in the plan (reference numbers from Bibliotheque Nationale Le[43] series): Boilleau (2687), Duplantier (2688), Scherlock (2689), Bremontier (2704), Joubert (2706), Sonthonax (2807), and Andrieux (2994); Duplantier, Scherlock, and Sonthonax supported compulsory *public* primary schooling with an eccentric interpretation nullifying the constitutional protection of private schools; two deputies opposed expansion of primary schools: Bailleul (2924), and Boulay de La Meurthe, in a speech reprinted in *Moniteur universel* (23 and 29 Germinal VII), XXIII, 826-828, 851; two deputies opposed reinforced primary schools: Sonthonax, and Andrieux; one favored them: Challan (2705); and three opposed stringent surveillance: Boulay, Andrieux, and Pison-du-Galland, in a speech reprinted in *Moniteur universel* (14, 15, and 16 Germinal VII), XXIII, 791-792, 794-796, 798-800.

38. *Opinion de Sonthonax* (Le[43] 2807), pp. 5-10.

39. Boulay, pp. 828, 826, 851.

40. Pison-du-Galland, 28 brumaire VI, pp. 4-6.

41. Boulay, 828; Pison-du-Galland, *Moniteur*, pp. 794-796.

42. *Opinion de Andrieux* (Le[43] 2994), pp. 3, 5, 10-12, 21-22, 25-26; for the Conseil d'instruction publique reports on textbooks, see AN, F[17A] 1011; for the final report and consequences of its work, see Albert Duruy, *L'Instruction publique et la Révolution* (Paris, 1882), pp. 391-411, 433-449.

43. Destutt de Tracy, *Observations sur le système actuel d'instruction publique* (Paris, an IX), pp. 1-5, 64-68; Garat favorably reviewed

Tracy's essay in *La Décade* (10 Messidor ix), p. 14, cited in Joanna Kitchin, *"La Décade"* (Paris, 1965), p. 190.

44. References to Boulay in *OP* ii, 429, place composition of the speech after 21 Germinal; other remarks (pp. 441, 445) apparently refer to Andrieux's comments on 1 and 11 Floréal; several opinions were reprinted on 4 Prairial in *Procès-verbaux des séances du Conseil des cinq-cents* (prairial VII), p. 96; cf. Kitchin, *"La Décade"*, pp. 199-201.

45. *OP* ii, 428-430, 443, 433-434.

46. Ibid., pp. 443 n. 1, 436-437, 443-444.

47. Ibid., pp. 449 n. 1, 439.

48. *Tribunat. Rapports fait par Fourcroy*, (30 Germinal x), pp. 3-6, 9; see Maurice Gontard, *L'Enseignement primaire en France de la Révolution à la loi Guizot (1789-1833)* (Paris, 1959), pp. 202-211.

49. Antoine Léon, "Promesses et ambiguités de l'oeuvre d'enseignement technique en France, de 1800 à 1815," *Annales historiques de la Révolution française* xlii (1970), 419-436; Margaret Bradley, "Scientific Education versus Military Training: The Influence of Napoleon Bonaparte on the *Ecole polytechnique*," *Annals of Science* xxxii (1975), 414-449.

50. Vermeil de Conchard, *Trois Etudes*, p. 35.

51. Ibid.

52. Archival sources as indicated confirmed the following account, which otherwise is based on Isser Woloch, *Jacobin Legacy: The Democratic Movement in the Directory* (Princeton, 1970), pp. 311-346; J. R. Suratteau, *Les Elections de l'an vi et le coup d'état du 22 floréal* (Paris, 1971), esp. pp. 329-336; Albert Meynier, *Les Coups d'état du Directoire* (Paris, 1927-1928), 3 vols., esp. ii, 68-75.

53. AN, F I. C. III. Seine 1. Electoral assemblies (an vi).

54. AN, AF III. 99 (438), p. 4.

55. Suratteau, *Les Elections*, p. 244.

56. AN, B¹ 17, Seine-Institut, an vi, Procès-verbaux de l'assemblée électorale de La Seine, p. 1; cf. Woloch, *Jacobin Legacy*, p. 331.

57. Woloch, *Jacobin Legacy*, pp. 340-341.

58. Procès-verbaux de l'assemblée électorale de la Seine, fol. 19v.

59. Suratteau, *Les Elections*, pp. 71, 231.

60. *Opinion de Cabanis sur les réunions s'occupant d'objets politiques*, miscatalogued; correct date is 6 Thermidor vii.

61. Cabanis, *Discours . . . sur le message du Conseil des anciens . . .* (1 Fructidor vii).

62. See Max Fajn, The "Journal des hommes libres de tous les pays," 1792-1800 (The Hague, 1975).

63. Opinion de Cabanis sur l'impôt du sel a l'extraction (11 Fructidor vi), pp. 7-8.

64. Commission du Conseil des cinq-cents. (25 Brumaire viii), pp. 2-6.

65. Meynier, Les Coups d'état iii, 80-81.

66. On Bonaparte's links with the Idéologues, see Antoine Guillois, Le Salon de Mme Helvétius (Paris, 1894), pp. 123-130; A. Vandal, L'Avènement de Bonaparte (Paris, 1902), i, 265-267, 284-291; Paul Bastid, Siéyès et sa pensée (2d ed., Paris, 1970), pp. 232, 237; Emmet Kennedy, A Philosophe in the Age of Revolution, p. 77; Adrienne Gobert, L'Opposition des assemblées pendant le Consulat (Paris, 1925), p. 29; for Bonaparte's letter, see Correspondance iii, 2392, cited in Maurice Crosland, The Society of Arcueil: A View of French Science at the Time of Napoleon I (London, 1967), p. 13.

67. Procès-verbaux des séances du Conseil des cinq-cents (19 Brumaire viii), pp. 337-347.

68. OP ii, 452-453.

69. Ibid., 457-459.

70. See Bastid, Siéyès, pp. 250-256.

71. Le⁴⁴ 48, Discours . . . 3 Nivôse viii, p. 3.

72. OP ii, 475.

73. Ibid., p. 481.

74. Ibid., pp. 465, 477-478.

75. Ibid., p. 463; see also Bernard Plongeron, "Nature, métaphysique, et histoire chez les idéologues," Dix-huitième Siècle v (1973), 375-412.

76. OP ii, 463-466.

77. Cited in Louis Villefosse et Janine Bouissounouse, L'Opposition à Napoléon (Paris, 1969), p. 92.

78. OP ii, 467-468.

79. Ibid., pp. 483-485.

80. See Louis Bergeron, L'Episode napoléonien: Aspects intérieurs 1799-1815 (Paris, 1972), for an excellent recent summary.

81. See Gobert, L'Opposition, p. 155; and, more recently, Jean Vidalenc, "L'Opposition sous le Consulat et l'Empire," Annales historiques de la Révolution française xl (1968), 472-488.

82. Messager des relations extérieures (12 January 1800), cited in

Emmet Kennedy, " 'Ideology' from Destutt de Tracy to Marx," *Journal of the History of Ideas* XL (1979), 354.

83. Gobert, *L'Opposition*, pp. 117, 175-178; Guillois, *Le Salon*, p. 144.

84. *Journal de Paris* (15 Pluviôse VIII), reprinted in *Mercure de France* (16 Pluviôse), cited in Gobert, *L'Opposition*, p. 141.

85. See Gobert, *L'Opposition*, p. 226; Guillois, *Le Salon*, p. 162; Jean Thiry, *Le Sénat de Napoléon (1800-1814)* (Paris, 1932), pp. 79-83.

86. Guillois, *Le Salon*, pp. 167-169; Gobert, *L'Opposition*, pp. 366, 373; for attendance at Senate at a particular session, see manuscript "Procès-verbaux du Sénat Conservateur," AN, CC 1-CC 4.

87. Jules Simon, *Une Académie sous le Directoire* (Paris, 1885), pp. 470-472; Aucoc, *L'Institut*, pp. 67-84, esp. pp. 74; 184.

NOTES TO CHAPTER XI

1. *OP* II, 531-539.
2. Ibid., p. 257, for comments on Stoics. Cabanis presumably knew Cicero's exposition in *De natura deorum* as well as the *Meditationes* of Marcus Aurelius.
3. Sergio Moravia, in *La Scienza dell'uomo nel settecento* (Bari, 1970), p. 70, calls the letter a "text of old age, very much overrated in importance."
4. *OP* II, 276-277, 269.
5. Ibid., pp. 258-259.
6. Ibid., pp. 265.
7. Ibid., pp. 259, 262-264.
8. Ibid., p. 295.
9. See Albert Mathiez, *La Théophilanthropie et le culte décadaire, 1796-1801* (Paris, 1903).
10. *OP* II, 263-265, 274-275.
11. Ibid., pp. 277-278, 285; cf. d'Holbach, *Système de la nature par Mirabaud* ([1770] London [Paris], 1774), I, 24n., 49-52.
12. *OP* II, 286-287, 291-294.
13. Ibid., pp. 294-295.
14. Archives de Broglie, cited in Robert de Luppé, *Les Idées littéraires de Madame de Staël et l'héritage des lumières (1795-1814)* (Paris, 1969), pp. 70-71.
15. E. Frédéric Dubois (d'Amiens), *Examen des doctrines de Cabanis Gall, et Broussais* (Paris, 1842), pp. 15, 17, 19, 23, 36, 48, 68, 75.

16. Joseph Tissot, *Anthropologie spéculative générale* (Paris, 1842), I, 426-428, 437, 439, 444-445.

17. Cabanis, *Rapports du physique et du moral*, ed. L. Cérise (Paris, 1843), pp. xxxiii-xxxvi, xl; a comment on Pinel's influence in Georges Gusdorf, *La Conscience révolutionnaire, les Idéologues* (Paris, 1978), p. 471 notes the foundation of a periodical of psychiatry, the *Annales médico-psychologiques*, in 1843. Interest in Cabanis's *Rapports* may also relate to the concerns of the "second generation" of Pinel's pupils.

18. Cabanis, *Rapports du physique et du moral*, ed. Louis Peisse (Paris, 1844), pp. lvii, 43n., 53n., 138-139n., 492n., 532n., 596-597n., 647n., 653-655n.

19. AN CC 240, fol. 907; Bibliothèque de l'Institut, MS 2327, letters of Mme Cabanis to Fauriel (in 1844, she still referred to her husband as "our angel"); see also Antoine Guillois, *Le Salon de Mme Helvétius* (Paris, 1894), pp. 223-231; Destutt de Tracy, "Discours de M. le comte de Tracy, prononcé dans la séance publique du 21 décembre 1808, en venant prendre séance à la place de M. Cabanis," *Recueil des discours, rapports, et pièces diverses, lus dans les séances . . . de l'Académie française, 1803-1819*, 1ʳᵉ partie (Paris, 1857), pp. 299-318.

20. Owsei Temkin, "The Philosophical Background of Magendie's Physiology," *Bulletin of the History of Medicine* xx (1946), 10-35; Georgette Legée, "Les Concepts de localisation et de co-ordination dans la neurophysiologie de Marie-Jean-Pierre Flourens (1794-1867)," *96ᵉ Congrès national des sociétés savantes, Toulouse, 1971, Sciences* (Paris, 1974), I, 123-151.

21. Erwin Ackerknecht, "Broussais, or a Forgotten Medical Revolution," *Bulletin of the History of Medicine* xxvii (1953), 320-343.

22. See the forthcoming University of Paris thesis for the *doctorat d'état* by Bernard-Pierre Lécuyer of the Université de Paris-v, "Naissance d'un savoir: Recherche sociale, état et société en France durant la première industrialisation (1800-1850)"; Ann Fowler La Berge, "The Paris Health Council, 1802-1848," *Bulletin of the History of Medicine* xlix (1975), 339-352.

23. Paul Janet, "Schopenhauer et la physiologie française: Cabanis et Bichat," *Revue des deux mondes*, 3ᵉ Période, xxxix (1 May 1880), 35-59.

24. Frank Manuel, *The New World of Henri Saint-Simon* (Cambridge, Mass., 1956), pp. 49-51, 58, 112-113, 118-119, 132-137, 158-159, 222, 231, 297-298, 328-329, 391-392, n. 5.

Appendix A
Correspondences in Ancient Greco-Roman Philosophy and Medicine

Qualities	Element	Humor	Temperament	Age	Season	Organ	Winds	Planets
warm and moist	air	blood	sanguine	childhood	spring	heart	east	Jupiter
warm and dry	fire	bile	bilious	youth	summer	liver	north	Mars
cold and dry	earth	black bile	atrabilious (melancholic)	maturity	autumn	spleen	west	Saturn
cold and moist	water	phlegm	phlegmatic (pituitary)	old age	winter	brain	south	Moon

Appendix B

Possible evidence of the early medical interests of Cabanis can be found in the "Versailles manuscript," an excerpt, actually Cabanis's reading notes, of the works of Hippocrates, Galen, and other authors (Origen, Jerome, Quintilian, and a seventeenth-century Spanish official and jurist Solade de Samoza), (described in Lehec, ed., *OP* II, 544-45). This manuscript, found in the papers of Mme Condorcet at the place of Cabanis's death, the château of Rueil-Seraincourt, was purchased by a Doctor Bérigny, physician at the Hôtel-Dieu de Meulan. Having proposed to write a rather casual and anecdotal notice on Cabanis, Bérigny met with the disdain of Mme Cabanis, who considered "feuilletons anecdotiques" unsuitable for "such a great subject." The manuscript attributed to Cabanis has the following tantalizing prefatory note:

> Ce travail écrit en entier de la main du D^r. Dubreuil qui a guidé mes premiers pas dans l'étude de la médecine a été fait par moi sous sa direction et avec sa coopération.
>
> Pierre Cabanis

The handwriting bears some resemblance to the script of authenticated letters (the earliest of these that I have seen is the letter of "22 mars an II" [1793]—the letter of 1781 cited by Lehec was clearly not written by P.J.G. Cabanis, who was still a medical student at the time; its handwriting is different from known samples). Yet, as Lehec remarks, it would be rather odd that Cabanis, at the time he began the study of medicine with Dubreuil (1777 or 1778) would have employed his mentor as a copyist.

There is little in the substance of the notes on Hippocrates and Galen (French, interspersed with Latin and Greek citations) that might distinguish this notebook from the work of any other physician or medical student who followed the order of the edition of Foes (Frankfurt, 1595) for Hippocrates and of a standard edition of Galen. Its view of Galen is more favorable than that later expressed in the published works of Cabanis.

The orthography of the manuscript, despite the idiosyncrasies of even the greatest eighteenth-century authors, would seem to place it earlier than the 1770s. Some examples: faict for fait, dict for dit, eust for eut, autheur for auteur, mesmes for mêmes, chasq for châque. Folios 21-425 also appear yellower than does the 20th folio, on which the prefatory note is written. Could then the note in the hand of Cabanis have originally been attached to another work? Could the note conceivably have been a nineteenth-century invention? Lacking new evidence, proof that the Versailles manuscript indeed contains reading notes of Cabanis is rather difficult.

Appendix C

The heirs of Whytt in the elaboration of the concept of the reflex were no more mechanist than he. Johann August Unzer (1727-1799), a pupil of the Stahlian Juncker at Halle, explained certain phenomena of sensation and motion by *vis nervosa* (Haller's term) independent of the soul in *Erst Grunde einer Physiologie der eigentlichen Thierischen Natur Thierischen Körper* (Leipzig, 1771). Unzer believed that impressions from external sense organs or internal nerve endings could be "reflected" at points of concentration of "animal forces," such as ganglia, bifurcations of nerves, or plexuses, and transformed into muscular movement. The Czech physician and anatomist Georg Prochaska developed Unzer's ideas in *De Fonctionibus Systematis Nervosi* (Prague, 1784; 2d ed., Vienna, 1800 in *Opera minorici . . .*). He compared the equally incomprehensible *vis nervosa* to Newton's *vis attractiva*, explained the irritability of the muscles by their dependence on the nerves and *vis nervosa*, and refused to admit that reflex phenomena were caused by ordinary "physical laws," even if they were spontaneous and automatic. He thought that ganglia and plexuses *may* have acted as ligatures, reflecting impressions too weak to penetrate to the brain. (See discussion in Canguilhem, *La Formation du concept de réflexe aux XVIIᵉ et XVIIIᵉ siècles* (Paris, 1955), 108-124, and *Unzer and Prochaska on the Nervous System* (London, 1851) especially 192, 223-224, 342-343, 391, 397, 400, 402-404, 427, 430-432, 436.) Cabanis does not cite these works in the *Rapports*, though he probably knew of the second edition of Prochaska, widely circulated in France.

Appendix D
"Cabanis" Manuscripts
of the Muséum National D'Histoire Naturelle

Ms 2038 is an incomplete translation of G. E. Stahl's *Experimenta, observationes, animadversiones, CCC numero, chymicae, et physicae* (Berolini, 1731) here entitled "Théorie chimique du feu, ou Les 300 Expériences, observations, et remarques de Stahl." The Museum also has a complete manuscript translation (MS 2037) of the same work, by an apothecary Hénault, dated 1749. The handwriting of MS 2038 does not resemble other samples of Cabanis's writing, so its authenticity remains questionable. However, there is an astounding similarity of the script to that found in portions of the "presumed" papers of abbé La Roche, Cabanis's neighbor in the villa of Mme Helvétius (MSS 2222-2223 in the Bibliothèque de l'Institut). Several possibilities emerge: La Roche himself translated Stahl; or a copyist employed by both La Roche and Cabanis transcribed the translation for one of them. There seems to be no special motivation for Cabanis to have translated this work of Stahl. Obviously, he was indebted to Stahl's medical works and he was certainly interested in chemistry as a medical student. Perhaps he shared Stahl's opinion that chemistry was worth pursuing for its own sake even if not for its immediate utility to medicine. Unlike Lamarck, however, Cabanis accepted the theory of the Chemical Revolution, so he would have no continuing fascination with a work outlining the phlogiston theory.

As a footnote to the interest of this manuscript, I would add that Stahl's remarks here on phlogiston as the "matter of fire" (fols. 11v., 13v., 18, 33), a phrase that occurs in the 1723 edition of J.-B. Sénac's anonymous exposition of Stahlian chemistry, *Nouveau Cours de chymie suivant les principes de Newton et de Stahl*, as well as in Rouelle's lectures, would suggest to me that Rouelle could have taken the notion of fire as a constituent of bodies, rather than merely an instrument of chemical change, from Hénault's translation of Stahl's experiments, available since 1749. The point is worth stressing, because in Rhoda Rappaport's otherwise excellent article on "Rouelle and

Stahl: The Phlogistic Revolution in France," *Chymia* vii (1961), 73-102, Sénac is charged with "confusing the instrument fire with the earthy element phlogiston." (p. 88). Miss Rappaport supports this contention by comparing Sénac's exposition with Peter Shaw's version of Stahl, the *Philosophical Principles of Universal Chemistry*, published in London in 1730 but actually based on Stahl's Jena lectures of 1684, which were compiled with Stahl's authorization as *Fundamenta Chymiae Dogmaticae et Experimentalis*, Nuremberg, 1723. Rouelle himself believed that Stahl considered these lectures the "folly of his youth." (Bibliothèque Nationale, Fonds français, ms 12303, fol. 50) and approvingly cited the *CCC Experimenta* (fols. 50ff.). How much more likely, then, that Rouelle used the most recent source of Stahl's views on the matter of fire, the *CCC Experimenta* (see fols. 50-52) than that Sénac transmitted to Rouelle an inadvertent distortion of Stahl's early lectures?

Ms 2039 consists of seven notebooks entitled "Leçons de chymie—Idées sommaires." Once again the script differs from known samples of Cabanis's handwriting as well as from that of ms 2038. There is no *prima facie* proof of Cabanis's authorship. This document has intrinsic value, then, not for any information conveyed about Cabanis, but as a sidelight to the impact of the Chemical Revolution. The notebooks appear to be transcriptions of the lectures of Hilaire-Marin Rouelle (1718-1779), Royal "demonstrator" in chemistry at the Jardin du Roi and successor of his more illustrious older brother, Gustave-François Rouelle (1703-1770). Aside from the numerous references in the notes to "Rouelle le jeune," the order of presentation parallels the sequence of H.-M. Rouelle's *Procédés chimiques du regne végétal, du regne animal, du regne minéral* (1774). The published work is merely a recipe-book for laboratory operations without the theoretical commentary customarily found in notes from the course of the elder Rouelle (cf. Museum ms 1202, F.F. mss 12303-12304 at the Bibliothèque Nationale, and mss 16-20 at the Ecole de Pharmacie). ms 2039, by contrast, contains a full commentary, with revisions and additions to the earlier lectures, references to the work of Jean D'Arcet, and expansion of precisely those subjects ("mucous bodies" in the animal kingdom) that interested the younger Rouelle. The manuscript may be dated by a reference to "feu M. Roux," (fol. 41r.) apparently Augustin Roux (1726-1776), who taught chemistry at the Paris Faculty of Medicine from 1771 until his death. The notes were most likely transcribed before the death of H.-M. Rouelle in 1779. Further study might reveal whether the interpolations, relative to the content of the lectures of the elder Rouelle, correspond to the interfoliated notes of the Bordeaux manuscript of G.-F. Rouelle's lectures. As Miss Rappaport notes, H.-M. Rouelle, D'Arcet, and Roux were planning to edit and update the lectures for publication as a textbook ("G.-F. Rouelle: An Eighteenth Century Chemist and Teacher," *Chymia* vi [1960], 89-90).

The most interesting differences between MS 2039 and the other known Rouelle manuscripts (all predating the death of G.-F. Rouelle) are the scattered references to "fixed" and "inflammable" air, terms not previously used. Stahl is still honored as the "creator of modern chemistry," however, and throughout the lectures subscribe to the phlogiston theory. A sample of the fascinating hybrid conceptions of a work written during the Chemical Revolution follows (fv. 28):

Mr. D'Arcet croit que la matière huileuse ou celle du feu / car on n'est pas bien sur que ce ne soit qu'une seule et même substance / s'y trouve [in inflammable air] dans un juste degré d'expansion. C'est par expansions que les corps deviennent combustibles. Il faut pour ainsi dire qu'ils deviennent aëriens pour brûler, peut-être n'y-a-t-il d'autre principe du feu, que cet état des corps de la nature qui peuvent le prendre. Hales nous avoit bien connu la distribution de l'air fixe et de l'air inflammable, en a gardé fort long-temps dans des vaisseaux fermés et les y a retrouvés tels qu'il les y avait mis.

Appendix E
Condensed Outline of Hygiene of J.-N. Hallé

Taken from *La Médecine éclairée par les sciences physiques*, ed. Antoine-François de Fourcroy. Vol. IV (1792), 225-235.

I. Public hygiene
   Knowledge of men according to:
   A. Climates and locations
   B. Assembly in common habitations [urbanization]
   C. Occupations, usage of air, food, other non-naturals
   D. Habits, customs and manners

II. Particularities of men
   A. Age
   B. Sex
   C. Temperament
   D. Travel
   E. Wealth or poverty

III. Private hygiene
   "Things men use," according to manner, measure, duration and continuity of use, matched with age, sex, temperament, habits, wealth and poverty.
   A. *Circumfusa*
      1. Air, sun, electricity, magnetism, weather, temperature, meteors
      2. Climate, soil, floods, waters, places, artificial changes
   B. *Ingesta*
      Foods, beverages, non-evacuating remedies
   C. *Excreta*
      Natural evacuations, artificial or medical evacuations
   D. *Gesta*
      Sleep and wakefulness, motion and rest
   Additions to Boerhaave's categories:
   E. *Applicata*
      Clothes, cosmetics, baths, frictions, amulets

F. *Percepta*
   1. Sensations: external senses, hunger and thirst, physical love, sympathy and antipathy
   2. Functions of soul: passive and active affections
   3. Functions of mind: intelligence, imagination, memory

IV. Rules of good hygiene, according to all categories in (I) and (II)
  A. Differences of healthy men and those with predispositions to illness.
    1. Epidemic and endemic predispositions
    2. Individual predispositions
  B. Knowledge of non-naturals and occasional causes of illness depending upon all categories of (III)
  C. Rules of conservation, preservation, and cure
    1. Epidemic and endemic illnesses
    2. Illnesses characteristic of individuals

Bibliography

This list of works cited (with several exceptions) will not attempt to duplicate either the nearly complete table of Cabanis's correspondence compiled by Claude Lehec (*Oeuvres philosophiques de Cabanis* [hereafter designated *OP*] II, 525-539) or his thorough bibliography (*OP* II, 541-562).

MANUSCRIPTS *(all libraries, except where noted, are located in Paris)*

Archives de l'Institut (Académie française)
Procès-verbaux de la classe d'histoire et de littérature ancienne. An XI-1808.
Dossiers: F.-G.-J.-S. Andrieux, Cabanis, Marie-Joseph Chénier, Dominque-Joseph Garat, N.-L. François de Neufchâteau, Constantin-François Chassebeuf de Volney. Assorted correspondence, dealers' catalogues of correspondence.
Procès-verbaux de la classe de langue et de [la] littérature française. An XI-1808.

Archives de l'Académie des sciences
Procès-verbaux de l'Académie royale des sciences. 1786-1793.

Archives de l'Académie des sciences morales et politiques
Procès-verbaux de la classe des sciences morales et politiques. 3 vols. Ans IV, V, and VI; ans VII and VIII; and ans IX-XI. Record of reading of memoirs, committee appointments, works received, essay prize competitions. Rather sketchy.

Archives de l'Assistance publique (rue des Minimes)
Archives Générales de l'Hôtel-Dieu. Registres 1160-1161.
MS 136. Conseil général des hospices. Collection des minutes des arrêtés, 1801.
MS 62. Période révolutionnaire. Hôpitaux. 1791-1793. La Commission des hôpitaux.

Archives de la Faculté de médecine (rue de l'Ecole de médecine)
MS 372. Société médicale d'émulation. Registre de présence aux séances.

Archives de l'Institut
Comptabilité. Registre indicatif des présences. Ans v-xi.

Archives départementales de la Seine
6 AZ 52 (printed). *Rapport sur la nouvelle distribution des secours proposés dans le Département de Paris par le comité de mendicité.* Paris, 1791.

Archives départementales de la Corrèze (Tulle)
Paroisse de Cosnac. Baptêmes, Mariages, Sépultures. 1747.
C. 178.
E. 35.
1.E.6. Letter of Treilhard to de Puymarets, 2 July 1772.
6.F.239. Letter of Cabanis to J.-B.-H. Serre, 17 April 1790.

Archives Nationales
AA[63] 140. Letters of Cabanis to Pollart, 20 Frimaire vi, André, 26 Fructidor xi, and J.-M. Degérando, 29 Nivôse xviii.
AF III. 99 (438). Interior Ministry circulars to departmental commissioners.
AJ[16] A[P1, 2, and 3] (temporary numbering). Procès-verbaux de l'assemblée des professeurs. Faculté de médecine. 3 vols. 1794-1808 consulted.
Procès-verbaux des séances du comité d'administration. 13 May 1796-18 August 1800. 2 vols.
AP 27. Papers of François de Neufchâteau.
BB[30] 25. Letters of Cabanis to Minister of Justice Gohier excusing himself from service on Revolutionary Tribunal. 23, 26, and 30 March, 2? and 23 April [1793].
B[I] 17. Seine-Institut. An vi. Procès-verbaux de l'assemblée electorale de la Seine.
CC 1-CC 4. Procès-verbaux du Sénat conservateur. 1799-1808 (portion consulted).
CC 14, fol. 224. Letter of Cabanis to Monge, 28 June 1806.
CC 240, fol. 907. Letters-patent of Cabanis.
F I.C. III. Seine 1. Electoral assemblies. An vi.
F[15] 133-134. Procès-verbaux du comité des hôpitaux. 15 April-3 October, 1791.

F¹⁷ᴬ 1011. Plaquette 1. Information on review of Volney's catechism by the Conseil d'instruction publique. Plaquette 3. Conseil d'instruction publique correspondence with D.-J. Garat. 1799-1800.

F¹⁷ᴬ 1014. Interior Ministry files on translations of public assistance memoirs.

F¹⁷ 1146. Clinics of the Ecole de médecine.

F¹⁷ 1344²⁷. Ecoles centrales—Seine. An ɪᴠ. 1344²⁸. Ecoles centrales—Seine. 1795-1802.

F¹⁷ 2273. Petitions to Interior Ministry on establishment of medical schools. 1795-1803.

F¹⁷ 2274. Interior Ministry policy on écoles centrales. 1795-1802.

F¹⁷ 2279. Ecoles centrales. Printed course summaries. 1795-1802.

F¹⁷ 2289. Papers of the Ecole de médecine.

H. 1503. Registres de la Société d'agriculture de Brive.

Bibliothèque de l'Arsénal

ᴍs 15087. Papers of Louis-Sébastien Mercier.

Bibliothèque de l'Institut

ᴍs 860. Papers of Condorcet. On Society of 1789.

ᴍs 885. Papers of Condorcet. On Probability in the Sciences. Fasc. ɪɪ. On Chain of Being. Fol. 218, fols. 245-263. "Sur la Persistance de l'âme." Opposes belief in immortality of soul. Interesting juxtaposition to *Letter to Fauriel*. Only conjectures that soul survives.

CABANIS CORRESPONDENCE

ᴍs 1256. Letter to Hennin, incorrectly attributed to Cabanis. Its date (1781) precludes possibility that Cabanis could have been issuing medical prescriptions. Probable author, a Dr. François-David Cabanis (1727-1794) of Geneva.

ᴍs 2128. "Mémoire sur l'habitude." Maine de Biran. Draft of first version. Pierre Tisserand ᴍs A.

ᴍss 2222-2223. Papiers présumés de l'abbé (Martin) Lefebvre de La Roche. Commentaries on Helvétius, Benjamin Franklin, sketch of life of Franklin, fragment of a letter complaining of relationship with Cabanis. Handwriting of copyist same as in Stahl translation attributed to Cabanis.

ᴍs 2327. Brief letters to Claude Fauriel, 6 Prairial xɪɪ (26 May 1804) and 1 Brumaire xɪɪɪ (23 October 1804); letters of Mme Cabanis to Fauriel.

MS 2475. Letter to A. Condorcet O'Connor.

MS 2714. Letters to "president" of Institut 1 Pluviôse VI [20 January 1798]; to Garnier-Deschener, 15 December 1807.

MS 4501. Letter to J.-M. Degérando.

MS 2954. Papers of François Thurot. Philosophy course outlines.

MS 2955. Papers of François Thurot. Notes on various philosophers.

MS 2958. Papers of François Thurot. Unpublished review of Mme Condorcet's *Lettres sur la sympathie* with Cabanis's handwritten corrections. Notes on "analysis."

MS 2959. Papers of François Thurot. *Logic* outline. General grammar course at Lycée des étrangers. 1797.

Bibliothèque historique de la ville de Paris
Dossier of Cabanis (no longer numbered). Contains Cabanis's printed medical theses, certificates of attendance at Faculty of Medicine in Paris, and various membership certificates in medical societies and scholarly organizations.

Bibliothèque municipale de Versailles
MS 96 (see *OP* II, 544-545). See discussion of manuscript in Appendix B.

Bibliothèque Nationale
N.A.F. 1390, fol. 203. Letter of Cabanis to Barbier, 16 Prairial XIII (5 June 1805).

N.A.F. 9192. Instruction publique pendant la Révolution. Collection Ginguené. Ecoles centrales, primaires, Ecole normale, polytechnique, etc.

N.A.F. 9193. Direction générale de l'instruction publique. Ans IV-VI.

N.A.F. 21881, 21896, 21897. Papers of Pierre-Claude-François Daunou. Extracts of memoirs read to *Classe d'histoire et de littérature ancienne*.

Fonds français 12302-12304. "Cours de chimie, ou leçons de M. Rouelle, démonstrateur au Jardin du Roy, recueillies en 1754 et 1755 . . . corrigées en 1757 et 1758."

Ecole de pharmacie
MS 16. "Notes sur la chimie d'après Mr. Rouelle." 1754.

MS 17. "Chimie de Rouelle." 1759.

MS 19. "Première Partie des leçons de chimie." 1757.

MS 20. "Seconde Partie des leçons de chimie."

Mairie du XVIe arrondissement
(1) Parent de Rosan collection.
—Vol. 20:
    Letters of Cabanis to Saltier, J.-M. Degérando, "président de l'Institut," Aldini, Paul Delaunay, Pierre-Louis Ginguené.
—Vol. 28: "Conseil général d'Auteuil, extraits."
    "Registres des déliberations (1790-1859) a l'hôtel de ville."
    "Auteuil, documents administratifs, copies séparées, 1790-1859."
(2) Collection de la Société historique d'Auteuil et de Passy, MSS 7652-7653.
MS 7654. Letter of Cabanis to Lebrun. 5 January 1793.
MS 7125.

Musée Ernest Rupin, Brive
Registres de la Société d'agriculture de Brive. 1743-1774.
Collection Labrousse. Correspondence of Cabanis, including a letter to Mme de Staël concerning *Delphine*, 28 Frimaire XI (19 December 1802).

Muséum national d'histoire naturelle
MS 1202. "Cours de chymie recueilli des leçons de Rouelle, apothicaire [A.-L. de Jussieu], Paris, 1767."
MS 2037. "Les Trois Cent Expériences, observations, et remarques phisiochimiques de George Ernée Staahl . . . par Mr. Hénault, apothicaire en 1749."
MS 2038. "Théorie chimique du feu ou les 300 expériences, observations, et remarques de Staahl," attributed to Cabanis.
MS 2039. "Leçons de chymie—Idées sommaires," attributed to Cabanis. See Appendix D.

PRINTED PRIMARY MATERIALS

PERIODICALS AND SERIALS

Annales de chimie.
Commentaires de la Faculté de médecine de Paris, 1777-1786. Edited by Steinheil. 2 vols. Paris, 1903.
Le Conservateur, journal politique, philosophique, et littéraire. Edited by Garat, Daunou, and Chénier. An VI.
La Décade philosophique, politique, et littéraire. 1794-1807.
Histoire et mémoires de la Société royale de médecine, années 1776-1790. 10 vols. Paris, 1779-an VI.

Journal de la Société de 1789. Edited by Condorcet, Dupont de Nemours, et al. 15 March-15 September 1790.

Journal of the Société de médecine (after 27 Pluviôse v [15 February 1797]), founded as the Société de santé on 2 Germinal IV (22 March 1796). Cabanis became a member in February 1797 after his appointment to the Ecole de médecine.

Magasin encyclopédique. XLV. An XI (1802).

La Médecine éclairée par les sciences physiques. Edited by Antoine-François de Fourcroy. 4 vols. Paris, 1791-1792.

Mémoires de l'Institut national des sciences et arts. Classe des sciences morales et politiques, an IV-an XI. 5 vols. Paris, an VI-1804.

Mémoires de la Société médicale d'émulation pour an V-an X. 6 vols. Paris, an VI-1806 (portion consulted).

Le Moniteur universel. (14, 15, 16, 23, and 29 Germinal VII). XXIII.

Philosophical Transactions [of the Royal Society]. Vol. 45. 1748.

Recueil périodique de la Société de médecine (Société de la santé de Paris, ans IV-V). 14 vols. Paris, an IV-1803 (portion consulted).

Réimpression de l'ancien moniteur. Vols. 13, 16, 29. Paris, 1847.

Le Républicain, ou le défenseur du gouvernement représentatif; par une société des républicains. July 1791. 4 nos. (Bibliothèque Nationale catalogue no. Lc² 673).

DOCUMENT COLLECTIONS

Aulard, F.-A., ed. *La Société des Jacobins.* 6 vols. Paris, 1889-1897.

Beauchamp, A. de, ed. *Enquêtes et documents relatifs à l'enseignement supérieur.* t. XXVIII. *Médecine et Pharmacie. Projets de lois, 1789-1803.* Paris, 1888.

Bloch, Camille, and Tuetey, Alexandre, eds. *Procès-verbaux et rapports du comité de mendicité.* Paris, 1911.

Brièle, M., ed. *Collection des documents pour servir à l'histoire des hôpitaux de Paris.* 4 vols. Paris, 1881-1887.

Debidour, A., ed. *Recueil des actes du Directoire exécutif.* Vol. IV. Paris, 1917.

Duguit, L., and Monnier, H. *Les Constitutions . . . depuis 1789.* Paris, 1923.

Guillaume, James, ed. *Procès-verbaux du comité d'instruction publique de l'Assemblée législative.* Paris, 1889.

———. *Procès-verbaux du comité d'instruction publique de la Convention nationale.* 6 vols. Paris, 1891-1907.

Institut de France. Académie des sciences. *Procès-verbaux des séances de l'Académie tenues depuis la fondation de l'Institut jusqu'au mois d'août 1835.* 10 vols. Hendaye, 1910-1924.

Lacroix, Sigismond, ed. *Actes de la Commune de Paris.* 16 vols. Paris, 1894-1942.

Procès-verbaux des sèances du Conseil des cinq-cents. Paris, ans VI-VIII (portion consulted).

Recueil de mémoires sur les établissements d'humanité. 17 vols. Paris, ans VII-XII. Sponsored by Interior Minister François de Neufchâteau; edited by Adrien Duquesnoy; translations of the literature on public assistance in Britain and Europe.

Recueil des discours, rapports, et pièces diverses, lus dans les séances . . . de l'Académie française, 1803-1819, 1re partie. Paris, 1847.

Séances des écoles normales recueillies par des sténographes et revues par les professeurs . . . Leçons . . . Débats (an III). 13 vols. 2d ed. Paris, an IX.

Tuetey, Alexandre. *L'Assistance publique à Paris pendant la Révolution.* 4 vols. Paris, 1895-1897.

————, ed. "Procès-verbaux du comité des hôpitaux, 15 avril-3 octobre 1791," *Bulletin d'histoire économique de la Révolution.* Paris, 1916, pp. 67-153.

WORKS OF CABANIS

Collections

Oeuvres complètes de Cabanis. Edited by François Thurot. 5 vols. Paris, 1823-1825.

Oeuvres philosophiques de Cabanis. Edited by Claude Lehec and Jean Cazeneuve. 2 vols. Paris, 1956.

Selections

Cabanis, choix de textes et introduction. edited by Georges Poyer. Paris, n.d. [1910]. An excellent brief biography and a helpful categorization (e.g. "Science and Method") of excerpts from the major works.

Editions of individual works (in chronological order)

An a pastu quies? Reims, 1784. Thesis for licentiate in medicine.

"Serment d'un médecin." *Feuille hebdomadaire de la Généralité de Limoges.* 10e année, no. 11. 27 April 1785.

Observations sur les hôpitaux. Paris, 1790.

Journal de la maladie et de la mort de Mirabeau. Paris, 1791.

Travail sur l'éducation publique, trouvé dans les papiers de Mirabeau l'aîne, publié par P.-J.-G. Cabanis. Paris, an VI (1798). 2d ed. Paris, an XI (1803). 3d ed. Paris, 1819.

Rapports du physique et du moral de l'homme. Paris, an X (1802). 2d ed. Paris, 1805.

———. Edited by L. Cérise. Paris, 1843.

———. Edited by Louis Peisse. Paris, 1844.

Coup d'oeil sur les Révolutions et sur la réforme de la médecine. Paris, an XII (1804).

Lettre (posthume et inédite) de Cabanis à M. F . . . sur les causes premières. Edited by F.-E. Bérard. Paris and Montpellier, 1824.

Addresses in the Council of Five Hundred and Commission of Council (in chronological order excluding some reprinted in *OP*) (Bibliothèque Nationale catalogue numbers)

Corps législatif. Conseil des cinq-cents. Rapport fait . . . sur un mode provisoire de police médicale. 4 Messidor VI (Le⁴³ 2075).

Discours prononcé le 26 messidor, anniversaire du 14 juillet, au sujet de l'adresse et de l'offrande des irlandais unis. . . . Paris, Thermidor VI (Le⁴³ 2141).

Discours de Cabanis en offrant au Conseil des cinq-cents la gravure du portrait de Mirabeau. . . . 13 Thermidor an VI (Le⁴³ 2205).

Opinion de Cabanis sur l'impôt du sel à l'extraction. 11 Fructidor VI (Le⁴³ 2275).

Rapport fait . . . sur l'organisation des écoles de médecine. 29 Brumaire VII (Le⁴³ 2450).

Opinion de Cabanis contre le projet de partage des biens communaux. 7 Pluviôse VII (Le⁴³ 2726).

Opinion de Cabanis sur les réunions s'occupant d'objets politiques. Paris, n.d. (Le⁴³ 1204). Misdated in *Catalogue de l'histoire de France* as 6 Thermidor V; actually 6 Thermidor VII.

Discours . . . sur le message du Conseil des anciens, relatif aux journaux calomniateurs des premières autorités. 1 Fructidor VII (Le⁴³ 3448).

Commission du Conseil des cinq-cents.

Opinion de Cabanis sur l'emprunt forcé. 25 Brumaire VIII (Le⁴⁴ 6).

Discours prononcé par Cabanis (on the new constitution). 3 Nivôse VIII (Le⁴⁴ 48).

Articles

"Note sur l'opinion de MM. Oelsner et Soemmering, et du citoyen Sue, touchant le supplice de la guillotine," *Magasin encyclopédique* V (1795), 155.

"Sciences, philosophie," in *Le Conservateur* no. 30 (9 Vendémiaire VI [30 September 1797]), pp. 236-238. This periodical was edited by Garat, Daunou, and Chénier.

Reviews in *La Décade philosophique* attributed to Cabanis

Claude-Louis Berthollet. *Essai de statique chimique* (10 Messidor XI), pp. 10-18.

Alexandre Corai. *Traité d'Hippocrate, des airs, des eaux, et des lieux* (30 Thermidor IX), pp. 325-332.

P. A. Latreille. *Histoire naturelle des fourmis* (10 Prairial x), pp. 385-395.

C.-F. Volney. *Traité du climat et du sol des Etats-Unis d'Amérique* (10, 20, 30 Frimaire XII), pp. 393-405, 449-464, 513-526.

Review of Frederick Morton Eden. *The State of the Poor*. 3 vols. London, 1797, in *Mercure français*. 20 and 30 Messidor and 20 Thermidor VI (8 and 18 July 1798 and 7 August 1798).

OTHER ADDRESSES IN THE COUNCIL OF FIVE HUNDRED AND IN OTHER LEGISLATIVE BODIES (Bibliothèque Nationale catalogue numbers)

Projet de résolution de Calès. 12 Prairial v (Le[43] 1017).
Projet de résolution de Vitet. 17 Ventôse VI (Le[43] 1816).
Opinion de [Jean-François] Barailon. 17 Germinal VI (Le[43] 1883).
Motion d'ordre de Vitet. 4 Messidor VI (Le[43] 2076).
Opinion de Vitet. 23 Nivôse VII (Le[43] 2683).

Education Debate

Rapport général fait par Roger-Martin sur l'organisation de l'instruction publique. 19 Brumaire VII (Le[43] 2438; redraft, Le[43] 2801, Pluviôse VII).
Rapport de Heurtault-Lamerville. 22 Brumaire VII (Le[43] 2440).
Rapport de Bonnaire. 23 Brumaire VII (Le[43] 2444).
Rapport fait par Hardy. . . . 1 Frimaire VII (Le[43] 2455).
J. A. Dulaure. *Sur La Surveillance et la police des écoles*. . . . 2, 7 Frimaire VII (Le[43] 2456).
Opinion de Jean-Edme Boilleau. 24 Nivôse VII (Le[43] 2687).
Opinion de J.-P.-F. Duplantier. 24 Nivôse VII (Le[43] 2688).
Opinion de Scherlock. 24 Nivôse VII (Le[43] 2689).
Opinion de Bremontier. . . . 28 Nivôse VII (Le[43] 2704).
Opinion de Challan. . . . 28 Nivôse VII (Le[43] 2705).

Opinion de Joubert. . . . 28 Nivôse vii (Le[43] 2706).

Opinion de Sonthonax. . . . 1 Ventôse vii (Le[43] 2807).

Motion d'ordre . . . par J.-Ch. Bailleul. 13 Germinal vii (Le[43] 2924).

Discours de Heurtault-Lamerville. . . . 14 Germinal vii (Le[43] 2928).

Opinion de Louvet. . . . 18 Germinal vii.

Opinion de André. 21 Germinal vii (Le[43] 2958).

Opinion de Andrieux. . . . 1, 11 Floréal vii (Le[43] 2994).

Tribunat. Rapport fait . . . par Thouret sur le projet de loi relatif à l'exercice de la médecine. 16 Ventôse xi.

Tribunat. Rapport fait par Fourcroy. . . . 30 Germinal x (Le[50] 104).

OTHER PRIMARY MATERIALS

Alembert, Jean le Rond d'. *Preliminary Discourse to the Encyclopedia of Diderot* (1751). Translated by Richard Schwab. New York, 1963.

Alibert, Jean-Louis. *Physiologie des passions, ou nouvelle doctrine des sentiments moraux.* Paris, 1825.

Bacon, Francis. *The Works of Francis Bacon.* Edited by James Spedding and Robert Ellis. 15 vols. London, 1858.

[Bailly, Jean-Sylvain]. *Discours et mémoires par l'auteur de "l'Histoire de l'astronomie."* 3 vols. Paris, 1790.

Barruel, Augustin. *Mémoires pour servir à l'histoire du Jacobinisme.* 5 vols. Hamburg, 1798-1799.

Barthez, Paul-Joseph. *Nouveaux Elémens de la science de l'homme.* Montpellier, 1778.

―――. *Nouveaux Eléments de la science de l'homme.* 2 vols. 2d edition, Paris, 1806.

Bernardin de Saint-Pierre, J.-H. *Oeuvres complètes de J.-H. Bernardin de Saint-Pierre.* Edited by L. Aimé-Martin. 12 vols. Paris, 1818.

Bichat, Xavier. *Recherches physiologiques sur la vie et la mort.* (1800). Paris, 1805.

Boerhaave, Hermann. *Praelectiones Academicae in Proprias Institutiones rei Medicae, edidit et notas addidit.* Edited by Albrecht von Haller. Göttingen, 1740.

Boissier de Sauvages, François. *Nosologie méthodique.* . . . (1763) 2 vols. Paris, 1770-1771.

Bonald, Louis de. *Oeuvres complètes de M. de Bonald.* Edited by Migne. Vol. iii. Paris, 1859.

Bonnet, Charles. *Oeuvres d'histoire naturelle et de philosophie.* 8 vols. Neuchâtel, 1779-1783.

Bordeu, Théophile de. *Correspondance.* Edited by Martha Fletcher. 4 vols. Montpellier, 1977-1979.

———. *Oeuvres complètes de Bordeu.* Edited by B.-A. Richerand. 2 vols. Paris, 1818.

Buffon, Georges-Louis Leclerc de. *Oeuvres philosophiques.* Edited by Jean Piveteau. Paris, 1954.

Chateaubriand. *Oeuvres complètes de Chateaubriand.* Vol. ii. Paris: Garnier, n.d.

Condillac, Etienne Bonnot de. *Oeuvres philosophiques.* Edited by Georges Le Roy. 3 vols. Paris, 1951.

Condorcet, Marie-Jean-Antoine-Nicolas Caritat de. *Oeuvres de Condorcet.* Edited by A. Condorcet O'Connor and M. François Arago. 12 vols. Paris, 1847-1849.

———. *Sketch for a Historical Picture of the Progress of the Human Mind.* Edited and translated by June Barraclough. London, 1955.

Condorcet, Mme (Sophie). *"Théorie des sentimens moraux" by Adam Smith . . . Lettres [dédiées] à Cabanis, sur la théorie des sentimens moraux.* Paris, an vi.

Cullen, William. *First Lines of the Practice of Physick.* 4 vols. Edinburgh, 1784.

———. *Médecine pratique.* Tranlated by E.F.M. Bosquillon. Paris, 1785.

———. *Physiologie de M. Cullen.* Translated by E.F.M. Bosquillon. Paris, 1785.

Degérando, J.-M. *Des Signes, et de l'art de penser considérés dans leurs rapports mutuels.* 4 vols. Paris, an viii.

Descartes, René. *Discours de la méthode* (1637). Edited by Etienne Gilson. Paris, 1930.

———. *Oeuvres de Descartes.* Edited by Charles Adam and Paul Tannéry. 13 vols. Paris, 1897-1913.

———. *Oeuvres philosophiques.* Edited by Ferdinand Alquié. 2 vols. Paris, 1963.

———. *Traité sur les passions de l'âme.* Edited by Geneviève Rodis-Lewis. Paris, 1965.

———. *Treatise of Man.* Edited by Thomas Steele Hall. Cambridge, Mass., 1972.

Destutt de Tracy, Antoine-Louis-Claude. *De L'Amour.* Edited by Gilbert Chinard. Paris 1926.

Destutt de Tracy, Antoine-Louis-Claude. *A Commentary upon Montesquieu's Spirit of Laws*. Philadelphia, 1811.

———. *Observations sur le système actuel de l'instruction publique*. Paris, an IX.

———. *Projet d'élémens d'idéologie à l'usage des écoles centrales*. . . . Paris, an IX (1801).

———. *Elémens d'idéologie. Deuxième partie. Grammaire*. Paris, an XI (1803).

———. *Elémens d'idéologie. Troisième partie. Logique*. Paris, 1805.

———. *Eléments d'idéologie*. 5 vols. Brussels, 1826-1827.

———. *Eléments d'idéologie*. Edited by Henri Gouhier. 2 vols. Paris, 1970. Reprint of 1817 edition, vols. I and II.

———. *Quels sont les moyens de fonder la morale chez un peuple?* Paris, an VI. Published first in *Mercure français*. 10, 20, 30 Ventôse VI.

———. *Traité sur la volonté et ses effets. Economie. Morale*. 2 vols. Paris, 1815.

Diderot, Denis. *Eléments de physiologie*. Edited by Jean Mayer. Paris, 1964.

———. *Lettre sur les aveugles*. Edited by Robert Niklaus. Geneva, 1951.

———. *Oeuvres complètes de Diderot*. Edited by J. Assézat and M. Tourneux. 20 vols. Paris, 1875-1877.

———. *Oeuvres philosophiques*. Edited by Paul Vernière. Paris, 1964.

———. *Rêve de d'Alembert*. Edited by Paul Vernière. Paris, 1951.

Dumas, Charles. *Principes de physiologie, ou Introduction à la science expérimentale, philosophique, et médicale de l'homme vivant*. 4 vols. Paris, 1800-1803.

Du Pont de Nemours, Pierre-Samuel. *Idées sur les secours à donner aux pauvres malades dans une grande ville*. Philadelphia and Paris, 1786.

Dupuis, Charles. *Origines de tous les cultes, ou religion universelle*. 4 vols. Paris, an III (1795).

Extrait des registres de l'Académie royale des sciences du 22 novembre 1786. Rapport des commissaires chargés, par l'Académie, de l'examen d'un projet d'un nouvel Hôtel-Dieu. 2d edition. Paris, 1787.

Fouquet, Henri. "Sensibilité, Sentiment." XV (1765). In *Encyclopédie, ou Dictionnaire raisonné des sciences et des arts et métiers*. 17 vols. Paris, 1751-1765.

Fourcroy, Antoine-François. "Action des médicaments." In *Ency-clopédie méthodique (Médecine)*. x (1787), 133-175.

Fray, J.-B. *Essai sur l'origine des corps organisés, et sur quelques phénomènes de physiologie animale et végétale*. Paris, 1817.

Galen. *Claudii Galeni Opera Omnia*. Edited by C. G. Kühn. Vol. i. Leipzig, 1821.

———. *De Usu Partium*. Edited by Margaret May. 2 vols. Ithaca, 1968.

———. *Oeuvres anatomiques, physiologiques, et médicales de Ga-lien*. Edited by Charles Daremberg. 2 vols. Paris, 1854-1856.

Garnier, Germain. *Rapport fait au conseil du département de Paris . . . 15 novembre 1791 . . . contenant l'exposé des travaux du Di-rectoire, et le compte de sa gestion* (Bibliothèque Nationale Cata-logue no. Lb⁴⁰ 183).

Gaub, Jerome. *Sermo Academicus de Regimine Mentis Quod Medicorum est. . . .* (1747) and (1763). In L. J. Rather. *Mind and Body in Eighteenth-Century Medicine*. London, 1965.

Guyton de Morveau. "Affinité." In *Encyclopédie méthodique (Chimie, pharmacie, métallurgie)*. i (1786), 535-539, 570.

Hales, Stephen. *Statique des animaux*. Translated by François Boissier de Sauvages. Paris, 1786.

Haller, Albrecht von. *First Lines of Physiology*. ([1747] Edinburgh, 1786 translation). Edited by Lester Snow King. New York, 1966.

———. "On the Sensible and Irritable Parts of Animals." Edited by Owsei Temkin. *Bulletin of the Institute of the History of Medi-cine* iv (1936), 651-699.

Helvétius, Claude-Adrien. *Oeuvres complètes*. 4 vols. Paris, 1795.

Hippocrates. *Hippocrate: Médecine grecque*. Edited by Robert Joly. Paris, 1964.

———. *The Medical Works of Hippocrates*. Edited by John Chadwick and W. N. Mann. Oxford, 1950.

———. *Oeuvres complètes d'Hippocrate*. Edited by Emile Littré. 10 vols. Paris, 1839-1861.

———. *The Works of Hippocrates*. Edited by W.H.S. Jones. 4 vols. London, 1939-1944.

Holbach, Paul Thiry d'. *Système de la nature, par Mirabaud* (1770). London (Paris), 1774.

Ingenhousz, Jan. *Nouvelles expériences et observations sur divers ob-jets de physique*. 2 vols. Paris, 1787-1789.

Lacaze, Louis. *Idée de l'homme physique et moral*. Paris, 1755.

Bernard-Germain-Etienne de la Ville-sur-Illon, comte de Lacépède.

Oeuvres du comte de Lacépède. Edited by M.A.G. Desmarest. 12 vols. Paris, 1826-1833.

Lamarck, Jean-Baptiste de. *Philosophie zoologique* (1809). 2 vols. Paris, 1873.

———. *Système des animaux sans vertebres.* Paris, an ix (1801).

La Mettrie, Julien Offray de. *Lamettrie's "L'Homme machine": A Study in the Origins of an Idea.* Edited by Aram Vartanian. Princeton, 1960.

Laplace, Pierre-Simon de. *Exposition du système du monde.* 2 vols. Paris, an iv (1796).

Le Camus, Antoine. *Médecine de l'esprit.* Paris, 1753.

———. *Médecine de l'esprit.* 2d ed. Paris, 1769.

Le Clerc, Daniel. *Histoire de la médecine.* The Hague, 1729. Reprint. Amsterdam, 1967.

The Leibniz-Clarke Correspondence. Edited by H. G. Alexander. Manchester, 1956.

Locke, John. *An Essay Concerning Human Understanding* (1690). Edited by A. C. Fraser. 2 vols. Oxford, 1894.

Maine de Biran. *Oeuvres de Maine de Biran.* Edited by Pierre Tisserand. 14 vols. Paris, 1920-1949.

Maistre, Joseph de. *Oeuvres complètes.* Vol. i. Lyon, 1884.

Maupertuis, Pierre-Louis Moreau de. *Oeuvres.* 4 vols. Lyon, 1756.

———. *Oeuvres* (Lyon, 1768). 5 vols. Reprint. Hildesheim, 1965.

Montesquieu. *Oeuvres complètes.* Edited by Daniel Oster. Paris, 1964.

Montlinot, Leclerc de. *Etat actuel du dépôt de Soissons, précédé d'un essai sur la mendicité.* Soissons, 1789.

Needham, John Turbervill. *Mémoires pour servir à l'histoire d'un polype d'eau douce.* Leyden, 1744.

Newton, Sir Isaac. *Mathematical Principles of Natural Philosophy* (1687). Edited by Florian Cajori. Translated by Andrew Motte. 2 vols. Berkeley, 1962.

Pinel, Philippe. *Nosographie philosophique, ou la méthode de l'analyse appliquée à la médecine.* 2 vols. Paris, an vi (1798).

———. *Traité médico-philosophique sur l'aliénation mentale, ou la manie.* Paris, an ix (1801).

Plan général de l'enseignement de l'Ecole de santé de Paris. Paris, an iii.

Richerand, Balthasar-Anthelme. *De La Population dans ses rapports avec la nature des gouvernemens.* Paris, 1837.

———. *Elements of Physiology*. Edited by James Copland. Translated by G.J.M. de Lys. New York, 1825.

———. *Nouveaux Elémens de physiologie*. an IX (1801). 2d ed. Paris, an x (1802).

———. *Nouveaux Eléments de physiologie*. Paris, 1833.

Rousseau, Jean-Jacques. *Du contrat social* (1762). Edition by Garnier Frères, Publishers. Paris, 1962.

———. *Emile* (1762). Edited by Michael Launay. Paris, 1966.

Roussel, Pierre. *Système physique et moral de la femme.* . . . Paris, 1775.

Sèze, Victor de. *Recherches phisiologiques et philosophiques sur la sensibilité ou la vie animale*. Paris, 1786.

Siéyès, Abbé. *Reconnaissance et exposition raisonnée des droits de l'homme et du citoyen*. Versailles, 1789. Draft Declaration of Rights. Speaks of needs of men as basis for rights.

Smith, Adam. *An Inquiry into the Nature and Causes of the Wealth of Nations* (1776). Ed. E. Cannan. 2 vols. London, 1904.

Stahl, G. F. *Oeuvres médico-philosophiques et pratiques de G. F. Stahl*. Edited by Théodore Blondin. 6 vols. Paris, 1859-1863.

Sydenham, Thomas. *The Works of Thomas Sydenham*. Edited by Greenhill. Translated by P. G. Latham. 2 vols. London, 1848.

Tenon, Jacques. *Mémoires sur les hôpitaux de Paris*. Paris, 1788.

Thurot, François. *Mélanges de feu François Thurot*. Edited by Thurot. Paris, 1880. Unpublished reviews, posthumously published lectures on grammar and logic.

———. *Oeuvres posthumes de M. François Thurot*. Edited by P.-C.-F. Daunou. Paris, 1837. Interesting reviews of *Rapports* and of Tracy's works.

[Volney] Constantin-François Boisgiray de Chassebeuf de. *La Loi naturelle* (1793). Edited by Gaston-Martin. Paris, 1934.

———. *Oeuvres complètes*. Edited by A. Bossange. VII. Paris, 1871.

———. *Les Ruines* (1791). Paris, 1871.

———. *Voyage en Egypte et en Syrie* (1787). Edited by Jean Gaulmier. Paris, 1959.

[Volney]. *Questions de statistique à l'usage des voyageurs*. Paris, 1813.

Voltaire. *Oeuvres complètes*. Edited by Louis Moland. 52 vols. Paris, 1877-1885.

Whytt, Robert. *Observations on the Nature, Causes, and Cure of Those Diseases which have been commonly called Nervous, Hypochondriac, or Hysteric.* . . . Edinburgh, 1764.

★ BIBLIOGRAPHY ★

BIBLIOGRAPHICAL AIDS AND REFERENCE WORKS

Caron, Pierre. *Manuel pratique pour l'étude de la Révolution française*. Paris, 1947.

Monglond, A. *La France révolutionnaire et impériale*. 9 vols. Paris, 1930-1963.

Puschmann, Neuburger, Pagel, eds. *Handbuch der Geschichte der Medizin*. 3 vols. Jena, 1902-1905.

Tourneux, Maurice. *Bibliographie de l'histoire de Paris pendant la Révolution*. 5 vols. Paris, 1894-1913.

Tuetey, Alexandre. *Répertoire général des sources manuscrites de l'histoire de Paris pendant la Révolution française*. 11 vols. Paris, 1890-1914.

MONOGRAPHS, ARTICLES

Abray, Jane. "Feminism in the French Revolution." *American Historical Review* LXXX (1975), 43-62.

Ackerknecht, Erwin. "Broussais, or a Forgotten Medical Revolution." *Bulletin of the History of Medicine* XXVII (1953), 320-343.

———. "Elisha Bartlett and the Philosophy of the Paris Clinical School." *Bulletin of the History of Medicine* XXIV (1950), 43-60.

———. *Medicine at the Paris Hospital*. Baltimore, 1967. Investigation of the work of Philippe Pinel, Xavier Bichat, and leading figures of the "clinical school." Introductory pages on Cabanis marred by inaccuracies.

Actes de la journée Maupertuis, Creteil, 1-12-73. Paris, 1975.

Adams, Thomas. "Mendicity and Moral Alchemy: Work as Rehabilitation." *Studies on Voltaire and the Eighteenth Century* CLI (1976), 47-76.

Alengry, Franck. *Condorcet*. Paris, 1904.

Alfaric, Prosper. *Laromiguière et son école*. Paris, 1929.

Allain, Ernest. *L'Oeuvre scolaire de la Révolution*. Paris, 1891.

Amiable, Louis. *Une Loge maçonnique d'avant 1789; Les Neuf Soeurs*. Paris, 1897.

Anderson, Lorin. "Charles Bonnet's Taxonomy and Chain of Being." *Journal of the History of Ideas* XXXVII (1976), 45-58.

Ariès, Philippe. *Centuries of Childhood: A Social History of Family Life*. Translated by Robert Baldick. New York, 1962.

Astruc, P. "Sur Dubreuil, maître de Cabanis." *Le Progrès médical*. Supplément illustré (24 January 1945), p. 45.

Aucoc, Léon. *L'Institut de France: Lois, statuts, et règlements*. Paris, 1889.

Baker, J. R. *Abraham Trembley of Geneva: Scientist and Philosopher, 1710-1784*. London, 1952.

Baker, Keith. *Condorcet: From Natural Philosophy to Social Mathematics*. Chicago, 1975.

———. "Condorcet's notes for a revised edition of his reception speech to the Académie française." *Studies on Voltaire and the Eighteenth Century* CLIX (1977), 7-68.

———. "Les Débuts de Condorcet au secrétariat de l'Académie des sciences, 1773-1776." *Revue d'histoire des sciences* (1967), 229-280.

———. "The Early History of the Term 'Social Science.' " *Annals of Science* XX (1964), 211-226.

Barnard, H. C. *Education and the French Revolution*. Cambridge, 1969.

Bastholm, E.B.M. "The History of Muscle Physiology." *Acta Historia Scientiarum Naturalium et Medicinalium* VII (Copenhagen, 1950), 219-225.

Bastid, Paul. *Siéyès et sa pensée*. 2d ed. Paris, 1970.

Becque, A., and Chuquin, N. "Un Philosophe toujours inconnu: L.Cl. de Saint-Martin." *Dix-Huitième Siècle* IV (1972), 169-190.

Bénétruy, J. *L'Atelier de Mirabeau*. Geneva, 1962.

Bérard, F.-E. *Doctrine médicale de l'école de Montpellier*. . . . Montpellier, 1819.

Bergeron, Louis. *L'Episode napoléonien: Aspects intérieurs 1799-1815*. Paris, 1972.

Berthier, Auguste-Georges. "Le Mécanisme cartésien et la physiologie du XVIIᵉ siècle." *Isis* III (1920), 21-58.

Biographie universelle ancienne et moderne [Michaud]. 45 vols. 2d ed. Paris, 1854-1865.

Bloch, Camille. *L'Assistance et l'Etat en France à la veille de la Révolution*. Paris, 1908.

Boas, George. *French Philosophies of the Romantic Period*. Baltimore, 1925.

Bouchet, Michel. *L'Assistance publique en France pendant la Révolution*. Paris, 1908.

Bourde, A.-J. *Agronomie et agronomes en France au XVIIIᵉ siècle*. 3 vols. Paris, 1967.

Bourgey, Louis. *Observation et expérience chez les médecins de la collection hippocratique*. Paris, 1953.

Bradley, Margaret. "Scientific Education versus Military Training:

The Influence of Napoleon Bonaparte on the *Ecole polytechnique.*" *Annals of Science* XXXII (1975), 414-449.

Breck, Allen D., and Yourgrau, Wolfgang, eds. *Biology, History, and Natural Philosophy.* New York, 1972.

Brunet, Pierre. *Maupertuis.* 2 vols. Paris, 1929.

Bulletin de la Société historique d'Auteuil et de Passy. Paris, 1892. Local history.

Burkhardt, Jr., Richard W. "The Inspiration of Lamarck's Belief in Evolution." *Journal of the History of Biology* v (1972), 413-438.

————. "Lamarck, Evolution, and the Politics of Science." *Journal of the History of Biology* III (1970), 275-298.

Burlingame, Leslie. "Lamarck." *Dictionary of Scientific Biography.* Vol. VII. New York, 1973, 584-593.

Cailliet, Emile. *La Tradition littéraire des idéologues.* Philadelphia, 1943.

Callot, Emile. *La Philosophie de la vie au XVIIIᵉ siècle.* Paris, 1965.

Candille, Marcel. "Les Projets de translation de l'Hôtel-Dieu de Paris hors de la cité." *Revue de l'Assistance publique à Paris* VII (1956), 743-752; VIII (1957), 239-263, 343-359, 433-449.

Canguilhem, Georges. "Cabanis." *Dictionary of Scientific Biography* Vol. III. New York, 1971, 1-3.

————. *La Formation du concept de réflexe aux XVIIᵉ et XVIIIᵉ siècles.* Paris, 1955.

————. *L'Idée de médecine expérimentale selon Claude Bernard.* Paris, 1965.

Carlson, Eric T., and Simpson, Meribeth. "Models of the Nervous System in Eighteenth-Century Neurophysiology and Medical Psychology." *Bulletin of the History of Medicine* XLIV (1969), 101-115.

Challamel, Augustin. *Les Clubs contre-révolutionnaires.* Paris, 1895.

Champeval, J.-B. *Dictionnaire généalogique des familles nobles et notables de la Corrèze.* Vol. II. Tulle, 1913.

Chancerel, J.-E. *Recherches sur la pensée biologique de Stahl.* Paris, 1934.

Chinard, Gilbert. *Jefferson et les idéologues.* . . . Baltimore, 1925. Correspondence of Jefferson with Cabanis and Tracy included.

————. *Volney et l'Amérique.* Baltimore and Paris, 1923.

Cobb, Richard. *Les Armées révolutionnaires: Instrument de terreur dans les départements, avril 1793-floréal an II.* Paris, 1961.

Coleman, William. "Health and Hygiene in the *Encyclopédie*: A Medical Doctrine for the Bourgeoisie." *Journal of the History of Medicine* xxix (1974), 399-421.

Colonna d'Istria, F. "Bichat et la biologie contemporaine." *Revue de métaphysique et de morale* xvi (1908), 261-280.

――――. "Cabanis et les origines de la vie psychologique." *Revue de métaphysique et de morale* xix (1911), 177-198.

――――. "Les Formes de la vie psychologique et leurs conditions organiques d'après Cabanis." *Revue de métaphysique et de morale* xx (1912), 25-47.

――――. "L'Influence du moral sur le physique d'après Cabanis et Maine de Biran." *Revue de métaphysique et de morale* xxi (1913), 451-461.

――――. "La Logique de la médecine, d'après Cabanis." *Revue de métaphysique et de morale* xxv (1917), 59-73.

――――. "La Psychologie de Bichat." *Revue de métaphysique et de morale* xxxiii (1926), 1-38.

――――. "La Religion d'après Cabanis." *Revue de métaphysique et de morale* xxiv (1916), 455-471. The five articles on Cabanis comprise the most concise of the available introductory analyses of Cabanis's thought.

Comte, Auguste. *Système de politique positive*. Vol. iv. Paris, 1854.

Contant, J.-P. *L'Enseignement de la chimie au Jardin royal des plantes*. Cahors, 1952.

Corlieu, A. *L'Ancienne Faculté de médecine de Paris*. Paris, 1877.

Cornet, L. "Un Protecteur de Théophile de Bordeu: Le Médecin Louis Lacaze (1703-1764)." *Bulletin de la Société des sciences, lettres, et arts de Pau*. 3ᵉ série. Vol. xxvi (1966), 55-63.

――――. "Théophile de Bordeu, le biologiste." *Bulletin . . . de Pau*. 4ᵉ série. Vol. i (1966) 123-125.

Crocker, Lester. "Cabanis." *Encyclopedia of Philosophy*. Vol. ii. New York, 1967, 3-4.

Crosland, Maurice. *The Society of Arcueil: A View of French Science at the Time of Napoleon I*. London, 1967.

Cumming, Ian. *Helvétius: His Life and Place in the History of Educational Thought*. London, 1955.

Damiron, Jean-Philibert. *Essai sur l'histoire de la philosophie en France au XIXᵉ siècle* (1828). Vol. i. Paris, 1834.

Darnton, Robert. *Mesmerism and the End of the Enlightenment in France*. Cambridge, Mass., 1968.

Daudin, Henri. *Cuvier et Lamarck: Les Classes zoologiques et l'idée de série animale (1790-1830)*. 2 vols. Paris, 1926.

———. *De Linne à Jussieu: Méthodes de classification et idée de série en botanique et en zoologie (1740-1790)*. Paris, 1926.

Daunou, P.-C.-F. *Notice sur la vie et les ouvrages de M. François Thurot*. Paris, 1833.

Davis, David B. *The Problem of Slavery in Western Culture*. Ithaca, 1966.

Dejob, Charles. *De L'Etablissement connu sous le nom de Lycée et d'Athénee et de quelques établissements analogues*. Paris, 1889.

Delasselle, Claude. "Les Enfants abandonnés à Paris au XVIIIᵉ siècle." *Annales ECS* xxx (1975), 187-218.

Delaunay, Paul. "D'Une Révolution à l'autre, 1789-1848. L'Evolution des théories et de la pratique médicales." *Scalpel*. Brussels, 1948.

———. "L'Evolution philosophique et médicale du bio-mécanicisme: De Descartes à Boerhaave, de Leibnitz à Cabanis." *Le Progès médical* (1927), cols. 1290-1293, 1338-1343, 1368-1384.

———. "La Médecine et les idéologues: L.-J. Moreau de La Sarthe." *Bulletin de la Société française d'histoire de la médecine* xiv (1920), 24-70.

———. *Le Monde médical parisien au XVIIIᵉ siècle*. Paris, 1906.

———. "Les Rapports intellectuels franco-européens principalement dans le monde des médecins et des naturalistes pendant la Révolution française et le premier Empire." *Scalpel*. Brussels, 1954.

Desaive, J.-P., et al. *Médecins, climat, et epidémies à la fin du XVIIIᵉ siècle*. Paris, 1972.

Desné, Roland., ed. *Les Matérialistes français de 1750 à 1800*. Paris, 1965.

Dewhurst, Kenneth. *Dr. Thomas Sydenham (1624-1689): His Life and Original Writings*. London, 1966.

Dictionary of National Biography. vi (1888; 1949 reprint), 356-357.

Dieckmann, Herbert. "Théophile Bordeu und Diderots *Rêve de d'Alembert*." *Romanische Forschungen* lii, no. 1 (1938), 55-122.

Dobbs, Betty Jo. *The Foundations of Newton's Alchemy: "The Hunting of the Greene Lyon."* Cambridge, 1976.

Dreyfus-Brisac, E. "Petits Problèmes de bibliographie pédagogique." *Revue internationale de l'enseignement* (1892), pp. 273-300. Discussion of authorship of Cabanis's discourses on education.

Dubois, E.-Frédéric (d'Amiens). *Examen des doctrines de Cabanis, Gall, et Broussais*. Paris, 1842.

Duchesneau, François. "Malpighi, Descartes, and the Epistemological

Problems of Iatromechanism." In M. L. Righini Bonelli and William R. Shea, eds. *Reason, Experiment and Mysticism in the Scientific Revolution*. New York, 1975.

———. "G.-E. Stahl: Antimécanisme et physiologie." *Archives internationales d'histoire des sciences* xxvi (1976), 3-26.

Dulieu, Louis. "Les Articles d'Henri Fouquet dans l'*Encyclopédie*." *Revue d'histoire des sciences* v (1952), 18-25.

———. "Le Mouvement scientifique montpelliérain au XVIIIᵉ siècle." *Revue d'histoire des sciences* xi (1958), 227-249.

———. "Paul-Joseph Barthez." *Revue d'histoire des sciences* xxiv, no. 2 (1971), 149-176.

Dupuy, Paul. *L'Ecole normale de l'an III*. Paris, 1895.

Durand, G.-L.-H. *Cabanis: Sa Vie, son oeuvre médicale*. Paris. Thesis. Faculty of Medicine. 1939.

Duruy, Albert. *L'Instruction publique et la Révolution*. Paris, 1882.

Fajn, Max. *The "Journal des hommes libres de tous les pays."* The Hague, 1975.

Farber, Paul. "Buffon and the Concept of Species." *Journal of the History of Biology* v (1972), 259-284.

———. "Buffon and Daubenton: Divergent Traditions within the *Histoire naturelle*." *Isis* lxvi (1975), 63-74.

Fayet, Joseph. *La Révolution française et la science, 1789-1795*. Paris, 1960.

Feugère, Anatole. "Raynal, Diderot, et quelques autres 'historiens' des deux indes." *Revue d'histoire littéraire de la France* xx (1914), 343-378.

Figlio, Karl. "Theories of Perception and the Physiology of Mind in the Late Eighteenth Century." *History of Science* xii (1975), 177-212.

Forado-Cunéo, Yvonne. *Les Ateliers de charité de Paris pendant la Révolution française (1789-1791)*. Paris, 1934.

Foucault, Michel. *Histoire de la folie à l'âge classique*. Paris, 1961.

———. *Les Mots et les choses*. Paris, 1966.

———. *Naissance de la clinique*. Paris, 1963.

———. *Surveiller et punir: Naissance de la prison*. Paris, 1975.

Foucault, Michel, Kriegel, Blandine, et al. *Les Machines à guérir (aux origines de l'hôpital moderne)*. Paris, 1976.

François, Y., and François, T. "Quelques Remarques sur les *Eléments de physiologie* de Diderot." *Revue d'histoire des sciences* v (1952), 77-82.

French, R. K. *Robert Whytt, The Soul, and Medicine*. London, 1969.

French, R. K. "Sauvages, Whytt, and the Motion of the Heart: Aspects of Eighteenth-Century Animism." *Clio medica* VII (1972), 35-54.

Furet, François, and Richet, Denis. *La Révolution du 9 Thermidor au 18 Brumaire*. Paris, 1966.

Gaulmier, Jean. "Volney et ses *Leçons d'histoire*." *History and Theory* II (1962), 52-65.

———. *Volney: Un Grand Témoin de la Révolution et de l'Empire*. Paris, 1959. Unfortunately Gaulmier's more scholarly work, *L'Idéologue Volney*, Beirut, 1951, was not accessible.

Gay, Peter. *The Enlightenment*. Vol. 2. *The Science of Freedom*. New York, 1969.

Gelfand, Toby. "A Clinical Ideal: Paris 1789." *Bulletin of the History of Medicine* LI (1977), 397-411.

———. "A Confrontation over Clinical Instruction at the Hôtel-Dieu of Paris during the French Revolution." *Journal of the History of Medicine* XXVIII (1973), 268-282.

———. "The Hospice of the Paris College of Surgery (1774-1793): 'A Unique and Invaluable Institution'." *Bulletin of the History of Medicine* XXVII (1972), 375-393.

———. "Medical Professionals and Charlatans. The *comité de salubrité enquête* of 1790-91." *Histoire sociale—Social History* (May 1978), pp. 62-97.

Germain, A.-C. *L'Ecole de médecine de Montpellier: Ses Origines, sa constitution, son enseignement*. Montpellier, 1880.

Gewirth, Alan. "Experience and the Non-Mathematical in Cartesian Method." *Journal of the History of Ideas* II, no. 2 (1941), 183-210.

Gillispie, Charles. "The *Encyclopédie* and the Jacobin Philosophy of Science." *Critical Problems in the History of Science*. Edited by Marshall Clagett. Madison, Wis., 1959.

———. "The Formation of Lamarck's Evolutionary Theory." *Archives internationales d'histoire des sciences* IX (1946), 323-338.

Ginguené, P.-L. "Cabanis." *Biographie universelle* [Michaud] VI (1843), 298-303.

Glass, Bentley. "Maupertuis, Pioneer of Genetics and Evolution." *Forerunners of Darwin: 1745-1859*. Edited by Glass, Temkin, and Straus. Baltimore, 1959.

Gobert, Adrienne. *L'Opposition des assemblées pendant le Consulat*. Paris, 1925.

Godfrey, James Logan. *Revolutionary Justice*. Chapel Hill, 1951.

Gontard, Maurice. *L'Enseignement primaire en France de la Révolution à la loi Guizot (1789-1833)*. Paris. 1959.

Goodfield, G. J. *The Growth of Scientific Physiology*. London, 1960.

Gottlieb, B. J. "Bedeutungen und auswirkungen des hallischen Professors and Kgl. Preussischen Leibarztes Georg Ernst Stahl auf den Vitalismus des XVIII. Jahrhunderts, insbesondere auf die Schule von Montpellier." *Nova Acta Leopoldina* (Halle) n.s. (1943), pp. 425-502.

Goubert, Jean-Pierre. "L'Art de guérir. Médecine savante et médecine populaire dans la France de 1790." *Annales ESC* xxxii (1977), 908-926.

Gouhier, Henri. *Les Conversions de Maine de Biran*. Paris, 1948.

——. *La Jeunesse de comte et la naissance du positivisme*. 3 vols. Paris, 1933-1941.

Granger, Gilles-Gaston. *La Mathématique sociale du marquis de Condorcet*. Paris, 1956.

Greenbaum, Louis. " 'The Commercial Treaty of Humanity': La Tournée des hôpitaux anglais par Jacques Tenon en 1787." *Revue d'histoire des sciences* xxiv (1971), 317-350.

——. "Health Care and Hospital-Building in Eighteenth-Century France: Reform Proposals of Du Pont de Nemours and Condorcet." *Studies on Voltaire and the Eighteenth Century* clii (1976), 895-930.

——. Jean-Sylvain Bailly, the Baron de Breteuil, and the 'Four New Hospitals' of Paris." *Clio medica* viii (1973), 261-284.

——. " 'Measure of Civilization': The Hospital Thought of Jacques Tenon on the Eve of the French Revolution." *Bulletin of the History of Medicine* xlix (1975), 43-56.

——. "Tempest in the Academy: Jean-Baptiste Le Roy, the Paris Academy of Sciences, and the Project of a New Hôtel-Dieu." *Archives internationales d'histoire des sciences* xxiv (1974), 122-140.

Guardia, J.-M. *Histoire de la médecine d'Hippocrate à Broussais et ses successeurs*. Paris, 1884.

——. *La Médecine à travers les siècles*. Paris, 1865.

Guédon, Jean-Claude, "Chimie et matérialisme: la stratégie anti-newtonienne de Diderot." *Dix-huitième siècle* xi (1979), 185-200.

Guelliot, O. "Cabanis à la Faculté de médecine de Reims." *Bulletin de la Société française d'histoire de la médecine* (1908), pp. 186-192.

Guerlac, Henry. "The Background to Dalton's Atomic Theory." *John*

Dalton and the Progress of Science. Edited by D.S.L. Caldwell. New York, 1968, pp. 57-91.

——. "Newton and the Method of Analysis." *Dictionary of the History of Ideas* III (1973), 378-391.

——. *Newton et Epicure*. Paris, 1963.

Guillois, Antoine. *La Marquise de Condorcet: Sa Famille, son salon, ses amis, 1764-1822*. Paris, 1897.

——. *Pendant la Terreur, le poète Roucher*. Paris, 1890.

——. *Le Salon de Mme Helvétius. Cabanis et les Idéologues*. Paris, 1894.

Gusdorf, Georges. *La Conscience révolutionnaire, les Idéologues*. Paris, 1978.

——. *Dieu, la nature, l'homme au siècle des lumières*. Paris, 1972.

——. *Introduction aux sciences humaines*. Paris, 1960.

——. *Naissance de la conscience romantique au siècle des lumières*. Paris, 1976.

——. *Les Principes de la pensée au siècle des lumières*. Paris, 1971.

Gutton, Jean-Pierre. *L'Etat et la mendicité*. . . . Lyon, 1973.

Guyénot, Emile. *L'Evolution de la pensée scientifique: Les Sciences de la vie aux XVIIe et XVIIIe siècles* (1941). Paris, 1957.

Haeser, Heinrich, ed. *Lehrbuch der Geschichte der Medicin und der epidemischen Krankheiten*. 3 vols. Jena, 1881.

Haigh, Elizabeth. "Glandular Secretion, Sensibility, and the Soul in the Work of Théophile de Bordeu." Paper, Canadian Learned Societies Conference, Edmonton, 1975.

——. "Vitalism, The Soul, and Sensibility: The Physiology of Théophile Bordeu." *Journal of the History of Medicine* XXXI (1976), 30-41.

Hall, Thomas Steele. "Descartes's Physiological Method." *Journal of the History of Biology* III (1970), 53-79.

——. *Ideas of Life and Matter*. 2 vols. Chicago, 1969.

——. "On Biological Analogs of Newtonian Paradigms." *Philosophy of Science* XXXV (1968), 6-25.

Hannaway, Caroline. "The Société Royale de Médecine and Epidemics in the Ancien Régime." *Bulletin of the History of Medicine* XLVI (1972), 257-273.

Hans, Nicholas A. "UNESCO of the 18th Century: La Loge des Neuf Soeurs and its Venerable Master Benjamin Franklin." *Proceedings of the American Philosophical Society* XCVII (1953), 513-524.

Harvey, E. N. *A History of Luminescence*. Philadelphia, 1957.

Heimann, P. M. "Voluntarism and Immanence: Conceptions of Nature in Eighteenth-Century Thought," *Journal of the History of Ideas* xxxix, no. 2 (1978), 271-283.

Heimann, P. M., and McGuire, J. E. "Newtonian Forces and Lockean Powers: Concepts of Matter in Eighteenth-Century Thought" *Historical Studies in the Physical Sciences* iii (1971), 233-306.

Helmreich, Jonathan. "The Establishment of Primary Schools in France under the Directory." *French Historical Studies* ii (1961), 189-208.

Hillemand, Constantin. "*Coup d'oeil* de Cabanis *sur les révolutions et sur la réforme de la médecine.*" *Le Progrès médical* (1932), no. 39, cols. 1626-1639, no. 40, cols. 1658-1673.

————. "*Du Degré de certitude de la médecine* d'après Cabanis." *Le Progrès médical* (1932), no. 2, cols. 66-77. no. 7, cols. 294-301, no. 19, cols. 823-832.

Hintzsche, Erich. "A. V. Hallers Korrespondenz mit Johann Stephan Bernard." *Clio medica* i (1966), 324-343.

Hippeau, Célestin. *L'Instruction publique en France pendant la Révolution.* 2 vols. Paris, 1881-1883.

Hodge, M.J.S. "Lamarck's Science of Living Bodies." *British Journal for the History of Science* v (1971), 323-352.

Hoff, Herbel, and Kellaway, Peter. "The Early History of the Reflex." *Journal of the History of Medicine* vii (1952), 211-249.

Hoffmann, Paul. *La Femme dans la pensée des lumières.* Paris, 1976.

————. "L'Idée de liberté dans la philosophie médicale de Bordeu." *Studies on Voltaire and the Eighteenth Century* lxxxviii (1972), 769-787.

Hubert, René. *Les Sciences sociales dans l'Encyclopédie.* Paris, 1923.

Imbert, Jean. *Le Droit hospitalier de la Révolution et de l'Empire.* Paris, 1954.

Ingrand, Henry. *Le Comité de salubrité de l'Assemblée nationale constituante (1790-1791).* Paris. Thesis in medicine. 1934.

Irsay, S. d'. *Albrecht von Haller. Eine Studie zur Geistesgeschichte der Aufklärung.* 2 vols. Leipzig, 1930.

Jackson, Stanley W. "Force and Kindred Notions in Eighteenth-Century Nerve Physiology." *Bulletin of the History of Medicine* xliv (1970), 397-410, 539-554.

Jacob, Margaret C. "John Toland and the Newtonian Ideology." *Journal of the Warburg and Courtauld Institutes* xxxii (1969), 307-332.

Janet, Paul. "Schopenhauer et la physiologie française: Cabanis et Bichat." *Revue des deux mondes*, 3ᵉ période, xxxix (1 May 1880), 35-59.

Jarcho, S. "Galen's Non-Naturals." *Bulletin of the History of Medicine* xliv (1970), 372-377.

Joussain, André. "Le Spiritualisme de Cabanis." *Archives de philosophie* xxi, no. 3 (1958), 386-409.

Juge, L.-Th. *Hiérologies et bébélologies*. 2 vols. Paris, 1839-1840. Cabanis as a Freemason, I, 307-313.

Kaiser, Thomas. "Liberalism and Repression in the Program and Thought of the Idéologues." Paper, American Historical Association Annual Meeting, San Francisco, 1978.

Keim, Albert. *Helvétius: Sa Vie et son oeuvre*. Paris, 1907.

Kennedy, Emmet. *A Philosophe in the Age of Revolution: Destutt de Tracy and the Origins of "Ideology."* Philadelphia, 1978.

———. "Destutt de Tracy and the Unity of the Sciences." *Studies on Voltaire and the Eighteenth Century* clxxi (1977), 223-239.

———. " 'Ideology' from Destutt de Tracy to Marx." *Journal of the History of Ideas* xl (1979), 353-368.

Kersaint, G. *Antoine-François de Fourcroy (1755-1809): Sa Vie et son Oeuvre*. Paris, 1966.

King, Lester Snow. "Attitudes towards 'Scientific' Medicine around 1700." *Bulletin of the History of Medicine* xix (1963), 124-128.

———. "Boissier de Sauvages and 18th-Century Nosology." *Bulletin of the History of Medicine* xl (1966), 43-51.

———. *The Growth of Medical Thought*. Chicago, 1963.

———. *The Medical World of the Eighteenth Century*. Chicago, 1958.

———. "A Note on the So-Called 'Moral Treatment'." *Journal of the History of Medicine* xix (1964), 297-298.

———. "Some Problems of Causality in Eighteenth-Century Medicine." *Bulletin of the History of Medicine* xxxvii (1963), 15-24.

———. "Stahl and Hoffmann: A Study in Eighteenth-Century Animism." *Journal of the History of Medicine* xix (1964), 124-128.

Kirkinen, Heiki. *Les Origines de la conception moderne de l'homme-machine: Le Problème de l'âme en France à la fin du règne de Louis XIV (1670-1715)*. Helsinki, 1960.

Kitchin, Joanna. *"La Décade" (1794-1807): Un Journal "philosophique."* Paris, 1965. Thesis at the Faculty of Letters, University of Paris.

Knight, Isabel. *The Geometric Spirit: The Abbé de Condillac and the French Enlightenment*. New Haven, 1968.

Koestler, Arthur. *The Sleepwalkers*. London, 1959.

Kors, Alan. *D'Holbach's Coterie: An Enlightenment in Paris*. Princeton, 1976.

Koyré, Alexandre. *Newtonian Studies*. Cambridge, Mass., 1965.

Koyré, Alexandre, and Cohen, I. B. "The Case of the Missing 'Tanquam': Leibniz, Newton, and Clarke." *Isis* LII (1961), 555-566.

Kuhn, Thomas. *The Structure of Scientific Revolutions*. 2d ed. Chicago, 1969.

La Berge, Ann Fowler. "The Paris Health Council, 1802-1848." *Bulletin of the History of Medicine* XLIV (1975), 339-352.

Labrousse, Ernest et al. *Histoire économique et sociale de la France, II (1660-1789)*. Paris, 1970.

Labrousse, François. *Quelques Notes sur un médecin-philosophe, P.-J.-G. Cabanis*, Paris, 1903.

Landrieu, Marcel. "Lamarck, le fondateur de transformisme: Sa Vie, son oeuvre." *Mémoires de la Société zoologique de France* XXI. Paris, 1909.

Le Bihan, Alain. *Franc-maçons parisiens du Grand Orient de France (fin du 18ᵉ siècle)*. 2 vols. Paris, 1967.

Lécuyer, Bernard-Pierre. "Naissance d'un savoir: Recherche sociale, état et société en France durant la première industrialisation (1800-1850)." Paris, 1975. MS outline.

Legée, Georgette. "Les Concepts de localisation et de co-ordination dans la neurophysiologie de Marie-Jean-Pierre Flourens (1794-1867)." *96ᵉ Congrès national des sociétés savantes, Toulouse, 1971, Sciences*, I. Paris, 1974.

Leith, James. "Modernization, Mass Education, and Social Mobility in French Thought, 1750-1789." *Studies in the Eighteenth Century* II. Canberra, 1973, 223-238.

Lemee, Pierre. *Julien Offray de La Mettrie*. Saint-Malo, 1954.

Lemoine, Albert. *Le Vitalisme et l'animisme de Stahl*. Paris, 1864.

Léon, Antoine. "Promesses et ambiguités de l'oeuvre d'enseignement technique en France, de 1800 à 1815." *Annales historiques de la Révolution française* XLII (1970), 419-436.

Le Roy, Georges. *La Psychologie de Condillac*. Paris, 1937.

Le Roy, Maxime. *Histoire des idées sociales en France*. 2 vols. Paris, 1950.

Lesky, Erna. "Cabanis und die Gewissheit der Heilkunde." *Gesnerus* XI (1954), 152-182.

Liard, Louis. *L'Enseignement supérieur en France 1789-1889*. 2 vols. Paris, 1888-1894.

Lindeboom, G.-A. *Hermann Boerhaave: The Man and His Work*. London, 1968.

Lovejoy, Arthur. *The Great Chain of Being: A Study of the History of an Idea*. Cambridge, 1936.

Luppé, Robert de. *Les Idées littéraires de Madame de Staël et l'héritage des lumières (1795-1814)*. Paris, 1969.

McGuire, J. E. "Force, Active Principles, and Newton's Invisible Realm." *Ambix* xv (1968), 154-208.

McRae, Robert. "The Unity of the Sciences: Bacon, Descartes, and Leibniz." *Journal of the History of Ideas* xviii, no. 1 (1957), 27-48.

Mackler, Bernard. *Philippe Pinel, Unchainer of the Insane*. New York, 1968.

Madinier, Gabriel. *Conscience et mouvement: Essai sur les rapports de la conscience et de l'effort moteur dans la philosophie française de Condillac à Bergson*. Paris, 1938.

Manuel, Frank. *The New World of Henri Saint-Simon*. Cambridge, Mass., 1956.

———. *The Prophets of Paris*. Cambridge, Mass., 1962.

Margerison, Kenneth. "P.-L. Roederer: The Industrial Capitalist as Revolutionary." *Eighteenth-Century Studies* xi (1978), 473-488.

Mathiez, Albert. *La Théophilanthropie et le culte décadaire, 1796-1801*. Paris, 1903.

Mayer, Jean. *Diderot, homme de science*. Rennes, 1959.

Metzger, Hélène. *Newton, Stahl, Boerhaave, et la doctrine chimique*. Paris, 1930.

Meynier, Albert. *Les Coups d'état du Directoire*. 3 vols. Paris, 1927-1928.

Mignet, M. *Portraits et notices historiques et littéraires*. 2 vols. Paris, 1877. Sketch of Cabanis, ii, 225-266. Also brief biographies of Destutt de Tracy, P.-C.-F. Daunou, abbé Siéyès, Charles-Maurice de Talleyrand, P.-L. Roederer.

Misch, Georg. "Zur entstehung des französischen Positivismus." *Archiv für geschichte der Philosophie* xiv (1900-1901), 1-29, 156-209.

Monin, H. "Le Discours de Mirabeau sur les fêtes publiques." *La Révolution française* xxv (1893), 214-231.

Moore, F.C.T. *The Psychology of Maine de Biran*. Oxford, 1970.

Morange, J., and Chassaing, J.-F. *Le Mouvement de réforme de l'enseignement en France 1760-1798*. Paris, 1974.

Moravia, Sergio. "Dall' 'homme machine' all' 'homme sensible'." *Belfagor* XXIX (1974), 633-648. Translated as "From *Homme Machine* to *Homme Sensible*: Changing Eighteenth-Century Models of Man's Image." *Journal of the History of Ideas* XXXIX (1978), 45-60.

———. "Filosofia e 'sciences de la vie' nel secolo XVIII." *Giornale critico della filosofia italiana* XXI (1966), 64-109.

———. *Il Pensiero degli idéologues*. Florence, 1974.

———. "Philosophie et médecine en France à la fin du XVIIIᵉ siècle." *Studies on Voltaire and the Eighteenth Century* LXXXIX (1972), 1089-1151.

———. *La Scienza dell'uomo nel settecento*. Bari, 1970.

———. *Il Tramonto dell'illuminismo: Filosofia e politica nella società francese (1770-1810)*. Bari, 1968.

Moreau de La Sarthe, Jacques-Louis. "Moral." In *Encyclopédie méthodique* CLXXIII (*Médecine*) x (1821), 250-276.

Mortier, Roland. "D'Holbach et Diderot: Affinités et divergences." *Revue de l'Université de Bruxelles* (1972), pp. 223-237.

Naville, Pierre. *D'Holbach et la philosophie scientifique du XVIIIᵉ siècle*. 1943. 2d ed. Paris, 1967.

Niebyl, Peter H. "The Non-Naturals." *Bulletin of the History of Medicine* XLV (1971), 486-492.

Nussac, Louis de. "La 'Venue' de Georges Cabanis: Son Nom et sa famille, son père et son berceau." *Bulletin de la Société scientifique, historique, et archéologique de la Corrèze* XLIV-XLV (1923), 243-270.

Ozouf, Mona. *La Fête révolutionnaire, 1789-1799*. Paris, 1976.

Pagel, Walter. *The Religious and Philosophical Aspects of Van Helmont's Science and Medicine*. Baltimore, 1944.

Paultre, Christian. *De La Répression de la mendicité et du vagabondage en France sous l'ancien régime*. Paris, 1906.

Payne, Harry G. *The Philosophes and the People*. New Haven, 1976.

Perkins, Jean. "Diderot and La Mettrie." *Studies on Voltaire and the Eighteenth Century* x (1959), 49-100.

Picavet, François. *Les Idéologues*. Paris, 1891. The indispensable classic study of the Auteuil circle almost completely ignores the medical aspects of Cabanis's thought. Excellent philosophical summaries. Rather diffuse because of unmanageable scope ("history of scientific, philosophical, and religious ideas and theories in France since 1789").

Picqué, Lucien, and Dubousquet, Louis. "L'Incident du salon de Mme Helvétius (Cabanis et l'abbé Morellet)." *Bulletin de la Société française d'histoire la médecine* XVII (1914), 281-296.

Pierson, C. Antoine. *Georges Cabanis, psychophysiologiste et sénateur*. Paris, 1946.

Plongeron, Bernard. "Nature, métaphysique, et histoire chez les Idéologues." *Dix-huitième siècle* V (1973), 375-412.

Pomeau, René. *La Religion de Voltaire*. Paris, 1956.

Ponteil, Félix. *Histoire de l'enseignement en France*. Paris, 1966.

Portier, Antoine. *L'Enseignement médical à Paris de 1794 à 1809*. Paris, 1925.

Poulbrière, J.-B., abbé. *Dictionnaire historique et archéologique des paroisses du diocèse de Tulle* (1890). Vol. I. 2d ed. Brive, 1964.

Prévost, A. *L'Ecole de santé de Paris (1794-1809)*. Paris, 1901.

Proust, Jacques. *Diderot et l'Encyclopédie*. Paris, 1962.

———. *L'Encyclopédisme dans le Bas-Languedoc au XVIIIe siècle*. Montpellier, 1968.

Purver, Margery. *The Royal Society: Concept and Creation*. London, 1967.

Ramsey, Matthew. "Medical Power and Popular Medicine: Illegal Healers in Nineteenth-Century France." *Journal of Social History* X (1977), 560-587.

Randall, J. H. "The Development of Scientific Method in the School of Padua." *Journal of the History of Ideas* I, no. 2 (1947), 177-206.

Rappaport, Rhoda. "G.-F. Rouelle: An Eighteenth-Century Chemist and Teacher." *Chymia* VI (1960), 68-101.

———. "Rouelle and Stahl—The Phlogistic Revolution in France." *Chymia* VII (1961), 73-102.

Rather, L. J. "G. E. Stahl's Psychological Physiology." *Bulletin of the History of Medicine* XXXV (1961), 27-49.

———. *Mind and Body in Eighteenth-Century Medicine: A Study based on Jerome Gaub's "De Regimine Mentis."* London, 1965.

———. "The 'Six Things Non-Natural': A Note on the Origins and Fate of a Doctrine and a Phrase." *Clio medica* III (1968), 337-347.

Régaldo, Marc. "*La Décade* et les philosophes du XVIIIe siècle." *Dix-huitième siècle* II (1970), 113-130.

———. "Matériaux pour une bibliographie de l'Idéologie et des

Idéologues." *Répertoire analytique de littérature française* I (1970), no. 1.

———. *Un Milieu intellectuel: La "Décade philosophique" (1794-1807)*. Thesis typescript offset, Lille, 1976. The limited number of copies has made this work inaccessible to me.

Richmond, P.N.A. "The Hôtel-Dieu of Paris on the Eve of the Revolution." *Journal of the History of Medicine* XVI (1961), 335-353.

Riese, Walther. *The Legacy of Philippe Pinel: An Inquiry into Thought on Mental Alienation*. New York, 1969.

———. "La Méthode analytique de Condillac et ses rapports avec l'oeuvre de Philippe Pinel." *Revue philosophique* CLVIII (1968), 321-336.

Roger, Jacques. "Buffon." *Dictionary of Scientific Biography*. Vol. II. New York, 1970, 579.

———. "Méthodes et modèles dans la préhistoire du vitalisme français: Lacaze, Fouquet, Menuret de Chambaud." *XIIe Congrès international d'histoire des sciences. Actes, III B*. Paris, 1971, pp. 101-108.

———. *Les Sciences de la vie dans la pensée française du XVIIIe siècle*. Paris, 1963.

Rosen, George. "Hospitals, Medical Care, and Social Policy in the French Revolution." *Bulletin of the History of Medicine* XXX (1956), 124-149.

———. "The Philosophy of Ideology and the Emergence of Modern Medicine in France." *Bulletin of the History of Medicine* XX (1946), 328-339.

Rosenfield, Leonora C. *From Beast-Machine to Man-Machine* (1940). 2d ed. New York, 1968.

Rothschuh, Karl. *Alexander von Humboldt et l'histoire de la découverte de l'électricité animale*. Paris, 1960.

Roule, Louis. *Lacépède . . . et la sociologie humanitaire de la nature*. Paris, 1932.

Rudé, George. *The Crowd in the French Revolution*. Oxford, 1959.

Rudolph, G. "Hallers Lehre von der Irritabilität und Sensibilität." In Karl Rothschuh, ed. *Von Boerhaave bis Berger. Die Entwicklung der Kontinentalen Physiologie im 18. und 19. Jahrhundert*. Stuttgart, 1964.

Salomon-Bayet, Claire. "L'institution de la science: Un Exemple au XVIIIe siècle." *Annales ESC* XXX (1975), 1028-1044.

Savioz, Raymond. *La Philosophie de Charles Bonnet de Genève*. Paris, 1948.

Schiller, Joseph. "Queries, Answers, and Unsolved Problems in Eighteenth-Century Biology." *History of Science* XII (1974), 184-199.

Schofield, Robert. *Mechanism and Materialism: British Natural Philosophy in an Age of Reason*. Princeton, 1970.

Schöner, Erich. *Das Vierschema in der Antiken Humoralpathologie*. supplement 4. *Sudhoffs Archiv für Geschichte der Medizin und der Naturwissenschaften*. Wiesbaden, 1964.

Scott, Samuel F. "Problems of Law and Order during 1790, the 'Peaceful' Year of the French Revolution." *American Historical Review* LXXX (1975), 859-888.

Seilhac, Victor de. *Scènes et portraits de la Révolution en Bas-Limousin*. Paris, 1878.

Semelaigne, René. *Philippe Pinel et son oeuvre au point de vue de la médecine mentale*. Paris, 1888.

Shryock, Richard. *The Development of Modern Medicine*. Philadelphia, 1936.

Simon, Jules. *Une Académie sous le Directoire*. Paris, 1885.

Smeaton, William A. *Fourcroy, Chemist and Revolutionary (1755-1809)*. London, 1962.

Smith, D. W. *Helvétius: A Study in Persecution*. Oxford, 1965.

Smith, Roger. "The Background of Physiological Psychology in Natural Philosophy." *History of Science* XI (1973), 75-123.

Staum, Martin S. "Cabanis and the Revolution: The Therapy of Society." *The Analytic Spirit: Festschrift for Henry Guerlac*. Edited by Harry Woolf. Ithaca, forthcoming.

———. "Cabanis and the Science of Man." *Journal of the History of the Behavioral Sciences* X (1974), 135-143.

———. "Medical Components of Cabanis's Science of Man." *Studies in History of Biology* II (1978), 1-31.

———. "Newton and Voltaire: Constructive Sceptics." *Studies on Voltaire and the Eighteenth Century* LII (1968), 29-56.

Stein, Jay. *The Mind and the Sword*. New York, 1961.

Stocking, George W. "French Anthropology in 1800." *Isis* LV (1964), 134-150.

Suratteau, J. R. *Les Elections de l'an VI et le coup d'état du 22 floréal*. Paris, 1971.

Tanner, J. M. "Earlier Maturation in Man." *Scientific American* CCXVIII (January, 1968), 21-27.

414

Taton, René, ed. *Enseignement et diffusion des sciences en France au XVIIIe siècle.* Paris, 1964.

————. *Histoire générale des sciences.* 3 vols. Paris, 1957-1961.

Temkin, Owsei. "Basic Science, Medicine, and the Romantic Era." *Bulletin of the History of Medicine* xxxvii (1963), 97-129.

————. "The Classical Roots of Glisson's Doctrine of Irritation." *Bulletin of the History of Medicine* xxxviii (1964), 297-328.

————. *Galenism: The Rise and Decline of a Medical Philosophy.* Ithaca, 1973.

————. "Galen's Pneumatology." *Gesnerus* viii (1951), 180-189.

————. "The Philosophical Background of Magendie's Physiology." *Bulletin of the History of Medicine* xx (1946), 10-35.

————. "The Role of Surgery in the Rise of Modern Medical Thought." *Bulletin of the History of Medicine* xxv (1951), 248-259.

Tencer, Marie. *La Psychophysiologie de Cabanis d'après son livre "Rapports du physique et du moral de l'homme."* Toulouse, 1931. Thesis at Faculty of Letters, University of Toulouse. Close analysis of the *Rapports* with some commentary on relationship to late nineteenth-century psychologists Paul Janet and Théodule Ribot. Attempts to align Cabanis as a precursor of "historical materialism."

Thackray, Arnold. *Atoms and Powers: An Essay on Newtonian Matter-Theory and the Development of Chemistry.* Cambridge, Mass., 1970.

Thiry, Jean. *Le Sénat de Napoléon (1800-1814).* Paris, 1932.

Thomson, Ann. "Quatre lettres . . . de La Mettrie." *Dix-huitième Siècle* vii (1975), 5-19.

Tissot, C.-Joseph. *Anthropologie spéculative générale.* . . . 2 vols. Paris, 1842-1843.

Tobey, Ronald. "The Medical Speculations of William Cullen." Unpublished master's thesis, Cornell University, 1966.

Toellner, Richard. "Anima et Irritabilitas: Hallers Abwehr von Animismus und Materialismus." *Sudhoffs Archiv* li, no. 2 (1967), 130-144.

————. *A. von Haller, über die Einheit im Denken des letzten Universalgelehrten. Sudhoffs Archiv.* Supplement 10. Wiesbaden, 1971.

Vandal, A. *L'Avènement de Bonaparte.* 2 vols. Paris, 1902.

Van Duzer, Charles. *The Contribution of the Idéologues to French Revolutionary Thought.* Baltimore, 1935. Johns Hopkins Studies in Historical and Political Science, LIII, no. 4. Chief concern is reports and laws relating to education in revolutionary assemblies.

Vartanian, Aram. "Cabanis and La Mettrie." *Studies on Voltaire and the Eighteenth Century* CLV (1976), 2149-2166.

———. "From Deist to Atheist: Diderot's Philosophical Orientation, 1746-1749." *Diderot Studies* I (1949), 46-63.

———. "The Enigma of Diderot's *Eléments de physiologie.*" *Diderot Studies* X (1968), 285-301.

———. "Trembley's Polyp, La Mettrie, and Eighteenth-Century French Materialism." *Journal of the History of Ideas* XI (1950), 259-286.

Vermeil de Conchard, Colonel. *Trois Etudes sur Cabanis d'après des documents inédits*. Brive, 1914.

Vernière, Paul. "L'Idée de l'humanité au XVIIIᵉ siècle." *Studium generale*. jg. XV, no. 3 (1962), 171-179.

Vess, David. *Medical Revolution in France 1789-1796*. Gainesville, Fla., 1975.

Vidalenc, Jean. "L'Opposition sous le Consulat et l'Empire." *Annales historiques de la Révolution française* XL (1968), 472-488.

Vignery, Robert J. *The French Revolution and the Schools: Educational Policies of the Mountain, 1792-1794*. Madison, Wis., 1965.

Villefosse, Louis and Bouissounouse, Janine. *L'Opposition à Napoleon*. Paris, 1969.

Voutsinas, D. *La Psychologie de Maine de Biran*. Paris, 1964.

Weiner, Dora. "Le Droit de l'homme à la santé—Une Belle Idée devant l'Assemblée constituante: 1790-1791." *Clio medica* V (1970), 209-223.

Westfall, Richard. *Force in Newton's Physics*. London, 1971.

———. "The Role of Alchemy in Newton's Career." In M. L. Righini Bonelli and William R. Shea, eds. *Reason, Experiment, and Mysticism in the Scientific Revolution*. New York, 1975.

Williams, L. Pearce. "Science, Education, and the French Revolution." *Isis* XLIV (1953), 311-330.

———. "Science, Education, and Napoleon I." *Isis* XLVII (1956), 369-382.

Wilson, Arthur. *Diderot*. New York, 1972.

Wilson, Leonard. "Erasistratus, Galen, and the *Pneuma.*" *Bulletin of the History of Medicine* XXXIII (1959), 293-314.

Wohl, Robert. "Buffon and His Project for a New Science." *Isis* LI (1960), 194-199.

Woloch, Isser. *Jacobin Legacy: The Democratic Movement in the Directory*. Princeton, 1970.

Yates, Frances. *Giordano Bruno and the Hermetic Tradition*. Chicago, 1964.

———. *The Rosicrucian Enlightenment*. London, 1972.

Young, R. M. "Animal Soul." *Encyclopedia of Philosophy*. Vol. II. New York, 1967.

Index

physical sensitivity, 177-179; and Pinel, 160-161, 245-249; political attitudes of, 295-297, 312-313; posthumous influence of, 307-310; and public assistance, 117-121, 136-146; and the radical Revolution, 147-150; on reflexes, 375; regimen and occupation, 227-232; and Richerand, 251-253; "secretion of thought," 92, 177-179; on sex, 213-217; de Sèze, 84-85; species variation, 182-189; spontaneous generation, 183-186; and Stahl, 73-75; on sympathy, 189-191; temperament, 217-219; Versailles manuscript, 373-374; and Whytt, 75, 78

Works

Coup d'oeil sur les révolutions et sur la réforme de la médecine, 8, 50, 81, 108, 151-164, 179, 267, 298; *Du Degré de certitude de la médecine*, 6-7, 103-108, 127, 152, 154, 156-157, 264, 267, 298; *Discours prononcé par Cabanis* (on constitution, an 8), 289-292; "Iliad" translation, 16; *Journal de la maladie et de la mort de Mirabeau*, 130-131, 298; *Lettre à F. sur les causes premières*, 7-8, 126, 179, 185, 223, 298-303, 305-307, 311; *Lettre à M. T. sur les poèmes d'Homère*, 298; *Note sur un genre particulier d'apoplexie*, 298; *Observations sur les affections catarrhales*, 298; *Observations sur les hôpitaux*, 114-116; *Quelques Principes et quelques vues sur les secours publics*, 136-146; *Rapports du physique et du moral de l'homme*, 5-6, 24-25, 32, 59, 105, 126, 153, 162, 173-244, 251-254, 305-308; *Travail sur l'éducation publique*, 125-130

Calès, Jean-Marie, 269-271
Cambacérès, Jean-Jacques-Régis de, 329
Canguilhem, Georges, 375
Carlyle, Thomas, 140
Carnot, Lazare, 287
Cérise, L., 202 203, 306
Chabannes, 14
Chain of Being, Great, 22-25, 29, 35-37, 67-71, 186-187, 189, 245, 265, 310-311, 322; and unity of nature, 70-71, 85, 92-93, 161-163, 205-206
Chamfort, Nicolas, 16
Chaptal, Jean-Antoine, 251, 294
Chastelet, Achille-François, marquis du, 131
Chastellux, François-Jean, marquis de, 17
Chateaubriand, François-René de, 171, 236, 294
chemical affinity, 180-181
Chénier, Marie-Joseph, 18, 122, 124, 148, 150, 284, 288, 293
Cicero, 248
Civil Code, 293
climate, 11, 27, 33-34, 45, 52-53. *See also* Buffon, Cabanis's *Rapports*, Condorcet, Volney
clinical observation, 83-84, 89, 101-102, 104-107, 160, 232. *See also* Cabanis on medical method, Hippocrates, Montpellier medicine
Colombier, Jean, 111
Committee on Mendicity, National Assembly, 113-115, 117, 132-133, 135, 142-143
Committee of Public Safety, National Convention, 149
Commune of Paris, 142-143
Comte, August, 107, 215, 255
Concordat of 1801-1802, 293
Condillac, Etienne Bonnot de, 4, 17, 24, 37-44, 51, 61, 79, 90, 103-107,

163, 309; in Cabanis, 227-235; in
central schools, 164-165, 266; in
Hallé, 381-382; in medical education, 96. *See also* Cabanis and
Hallé

iatrochemistry, 55
iatromechanism, 325-326
iatrophysics, 55-58, 67, 72, 79,
81-82, 202, 208
Idéologues, 4-5, 9, 10-13, 17, 63,
170-171, 215, 244, 264-265, 303,
306, 308-310, 315; and Alibert,
249-251; Baconian method, 38;
Bonaparte, 292-295; on central
schools and higher education,
164-165, 273, 276-280; and Condillac, 39, 41; coup of Floréal,
283-285; on free will, 299-301; inconsistencies, 242-243; in Institute, 166-168; and Maine de Biran,
259-265; on materialism, 237; origins of term, 170-171; and Pinel,
160, 246; politics of, 168; *Rapports*
of Cabanis, 235-236, 240; Revolution of 1789, 122-124; and
Richerand, 252; Romantics, 236-
237. *See also* Cabanis, Destutt de
Tracy, and individual associates
Ideology, 129, 162, 173-176, 237-
239, 242, 252-254, 259, 264-265,
308, 316
Imperial University, 281, 294
Ingenhousz, Jan, 182
insanity, treatment of, 137. *See also*
Pinel and Cabanis on public assistance
Institute, National, 3, 29, 185, 187,
245, 287, 308
Institute, National, Class of Moral
and Political Sciences of, 3, 84,
130, 136, 138-139, 165-168, 174-
176, 183, 215, 235, 259-260, 264,
292, 294-295

intelligence, principle of universal,
84-85, 87, 184-185, 301-302, 307,
311
irritability, muscular, 63-65, 70,
76-77, 81, 193-194, 328
Itard, Jean, 358

Jacobin Club, 124, 148
Jacobins, neo-, 12, 141, 269, 276,
282-283, 284-285, 286, 288, 292,
295
Jacquemont, Frédéric-François, 173
Jardin royal des plantes, 27, 100
Jerome, Saint, 373
Joubert, Barthélemy-Cathérine, Gen-
eral, 287
Jussieu, Antoine-Laurent de, 132

Kant, Immanuel, 162, 346
Kepler, Johannes, 20
King, Lester Snow, 67

Lacaze, Louis, 83-84, 178, 195, 218,
259
Lacépède, B.-G.-E. de la Ville-sur-
Illon, comte de, 16, 18, 182, 187-
188
Lachèze, 123
Lacuée, Jean-Gérard, 136
Lafayette, M.-J.-P.-Y.-Roche Gilbert
du Motier, marquis de, 124, 131,
142, 150
La Harpe, Jean-François de, 236
Lakanal, Joseph, 160
Lalande, Jérôme, 18
Lamarck, Jean-Baptiste de, 23, 182-
183, 185-189, 224, 377
Lameth, Alexandre and Charles, 131
La Mettrie, Julien Offray de, 9, 25,
29, 33, 60, 66-71, 78, 90-91, 175,
211, 329
Lamourette, Antoine-Adrien, 125
Lancelin, P.-F., 173
Langlois, J.-E., 95

Turgot, Anne-Robert-Jacques, baron
de, 14-17, 110, 113, 117, 192, 300

unity of nature, 3-4, 24, 161. *See also*
Great Chain of Being
unity of sciences, 3-4, 37-41, 70,
83-84, 93, 108, 151-154, 310
Unzer, Johann August, 194, 375

variation in species. *See* Buffon,
Cabanis, transformism
Vartanian, Aram, 67, 329
Vauquelin, Louis-Nicolas, 102
Venel, Gabriel-François, 16, 30, 83,
95, 181
Vermeil de Conchard, 267
Versailles manuscript of Cabanis,
373-374
Vicq d'Azyr, Félix, 100-102, 129,
134, 151, 154, 156, 309
Villermé, Louis-René, 309
Vilna, 15
vitalism, 9, 50, 54, 63-64, 72-73,
84-86, 89-90, 179, 205-206, 258-
259, 302, 305. *See also* Montpellier
medicine and Bichat

vital principle, 72, 79-80, 86-90, 95,
103, 208, 302-303
Vitet, Louis, 269-271
Volney, Constantin-François Chassebeuf de Boisgiray de, 17-18, 122,
132, 145, 150, 165-170, 175, 298;
and climate, theory, 220-223,
225-226, 249; ethics, 200, 211; Institute and Senate, 292, 294
Volta, Alessandro, 178
Voltaire, François-Marie Arouet de,
16, 18, 22, 30, 107, 127

Warsaw, Academy of, 15
Weismann, August, 28
Whitbread, Samuel, 141
Whytt, Robert, 66, 75-78, 81, 84,
87-88, 91, 192-193, 195, 197, 375
Willis, Thomas, 55
Winslow, James, 75
Woloch, Isser, 284

Zabarella, Giacomo, 38
Zimmermann, Johann Georg, 64, 217

THIS BOOK HAS BEEN PRINTED ON 50LB WARRENS 1854 TEXT
WITH THE TEXT BEING COMPOSED IN 10PT V-I-P ALDUS
THE DISPLAY WAS SET IN 36PT CENTAUR ROMAN ON
A FORMAT DESIGNED BY BRUCE CAMPBELL
COMPOSITION AND PRINTING BY
THE SKILLED CRAFTSMEN OF
PRINCETON UNIVERSITY
PRESS

★

MCMLXXX